W9-CIN-814

Encyclopedia of
Natural Health and Healing
for Children

NOTE:

Even though the natural medicines suggested in this book are generally or usually safe, it is impossible to know how a child will react to a specific remedy or treatment. In many cases of illness, one form of treatment would be insufficient and should be used in conjunction with others, such as conventional medicine, herbs, diet, massage or acupuncture. For this reason the information presented here is not intended to replace or be a substitute for the advice of qualified practitioners but designed to help you make informed choices about your children's health.

If you have any doubts about an illness or its treatment, you should consult a professional practitioner or doctor. The author and publisher do not accept responsibility for any effects arising from the treatments and remedies in this book.

How to Order:

Single copies may be ordered from Prima Publishing, P.O. Box 1260BK, Rocklin, CA 95677; telephone (916) 632-4400. Quantity discounts are also available. On your letterhead, include information concerning the intended use of the books and the number of books you wish to purchase.

Encyclopedia of Natural Health and Healing for Children

Marcea Weber

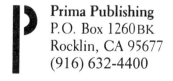

Prima Publishing
P.O. Box 1260 BK
Rocklin, CA 95677
(916) 632-4400

In this book one gender is not favoured over the other, however for practical purposes gender allocation is as follows:
Sections 1 and 2 — he
Section 3 — she

© 1992 Marcea Weber

All rights reserved. No part of this book may be reproduced or transmitted in any form or by any means, electronic or mechanical, including photocopying, recording, or by any information storage or retrieval system, without written permission from Prima Publishing, except for the inclusion of quotations in a review.

Library of Congress Cataloging-in-Publication Data

Weber, Marcea.
    Encyclopedia of natural health and healing for children / Marcea Weber.
        p.   cm.
    Originally published: Australia : Simon & Schuster, 1992.
    Includes bibliographical references and index.
    ISBN 1-55958-435-1 :
    1. Pediatrics—Popular works. 2. Children—Diseases—Alternative treatment. 3. Naturopathy. 4. Herbs— Therapeutic use. I. Title.
RJ61.W366 1994
615.5′35—dc20   93-23572
                                                      CIP

        97 AA 10 9 8 7 6 5 4 3

Printed in the United States of America

NATURAL HEALTH AND HEALING FOR CHILDREN

First published in Australasia in 1992 by
Simon & Schuster Australia
20 Barcoo Street, East Roseville NSW 2069

To all the world's children,
May they grow and flourish with our love

FOREWORD

Whenever we have something go wrong with either ourselves or our children, we are faced with the decision of what to do about it. Should we immediately consult a practitioner, try to do something about it ourselves, or do nothing and allow the body to heal itself? These questions may be as daunting at times for the practitioner as they are for the parents, and all of us must do whatever we feel is best for our children at the time.

In this book, Marcea Weber provides options for those parents wanting to try remedies which can be administered at home, whilst being very clear and helpful in suggesting times when a practitioner is best consulted.

Many of us learn about complementary therapies by attending a practitioner of a particular discipline such as herbal medicine or homoeopathy, and learning what works best for our own children with the practitioner's guidance. We then become increasingly confident of managing the simpler problems ourselves, without recourse to more invasive intervention.

Both western medicine as practised today and alternative or complementary therapies have advantages and disadvantages. In *Natural Health and Healing for Children*, Marcea Weber concentrates on the natural healing methods which attempt to augment the body's own healing powers, reasoning that much of the time, western medicine pays more attention to the removal of the symptoms than to the underlying causes of the disease. Much can be learnt of the current disease, and how to prevent another, by the gentler and perhaps slower approach offered by natural medicine.

It is important that people such as Marcea Weber continue to offer alternatives to conventional therapy, so that the choice of remedy and practitioner always rests with the person with whom responsibility ultimately lies. In the case of children this is the parents. All parents ultimately do the very best they can for their children, and one of the advantages of having parents become more familiar with therapeutics is the added confidence they bring to the healing of their own children. This added confidence is detected by the child and is a major factor in recovery, as is the willingness of us as parents to acknowledge that we are doing our best. This book goes a long way to helping us do that.

Dr John Harrison MB.BS.
Author of *Love Your Disease — It's Keeping You Healthy*

ACKNOWLEDGMENTS

I would like to thank the nine people who helped me put this book together, advising, recommending, and sharing their knowledge of children's health and well-being. In addition, the input and neverending support and confidence of friends, family and established practitioners of both orthodox and natural medicine have greatly contributed to getting this book to you.

I wish to acknowledge Allison Bramwell and Cozette Dean, two teenage girls who came into my life just when I needed help around the house and with my son and newly-born daughter. They also worked directly with me on this book and entered some of the manuscript and corrections into the computer. Caroline Jones, looked after my daughter with great devotion and love each week, enabling me to work on the book with some consistency and without interruption.

Renay Larsen persevered night after night after the children had gone to bed, feeding the corrections into the computer and giving me the benefit of her own experience as the mother of two young children.

Additional support came from Catriona Macmillian and Erik Wilkie, who always found the time to read, correct and listen to me when I was feeling unsure and doubtful.

Thanks to Allison Wheeler, a friend and former student, who believed in and shared my dream for this book and wrote the very first sample copy about baby massage when I was looking for contributors and feedback.

My friend and medical consultant Janet Widmer, who shares many of my views about healing, was always able, despite a demanding and busy schedule as a doctor and mother of two young children, to find the time to read, correct and share her medical knowledge and judgement with me.

My teachers, Herman and Cornelia Aihara, Michio and Aveline Kushi, and the late Masahiro Oki opened my eyes to the traditional ways of healing and how they could be applied to everyday home life.

Daniel my husband, who believed in my work from the start and always supported and encouraged me to carry on.

Last but not least, is Amanda Shipton, a friend who contributed not only her knowledge of home remedies and healing, but literally stood by me and encouraged me when I was too tired or too pregnant to think, let alone write.

CONTENTS

Appendices 237

Index 269

THE AUTHORS

Marcea Weber became interested in the relationship between health and diet when she herself alleviated a chronic back problem with a change in diet and lifestyle. She earned a B.A. in Speech Pathology and then went on to study nutrition, as she had a profound interest in the link between diet and disease.

Later she studied macrobiotic philosophy which led her towards Chinese herbalism. The use of Chinese herbs has played an important part in maintaining her health and it was also responsible for allowing her to conceive and give birth to her two children after the medical profession had given up hope of her ever having children at all.

Her experience with the various ailments of her children made her aware of the general lack of knowledge about the home nursing of children. This book was written not only to encourage parents to take more responsibility for their children's health, but as a reference for herself.

Marcea Weber has also written a number of books on natural foods, macrobiotic cuisine and philosophy, and sugarless desserts and is a regular contributor to various journals and magazines. She has appeared on television shows as a nutritional advisor and cooking demonstrator using natural foods and has had her own cooking schools in England, America and Australia.

· She lectures in philosophy, Chinese medicinal foods, nutrition, macrobiotic philosophy and healing.

She is currently living in the Blue Mountains, New South Wales with her husband and two young children.

Airdre Grant B.A., Dip Ed, was born in New Zealand, and trained as a macrobiotic counsellor and cook at the Kushi Institute in Boston, Massachusetts. A mother of two daughters, she now lives in Sydney with her family. Airdre teaches macrobiotic cooking and lectures extensively in philosophy, food energetics and food and healing. She practises as a macrobiotic and nutritional counsellor with a special interest in children's and women's health.

Rosalba Belford is a qualified naturopath, osteopath and acupuncturist and has many years' experience both lecturing and practising these disciplines. She is one of a handful of natural therapists who has completed three years of post-graduate training in Paediatrics. The approach she favours is based on an integration of orthodox medicine and natural therapy.

Her experience has shown that the most rapid recovery of children comes from a combination of natural healing techniques. She lives and practises in Sydney.

Hans Wohlmuth M.N.H.A.A., M.A.T.M.S. received his naturopathic training in Denmark from a number of prominent European natural healers. He has since specialised in medical herbalism and is the author of a book (in Danish) about growing and using medicinal plants. He now lives in Sydney with his family and lectures on botany and herbal medicine at Nature Care College, where he also has his practice.

Amanda Shipton lives in the Blue Mountains with her husband and her three children. Born and raised in East Africa, she came to Australia in the late 1970s, and gained experience in journalism and editing while working for the Herald and Weekly Times in Sydney for nine years. She became interested in herbalism and homoeopathy after the birth of her first child and has an increasing interest in healing her children using natural medicines.

'It is very distressing not to know how to comfort and help your sick child. Hopefully this book will encourage parents to begin to take their children's health back into their own hands as opposed to leaving it all up to the doctor.'

Tony Reid first became interested in oriental medicine in the early 1970s after reading Georges Ohsawa and Michio Kushi. He then went on to study Western medical sciences, completing studies in Anatomy, Physiology, Biochemistry, Pathology, Bacteriology and Pharmacology before becoming interested in acupuncture, Chinese herbalism, Indian yoga and Ayurveda. He studied these extensively in Australia and India. He has taught at the East-West Centre, Nature Care College and The N.S.W. College of Naturopathic Sciences.

At present he has a practice in Sydney, is involved in the production of data-base software for acupuncture and Chinese herbal medicine, and also teaches at the Sydney College of Traditional Chinese Medicine and the College for East-West Studies (Melbourne).

Dr Janet Widmer, Bachelor of Medicine, Bachelor of Surgery, Diploma of Royal Australian College of General Practitioners, Fellowship of Royal Australian College of General Practitioners.

Dr Widmer is a graduate of the University of Sydney and has post-graduate experience in obstetrics and gynaecology and general practice. She has worked in Australia and the United Kingdom. She is currently involved in full-time family practice.

She uses various modalities of treatment in her practice including acupuncture. She is also actively involved in post-graduate medical education. Currently she lives in Australia with her husband and two young children.

Rebecca M. Ridge has a Master's degree in Rehabilitation Counselling from the University of South Florida and a B.A. in Child Psychology from the University of Minnesota. She is a licensed massage therapist specialising in Craniosacral Therapy (advanced training through the Upledger Institute), Counterstrain, and Reflexology. As an international infant massage instructor she teaches infant massage classes to parents and caregivers at baby health clinics in Sydney. She also teaches reflexology and counterstrain to adults at Nature Care College in Sydney, offering workshops in specialised and integrative massage therapies. She has a private practice in integrative body/mind therapies in Sydney, Australia and in Tampa Florida, U.S.A. As a counsellor she facilitates groups in 'Growing through Grief and Surviving a Suicide'.

'Teaching our children how to love and care for their bodies, I believe is one of the most precious gifts we can give them for a healthy future.'

Diane McCombe N.D., D.B.M., Dip. Hom. Med. and **Peter Tumminello** N.D., D.B.M., Dip. Hom. Med. are professional homoeopathic practitioners and have been teachers of homoeopathy for the past six years at a number of institutions in Sydney. Diane specialises in the use of homoeopathy in pregnancy and childbirth and Peter has written a Homoeopathic text 'Repertory of the Child's Mind and Behaviour'. They are now directors of the Sydney College of Homoeopathic Medicine which runs professional courses in homoeopathic practice.

INTRODUCTION

I believe that my longtime interest and use of natural healing methods actually took root and began with the memories of my mother handing me a glass of salt water and telling me to gargle with it each time I complained of a sore throat. It turned out to be my solution to painful swelling, and ever since I have openly embraced and used home remedies, as well as herbs, massage and other natural healing techniques, on myself. Though my mother was trained as a nurse, she still saw the benefit of incorporating her mother's wisdom (and perhaps even her grandmother's and grandfather's wisdom) to heal with traditional medicines.

I have written and taught about natural health and healing using natural remedies from various sources since 1968. However, when my first child was born in 1985, my dedication and application of natural healing took a new direction. Even though I had used natural remedies on myself, friends and patients for the past 25 years with positive results, I must admit I was a bit apprehensive about administering remedies to my children.

So I continued to study and further explore naturopathic, homeopathic, Chinese medicine and massage and how to use them with children. Friends who were also parents began to ask me questions about healing children with natural remedies as they became fed up with useless medications and constant, unnecessary visits to the doctor. They urged me to collect all the information I was casually passing onto them into one book.

I liked that idea myself, as all too often I felt frustrated when my children got minor ills and fevers but I had no one easy reference to use. I decided that I would like to give specific advice on common childhood illnesses and to share my knowledge about how I know when a child is seriously ill, how to deal with simple childhood sickness that doesn't require medical attention, how to determine when you should call your doctor,

and how to tell that the suggested treatment prescribed for your child is safe.

With this basic information at your fingertips, all parents can assume a greater role in maintaining the health and well-being of their children. However, this does not mean that you become the doctor each and every time your child gets ill; rather, it means that you use your common sense and intuition and choose what is best each time. As parents, we want the very best for our children. We don't like to see them sick, but when they are, we can play an active role in supporting them toward a speedy recovery. This means taking responsibility by choosing and administering an appropriate treatment when they come down with simple ailments. There will be times when you need to consult a general practitioner (GP). Still, don't believe that only a qualified medical doctor can heal your children every time they get minor ills. There needs to be a delicate balance between the two extremes. The caveat to remember is, Never take any unnecessary risks with the health of your child.

By going about healing in this way, you're giving your family an opportunity to strengthen their immune system and natural body defenses with as little interference and intervention as possible. Unfortunately, over the past 40 to 50 years we have chosen to relinquish our power to heal our families, friends and selves to the medical establishment. And now, we have very little trust in our own healing ability.

Just remember that every situation and every child is different; they all have their own strengths and weaknesses. Choose the healing approach that is best suited for your child, remembering that everything always changes, and what is true for your child one day may not be true another.

First-time parenting especially can be confusing, as you are bombarded with plenty of well-meant but often confusing and even conflicting advice from friends and relatives. Trusting ourselves is like taking a giant step into the unknown. We are so used to visiting the doctor and listening to his or her diagnosis, receiving medication and following the prescribed advice, that doing it any other way at first seems unnatural. We feel incapable of understanding and healing our children's illnesses. But what is truly unnatural is administering chemically-based drugs and toxic medical procedures to infants and children when the situation is not serious or life-threatening.

If you can, it's wise to follow your instinct, intuition, gut feeling, or whatever you call it. Do not be persuaded by fear to administer unnecessary medications. Babies respond so quickly and are so sensitive to everything around them, especially parents, that the more gentle the approach, the better. Unless you are dealing with a serious illness, in which case you should consult a doctor (see Appendix 1), very little can go wrong. If you feel unsure, keep in touch with a practitioner of natural medicine.

When you begin to understand how natural medicines work, and how to choose the appropriate one for your child's age, condition and complaint, you will soon see how beneficial natural medicines are. For example, they actually deal directly with the cause, rather than just the symptoms, and therefore support the total health and well-being of your child. Natural remedies such as herbs and plants have been around for thousands of years and were often made into drinks called potions. Other mixtures were made into lotions or oils. They have been proven time and again to be safe and effective. Home treatment with natural, "traditional" medicine and perhaps the support of a natural practitioner such as a homeopath, naturopath or Chinese herbalist, is a perfectly acceptable option for treating the health of your family—provided you understand when you need orthodox medical assistance. (The word *orthodox* is interchangeable with the words *allopathic, conventional, Western,* or *traditional.* The word *natural* is interchangeable with the words *alternative, traditional,* or *holistic.*)

As you take on more responsibility for your child's well-being, you will begin to develop a "sixth sense" for determining what is troubling him or her. Parents who monitor and provide medical treatment at home can achieve greater bonding with their children. If your child feels confident with you looking after him or her, healing can take place much faster.

How To Use this Book

I've set out to give you a new and larger perspective on what is possible in the world of children's health and healing. I have included all the basic and essential information you will need in order to look after children between birth and twelve years when they are suffering with common, minor ailments. (At the age of twelve, most children have reached a developmental plateau, and it is best to consult a qualified practitioner when they become ill. However, this book can still be used as a reference guide since in some cases the only adjustment you need make is the dosage.)

This book is not intended as the be-all and end-all of manuals on children's health and healing, nor is it intended to be the only book you'll need to refer to. I want the ideas and suggestions presented here to form the basis of your knowledge, so that you feel confident enough to rely on yourself for treating minor complaints, and are able to recognise when you need further support. It is not meant to replace a qualified practitioner, but rather to help you reclaim some of the responsibility for healing your child. You can then regard health professionals as consultants (except, of course, in emergency situations when they *are* the experts). By taking appropriate care of your child when he has common, minor illnesses you also help to reduce the strain on the medical system, freeing it to cope better with more serious complaints.

Encyclopedia of Natural Health and Healing for Children is divided into three sections: the first section examines some of the different ways of healing that are available; the second section looks at preventative care and how you can best nurture the health and well-being of your child on a daily basis; and the third part is an A–Z list of complaints with three or more different natural therapy suggestions for each complaint.

Before choosing a therapy for a specific complaint, you should read the first section about all the different natural therapies offered. This will give you a good idea about where the therapies come from and their approach to treating sickness and health. You can then go on to read the specific complaint that you need to deal with, making sure that you carefully read the whole entry. Before you administer a remedy it's a good idea to read the Materia Medica, which explains each remedy and how it acts upon the body. After you have administered a remedy, closely watch your child's reaction to it.

Sickness Is Not Always So Terrible

All children will become ill at times during their early years; it is unavoidable. It is essential for them to experience the common illnesses of our society in order for them to develop and strengthen their immature immune systems. (However, clean air, pure water, exercise, nutritious food, laughter and plenty of love can help to support a child's growing body and keep them more resistant.) It has been estimated that an average child will become sick, in varying degrees, about eight times a year. The way that you decide to treat that sickness can have a profound effect upon the future health and well-being of your child. Remember: every child is different, every illness is different and every parent is different. How you choose to treat your child is up to you. After all, you know more about your child than anyone else.

According to Robert Mendelsohn, MD, author of *How to Raise a Healthy Child ... in Spite of Your Doctor*, 'the vast majority of childhood illnesses do not require medical attention and that when they receive it needlessly, the treatment given may do more harm than good'. I know it is easier to experiment on your own health and that making decisions for that special little person in your life seems like quite another issue. However, keep in mind that most childhood illnesses respond to normal bodily defences that could be hampered by medical treatment. By using sound, life-supporting therapies (as described in this book), wholesome nutrition and your own commonsense and wisdom, you will support your child in living a healthier life.

This book has not been written to dismiss modern medicine, but rather to show that it can be fused with natural methods of healing. We need to learn about all the various treatments available so that we can choose what is most appropriate for each particular situation.

You should never, ever, take any risks when it comes to the health and well-being of your child. If you are concerned, and do not feel that the remedies suggested are doing the job fast enough or thoroughly enough, then consult a practitioner of either orthodox or natural medicine as soon as possible.

SECTION I

Natural Health and Healing

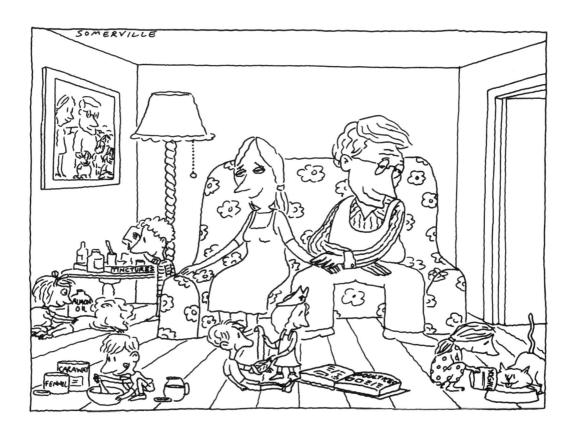

THE ROAD TO NATURAL MEDICINE

The Problems of Modern Medicine

Before 1900, most healing was done at home. It was not easy to get a doctor and if one was available they were summoned only for the most serious of illnesses. Every family had its own home medical books and supply of home remedies, using herbs, which were grown in the garden or which grew wild in the countryside. These were picked and used fresh, dried and hung in bunches in a cool place, turned into salves and ointments or waters, steeped in oils and distilled with brandy. These herb remedies and patent medicines, such as croup water, were the basis of domestic medicine and were all utilised before the doctor was called. It was the break down of the extended family and the consequent loss of knowledge that eventually led to the doctor becoming the sole provider of medical care.

Over the last 100 years, most of the more dangerous diseases of previous centuries, such as smallpox, diptheria and cholera, have been virtually wiped out by radical improvements in hygiene and diet. Great strides have, of course, also been made in the medical profession itself, in terms of knowledge, scientific equipment and drugs such as antibiotics. It is interesting to note that many of the traditional medicines have become the basis for modern drugs, so proving their effectiveness. For example, the cinchona plant was traditionally used by Peruvian Indians as a remedy for fever. It was taken to the West by Jesuit priests in 1739 and from the plant, quinine was isolated. This is the best known cure for malaria. Sassafras is another example. It was used by the American Indians, adapted for use by the English settlers and eventually exported to Europe as a cure for colic and for the relief of venereal disease. The aromatic oil safrole has been isolated from sassafras and is used as an antiseptic agent in dentistry.

With all the amazing medical advances, it has been tempting to sit back and place all our faith in orthodox medicine. A closer look, however, reveals some real problems. In the 1970s and '80s more money has been spent on health-care and research than ever before. Taking care of the sick has become one of the world's largest and fastest growing industries, but there has been virtually no improvement in the quantity or quality of life in the developed countries of the world during this time. Professor René Dubos of the Rockefeller University in New York in the 1960s made a startling discovery. He pointed out that all of the new drugs, surgical procedures and vaccines had not made people any healthier. In almost every respect they were unhealthier than their parents, and even dying younger than they had been ten years before.

Discontentment with doctors has also increased over the past few years. But the medical profession is being pulled and pushed in different directions at the same time. Doctors are being asked to act more responsibly to a patient's needs by making more home visits, spending more time with them, treating them holistically and listening more carefully to their needs. At the same time, doctors are put under pressure to study more, keep up-to-date with all new developments, and give more frequent but shorter consultations. A survey taken in England in 1980 showed that the proportion of people who still trusted their GPs had fallen from over 50 per cent to under 40 per cent in a single year.

What has happened? Up until the 1960s there was very little doubt, if any, that scientific medicine was winning the battle against disease by leaps and bounds. Epidemics were few and far between, diagnostic techniques were rapidly advancing, and with the discovery of the sulpha drugs (for example, sulpa methoxazole), anti-biotics and penicillin, infections were definitely under control. The introduction of cortisone and steroids promised that arthritis and other related disorders would soon be under control,

---

THE PLACEBO EFFECT

Frog sperm, crocodile dung, human sweat, spiders, earthworms, human and animal excrement are just a few materials which have been successfully used by doctors throughout the ages to cure illness. The placebo effect is the magic pill or potion that works because the doctor says it will and the patient believes the doctor. In _The Handbook of Psychotherapy and Behaviour Change_ by Drs. Arthur Shapiro and Louis Morro, they believe that between 50 and 80 per cent of all symptoms are emotional rather than physical in origin.

---

the Salk and Sabin vaccines were successfully immunising against poliomyelitis and surgery was taking care of any other maladies.

One of the difficulties is that the diseases from which we suffer today are very different from the diseases that were responsible for illness forty or fifty years ago. Prosperity, running water, better sanitation, sewage disposal facilities, better heating facilities and the discovery, production and distribution of effective medicines have all made a tremendous difference. They have conquered the old diseases but are struggling in the battle against the new.

When the new medicines were introduced in the 1940s and '50s showing such spectacular results, there wasn't any reason to question the concept of disease as an organic, physical process having resulted from one cause. A few doctors tried to convince their colleagues of the importance of considering the psychosomatic history of the patient in the process of diagnosis, but were largely ignored. Medicine became aggressive, interventionist and very highly specialised. This particular way of healing, however, was not adequately addressing the so-called 'modern' diseases, such as allergies, that were supposedly being caused by environmental pollution.

Research since the 1960s has indeed revealed that the concept of disease as an organic process is only part of the picture. Even though toxins, viruses and bacteria do play a role in the cause of disease, there is more than one cause for some diseases. Cancer and heart disease, for example, are said to be caused by a number of 'risk factors' which have to do mainly with lifestyles.

Too much fat in the diet, smoking, not enough exercise, and so on, are all factors that contribute to the cause of 'modern' diseases. Personality and stress also have a great deal to do with illness. Up until quite recently, most orthodox medical practitioners would have ignored this interpretation of disease or vehemently argued against it. More and more, however, a person's lifestyle, diet and personality are being taken into consideration when the medical profession is trying to determine the causes of disease. But the problem remains that orthodox practitioners are still dispensing enormous quantities of drugs and concentrating more on cure rather than cause and prevention.

The Advantages of Natural Medicine

In response to the problems encountered by orthodox medicine, a new breed of 'therapies' has appeared. At first they were hardly noticed and not taken very seriously, but these so-called 'unorthodox' or 'alternative' forms of treatment finally began to be heard. They were slow to catch on, but as time went by, and more and more people became fed up with a lack of results with conventional medicine, they began to seek out various alternatives. Homoeopathy, Chinese herbs, naturopathy, massage and acupuncture were particularly attractive as they treated the whole person rather than parts of an individual. Some natural therapies are as ancient as the hills, dating back thousands of years, while others are relatively modern.

One great advantage of natural medicine is the concept of Holistic health-care. It is very often thought to be a particular kind of treatment, like homoeopathy or acupuncture. It actually describes a philosophy rather than any particular type of medical practice. Any practitioner, whether they be a GP or another kind of health-care practitioner, can practise holistic medicine — treating the whole person rather than just the parts. It is nothing new, as the Greeks and various other cultures practised their own form of holistic medicine several thousand years ago. The functioning of all our body's structures and organs is intimately intertwined. The well-being of each part of the body will ultimately affect and depend upon what is going on everywhere else. With children, it is impossible to separate their physical, emotional and psychological development. What affects one particular part of growth, ultimately will affect the other. This may seem strange at first, but as you become familiar with treating parts of the body that may seem unrelated to the problem (for example treating the fingers for different intestinal or lung complaints) the results will speak for themselves. Treating the body and mind as one will bring more rapid and successful healing.

Over the years, holistic medicine has brought together many different kinds of healing. But a holistic health-care practitioner doesn't have to practise more than one discipline. What is important is that the practitioner sees her patient as a whole human being, that she is aware of the limitations of the type of healing she herself practises, that she is prepared to refer her patients to other practitioners who practise other forms of healing when necessary, and last but not least, that she is prepared to let her patients partake in the responsibility for their own healing process. This is a very exciting concept in that it brings the patient and practitioner closer together. They share the responsibility of healing, incorporate the self-healing powers of the patient together with the healing powers of nature, and try to meet the needs of the individual on a physical, mental and spiritual level. Any practitioner who is aware and willing to treat the whole patient rather than regarding him as a sick kidney or heart, can sincerely describe herself as a holistic practitioner.

HEALING

The most fundamental and successful way to heal your child is when you and your child *will it* to be so. Positive thoughts and visualising your child being healthy and happy and running around playing with other children can make all the difference.

There are many other reasons why people consult natural practitioners, but the most common reason is a dissatisfaction with what orthodox medicine has to offer.

We have developed such modern and sophisticated tools to deal with heart-attacks, cancers, and immune disorders and yet, these problems, along with allergies and diabetes, are becoming more common every day. We live in heated or air-conditioned buildings completely out of touch with the natural environment and still we are riddled with infections despite all the care taken with germ-free environments. We test more medicines more thoroughly than ever before and yet the incidences of doctor-induced diseases are on the rise. People are becoming more alarmed by the high incidence of side-effects thought to be associated with the use and abuse of modern medicine and surgical techniques. They are also discontented with the lack of personal interaction shown by many orthodox practitioners, and so are more attracted to the informality and sympathetic manner of many natural practitioners.

How To Choose Treatments

Start with the remedy you feel most comfortable with or which is the most practical for you. One remedy at a time is best, except for massage which you can add at any time. Massage usually helps the other remedy that you have chosen to work more quickly. If you find that the remedy that you have chosen is not working, then change to another or consult a practitioner. Remember, there is no one set of rules or formula that you must follow when it comes to looking after your child. Rules about babies simply don't work. Babies and children are individuals. It is simplistic to think that they can all be treated in the same manner. Some children react positively to one kind of treatment — others with the same problem may not respond at all to that treatment. Don't force your child to take something just because it's good for him. Find the remedy that works for both of you and always treat your child with respect and understanding.

Of course your choices will depend upon the stage that your child is developmentally, how old he is, as well as his apparent individual constitution. It's important to seek out the therapy which will be successful in supporting his well-being and making him feel comfortable at the time.

Healing in general is a very individual thing. Some people prefer conventional medicine, some natural medicine and some a combination of the two. You should always use what you feel most comfortable with and learn to trust your own judgement. If you really believe in the treatment that you have chosen, and apply common-sense along with plenty of tender loving care, it can sometimes make all the difference between a speedy recovery and a lingering illness.

When I was a child, my mother (who was

a nurse up until the time she had children of her own), chose to use a combination of conventional medicine and home remedies when treating our minor illnesses. If the home remedies didn't work and the illness lingered too long, or fevers went too high, the local GP would be called in and antibiotics were usually recommended.

Very often I find that even though parents will use natural therapies for themselves, they are reluctant to use them for their children. It seems that one of the reasons for hesitation is the common belief that there is an element of risk involved with natural medicines and therapy. Let me assure you that you will never harm your child by choosing a remedy from this book. The purpose of the book is to give you a chance to raise healthy children, without abusing and over-using drugs that can end up weakening their immune systems.

It is also important to realise that how your child takes care of himself when he grows up will be influenced by how you take care of him when he is young.

Becoming more involved in maintaining the health and well-being of your child does not mean that you should become the doctor. Remember, there are certain skills that doctors learn that parents should not take upon themselves. There are things which are best left up to the medical profession. However, if you are aware of the possible alternatives and are willing to incorporate other ways of healing along with those you already believe in, then you will undoubtably give your child a good foundation from which to grow and understand about health and sickness, without inappropriate medical interference.

There are so many natural therapies available that it is not possible to describe every single one. If you feel that you are ready to explore more, please consult the suggested reading list at the end of the book.

CAUTION

Seek professional help if your child:
- **develops a fever of above 40°C (104°F)**
- **becomes more and more tired and uninterested**
- **wheezes or has difficulty breathing**
- **has pain in the chest**

A Guide to Choosing a Health-care Practitioner

- Our bodies are capable of responding to a mixture of many different treatments, both orthodox and natural. We should be open to use a mixture of all the available and appropriate therapies whenever necessary.
- Some doctors believe that all natural therapies are useless and unethical. Some natural therapists have claimed that their particular modality holds all the answers. Some natural therapists are not reputable, reliable or safe. Ensure that the health-care practitioner you have chosen has had proper training and has a good reputation.
- If you are choosing to have an orthodox medical practitioner look after some of you child's health-care needs, take the time to interview several until you find one who you feel will treat your child in his best interest and one that can handle any emergencies consistent with your beliefs and desires.
- Select a practitioner of natural medicine who has a clear sense of which orthodox medical procedures are necessary in case of emergency and who knows when it is time to use the orthodox methods that are effective and known to work in a high percentage of cases.
- If you choose to consult only a practitioner of natural medicine you should be confident that this individual is capable of handling what ever condition may occur or that they are at least able to recognise their limitations and are willing to refer the child to someone else when necessary.
- You should consider the following questions when selecting a health practitioner for your family:

  When they ask a question, do they listen to your reply?

  Do they make themselves available if you feel that it is an emergency?

  Was there adequate time spent in listening to you about the physical and emotional condition of your child?

  Are they warm and friendly to your child?

  Do they value intimacy and are they comfortable with human emotions and closeness?

  How comfortable do you feel after a consultation?

  Are they very quick to hand out prescriptions or do they sometimes admit that nothing needs to be prescribed?

Do they explain the side-effects and ha-zards of the medications (if necessary) that are prescribed?

Do they give both sides of the picture when it comes to immunisation? (see pages 69-72)

Do they guide you with suggestions about how to maintain the health and well-being of your child?

Do they consider diet as being part of the treatment when applicable?

Do they take a complete history during your first visit?

Do they ask you about your observations about your child's physical and emotional condition?

- Be patient with yourself, as it takes time to find the person you can trust and who can respond to you and your family's needs. Remember that doctors and health-care practitioners are only support systems. It is you who plays the major role in preserving the well-being of your child.
- If you are seeing a practitioner of natural therapies be sure to tell your doctor and vice-versa as sometimes prescribed drugs and herbs may not go well together.

- When consulting a practitioner remember the following:

  If you don't understand the terminology used, ask for a simpler explanation.

  Be clear about the symptoms.

  Don't be afraid to seek a second opinion. Ask if there is anything that you can do to assist the healing (food, bathing, mas-sage, etc.) at home.

- If a condition is not life-threatening you do have a choice of how to treat it (see Appendix 1: Scale of Intervention). Approximately 80 per cent of all non-life threatening conditions just disappear with time as the body heals itself. But orthodox medical practitioners should always be consulted immediately for the following:

  Poisoning

  Loss of consciousness

  Seizures

  Massive bleeding

  Trauma (from burns, accidents, electrocution, hypothermia, etc.)

  Broken bones

  Head or neck injuries

  Life-threatening diseases

ANTIBIOTICS AND OTHER MEDICATIONS: FRIENDS OR FOES?

Medicine should be concerned with two things: healing and comforting. Sometimes, just changing a child's environment from a stressful one to a less stressful one is enough to relieve the symptoms of an illness. At other times, for example with asthma or chronic ear infections, it may be necessary to use more sophisticated means such as drugs to attack the problem. So, sooner or later, you will be faced with the dilemma of whether or not you should give your children antibiotics or other forms of medication.

Before antibiotics were discovered most children with problems such as ear infections and tonsillitis got better without complications. Some, of course, did not, and went on to develop conditions such as chronic ear infections which can produce deafness and throat abcesses which can predispose children to rheumatic fever (which can, in turn, cause heart disease). Most infections, however, are not life-threatening, do not pose a serious threat and do *not* need antibiotics. When I consult my GP about a childhood illness for which antibiotics are usually prescribed, she often suggests that we try something else first. (Antibiotics may be unnecessary and should only be used as a last resort.) Few would argue that antibiotics are an excellent way to kill large numbers of bacteria. The trouble is that not all bacteria are bad and sometimes a course of antibiotics is like a bombing raid in which the good guys get it just as much as the bad guys!

These days there is a huge number and variety of powerful antibiotic drugs available with new ones being continually developed. Such drugs play a vital role in medicine worldwide and can save lives. However, there is no doubt that medication is over-prescribed, particularly in general practice, and that more and more people are becoming concerned about this. Antibiotics, for example, are often given as a preventative measure without any investigation of the presence or type of bacteria. They are also prescribed without consideration of the individual. We all react differently to changes in our circumstances and environment, including sickness. When we first become ill, there may not be any obvious physical symptoms, but because the life force is being disturbed, we feel unwell. Children, especially, may exhibit only emotional imbalances at first, for example, unusual irritability or clinging behaviour. It is also important, therefore, to take an individual child's emotional state into account as well. So what will determine the course of the illness is not its nature but the type of person who is ill.

What also often gets overlooked is that our bodies do have their own natural defence mechanism — manufacturing antibodies to zero in on the invading bacteria and render them harmless.

A New Look at Antibiotics

Since the introduction of antibiotics a few decades ago, they have come to be regarded as the panacea of life-saving drugs. In the early days when antibiotics were used appropriately they truly were 'magic bullets' able to control many infectious bacterial diseases. In the 1940s they were regarded as miracle drugs for the infectious diseases that had killed more soldiers and civilians in the two World Wars than had bombs and real bullets. By 1950 numerous antibiotics were being raved about as the cure-all for virtually any kind of bacterial problem. Eventually antibiotics were being prescribed for a large number of diseases. The almost 'magical' reputation has led to the idea that antibiotics will make almost anything better faster and this has contributed to their overuse and abuse. Because antibiotics were so effective in treating life-threatening infectious diseases like pneumonia, their use has been over-generalised to treatable and untreatable diseases alike.

Antibiotics originally intended for bacterial diseases are sometimes prescribed for the common cough, cold, flu, and even measles, mumps and chickenpox, which are all viral in nature and will not respond to antibiotics. Some kinds of food poisoning and pneumonia, tonsillitis, boils and whooping cough, to name just a few, are bacterial in nature so respond to antibiotics. By killing off the disease-causing bacteria, antibiotics do in fact give the body's own immune system time to produce enough antibodies to fight the infection. But, when antibiotics destroy or inhibit bacteria they also take with them great numbers of relatively benign or even beneficial bacteria. Even Alexander Fleming who discovered penicillin (one of the first antibiotics) in 1928 cautioned against using the miracle medicine for every illness. He realised that penicillin did not kill all bacteria and that perhaps those that survived would be likely to resist more doses.

Our health depends a great deal on the presence of bacteria such as *Lactobacillus acidophilus* and *L. bifidus* in our gut and in the vaginal mucous membranes. These lactobacilli have the ability to ward off other bacteria protecting us from infection, by secreting small quantities of antibiotic-like substances, including hydrogen peroxide, benzoic acid, lactic acid, acetic acid, acidophilin and others. These bacteria are helpful when our intestines come in contact with harmful food-born bacteria. Antibiotics can inhibit these 'good' bacteria, and what is even worse is that the 'bad' bacteria usually recover first. Another problem is that many previously controllable infectious organisms have gradually changed their configuration to become resistant to antibiotics. New strains of antibiotics have to be developed all the time to combat these now resistant bacteria and all the new bacterial infections which have evolved over the last few decades.

Using Antibiotics

There are times when a child has an infection that needs to be handled immediately with antibiotics because his body defences and immune responses are too low. Serious damage can be avoided when antibiotics are used properly, infrequently and in the right circumstances. Please note however, that even though the infection may be destroyed, antibiotics will not restore balance in the body. If you are following a course of antibiotics to combat the infection, please do so in conjunction with natural medication to help strengthen the child's immune system.

What To Ask Your Doctor Before Accepting Antibiotics

- Is the complaint viral or bacterial in nature?
- Will it get better without antibiotics?
- Are there any known side-effects with the medication prescribed?

Types of Infection

- Bacterial infections like pneumonia, meningitis and septicaemia and all bone infections usually need antibiotics.
- Viral infections like measles, chickenpox, mumps, german measles, nearly all coughs, colds and throat infections usually do not respond to antibiotics except when bacteria complicate a viral illness.
- Harmless bacterial infections like ear infections, sticky eyes, urinary infections which are unpleasant may need antibiotics but not necessarily. It depends upon the child. Some may be better off without treatment.

Sometimes it is rather difficult for your doctor to ascertain without tests whether an illness needs medication. The correct way to prescribe antibiotics is for the doctor to take a throat swab or other specimen which she then sends away to the laboratory for analysis. Then the infection can be identified and its antibiotic sensitivity assessed so that the practitioner knows which drug to recommend.

How To Support the Body When Administering Antibiotics

If you have to give antibiotics to your child there are some ways to support his well-being at the same time, using natural remedies to strengthen his system.

- Administer small amounts (1 teaspoon per day for three weeks) of Acidophilus culture yogurt to help restore the intestinal bacteria (2 hours before or after administering antibiotics). For an infant (a child under 2 years), 1/3 of a teaspoon per day is recommended.
- If you are familiar with Miso soup it is also very beneficial for restoring the intestinal flora. Give 1 cup daily using 1/2 teaspoon of shiro (white) miso for children over the age of 4 and 1/4 teaspoon for 1–3 year olds.

Side-effects of Antibiotics

Antibiotics do have associated side-effects, some of which may cause irreversible damage. This is another reason why antibiotics should be the last choice for treating bacterial infections. All antibiotics are unsafe during pregnancy as they can cross into the baby's blood stream through the placenta. Between 25 and 75 per cent of the mother's concentration of penicillin or Tetracycline crosses into the baby. The common side-effects include:

- liver damage
- allergies
- destruction of valuable intestinal bacteria
- vitamin K deficiency
- interference with the absorption of nutrients
- can induce thrush
- diarrhoea due to a disturbance in the beneficial types of bacteria in the intestines
- skin rashes
- phlegm — even though the infection may clear up, there may be some phlegm left behind — if the phlegm remains it is more than likely that the child may get another infection very soon after the first one has cleared up.

DIARRHOEA

In small children, diarrhoea can be caused by a number of things but usually it is viral or bacterial. If it happens suddenly, causes a brief fever and stops just as suddenly, you can be pretty sure it was a viral infection. However, if the fever lasts for more than 24 hours and the child suffers from stomach cramps and sometimes bleeding stools, then a bacterial infection is more than likely to be the cause.

Colds and Flu

Children seem to be more susceptible to the common cold, flu, sore throat and cough than adults and more likely to be treated with medication for them when they occur. Even though medication may relieve cold symptoms, none of the drugs really *cure* the problem. The fact of the matter is that without medication a common cold usually lasts between four and seven days, and with treatment it usually lasts about seven. Because colds are viral in nature and are transmitted through the air by cough-

ing and sneezing, grandmothers' and mothers' warnings that cold weather and not enough clothing are responsible for winter ills are usually poo-pooed. However there may be a grain of truth in the fact that if children bundle up when they go outdoors in the cold, they probably have higher resistance to the viruses and other bugs that may be travelling around at that time because their bodies are not additionally stressed by trying to keep warm.

If you feel that you want to take your child to an orthodox practitioner for the common cold or flu, don't accept antibiotics. Not only will they not cure the problem, but can produce some nasty side-effects.

Whose Responsibility Is It Anyway?

During recent years, many thousands of people in Australia and the USA have died as a result of taking medication prescribed for a fairly mild condition. Such was the case with thalidomide which tragically proved that certain medications, thought to be safe can, in fact, be dangerous. Of all the new illnesses discovered in the last few years, many are actually drug-induced (iatrogenic). For example some forms of anaemia, some types of gastrointestinal ulceration and malabsorption.

It is not my intention to attack the medical and pharmaceutical professions, however, it is necessary to look not only at their achievements but also at their failings. While many orthodox medical practitioners may indeed be too quick to prescribe drugs for children and too lax in deciding whether the risk of the illness really justifies the risk of taking the medicine, perhaps we are too ready to use our children as guinea pigs. Ultimately, we as parents, make the decision as to whether or not our children take medication. More often than not we are so anxious that our children recover health quickly that we administer the medicine regardless of whether or not they really need it. We are generally too shy to ask about the side-effects and the testing that should have been done before it was administered. Medicines can be one of our most useful tools if we use them mindfully. If they are used carelessly they can be one of our greatest hazards.

NATUROPATHIC MEDICINE AND HERBALISM

Naturopathic Medicine

A mixture of traditional folk wisdom and modern healing techniques, naturopathic medicine is based on the healing power of nature. Symptoms are viewed as signs that the body is attempting to heal itself so treatments are designed to address the underlying cause of the illness, rather than the symptoms. Naturopathy is a form of holistic medicine, concerned with treating the person as a whole. Part of naturopathic treatment is based on making adjustments in diet, lifestyle, exercise, breathing and so on to make sure that the fundamental cause of the illness is healed.

The idea that toxins accumulate in the body from many different sources and give rise to lymph and blood disorders which make the body more vulnerable to infection is one of the foundations of naturopathic philosophy. There can be a slow accumulation of toxins in the system due to poor diet, lack of rest, pollution and lack of exercise. Naturopathy is concerned with adjusting lifestyle to rid the body of the toxins.

The aim of naturopathy is to treat the patient, not the sickness. There are, of course, some standard remedies which are used for particular problems. All the remedies are designed to stimulate the body's own defences to produce the desired effects and most of the dosages are kept very low, so side-effects would be rare indeed. Some of the remedies indicated will simply boost natural body chemicals that may be deficient for one reason or another rather than aiming to actually cure anything. Much of the emphasis in the naturopathic treatment of children is placed on increasing the vitality of the child so that he will be enabled to throw off the disease.

Diet is also an important aspect of naturopathy. If you take your child to a naturopath, she will probably discuss diet and may prescribe therapies which include minerals, vitamins and herbs which contain the vitamins and minerals in fairly concentrated amounts and in a form which children can very easily assimilate. Because herbs are living, active, organic substances, they are not at odds with the physical composition of children's bodies like chemical drugs made from inert materials. There may be other forms of healing such as osteopathy or massage that a naturopath may choose to use according to the symptoms presented and the individual child.

Naturopathy recognises three components of disease states or indifferent health:
- Circumstantial components such as environmental factors, for example, pollution.
- Physical components such as bacteria, viruses and germs.
- Emotional components.

Naturopathic practitioners are more than willing to hear what the patient's view is of the illness and what he has done to remedy it. They work on the principle that acute disease is simply a manifestation of the body's healing forces. So there is no sense in just suppressing the symptoms because the cause will be left untreated and will eventually return.

Naturopathy works well for acute conditions such as digestive and liver problems, colds, sore throats, colitis and bronchitis but can also be applied to more chronic conditions such as asthma and tuberculosis.

Herbalism

To the medical herbalist, a herb is any plant that has medicinal value, and there are at least 350,000 known species of plants, There are probably hundreds of thousands of medicinally valuable plants that we still know nothing about.

When I was a kid growing up in New York City, for many years at the beginning of every spring I would see this same little old lady leave our apartment building with an empty shopping bag under her arm. When she returned several hours later it was full up to the brim with dandelion flowers, dock sorrel, chicory and whatever else she could find growing along the roadside or in the bushy areas of the parks. I was always curious about what she was going to do with it all, but I was never game enough to ask.

Many years later, I was served a salad with several greens that I couldn't identify. I asked the waiter what they were and, lo and behold, they turned out to be dandelion greens and chicory, immediately triggering my memory of that little old lady and her bag of 'weeds'. This wise woman had been gathering her food from the wild, eating the plants that so many of us curse when we are tending our gardens. Dandelion root is in fact used as the basic ingredient for dandelion coffee and a daily ration of this beverage is recommended for anyone who has had liver ailments (such as hepatitis) or general liver weakness.

People have been using herbal medicines as long as they have been writing. The Chinese started recording their herbal drugs as far back as 3000 BC.

Herbal medicines are used throughout this book in conjunction with other naturopathic remedies, not to cure diseases, but to restore the body's balance to normal. However, you should not be surprised to find that once a child begins to take herbal medicine, symptoms will no doubt begin to disappear.

Herbal medicines are ideally suited to treat a variety of children's complaints because they are effective and generally have no unpleasant side-effects. All the herbal medicines mentioned in this book are entirely safe when used according to the directions given.

While there is no minimum age for children below which they shouldn't be given herbal remedies, the question of allergy should be taken into consideration. Any substance, other than the mother's milk, given to a baby under six months old carries with it an increased risk of provoking an allergic response in the child. This especially applies to such things as cow's milk and foods containing wheat, but may also be encountered with herbs, although it is very rare.

The recommended dosages of 'western' herbs in this book are provided for children one year old and up. Children under the age of one may be given herbs such as Fennel, Lemon Balm and Catmint. If younger than six months, it is suggested that a compress of the herb be applied to the abdomen or over the affected area rather than giving the herb internally. If the baby is being breastfed, many plant constituents will appear in the milk, if the mother takes the herb.

If you have any doubts, contact a qualified herbalist or naturopath.

There are a number of different ways herbs can be prepared and administered.

HERBAL DOSES FOR CHILDREN
Take age of child at next birthday. Divide this by twenty-four. This will give you the fraction of the recommended adult dose.

Preparation
INFUSION
An infusion is prepared just like a cup of tea. The dried herb is placed in a teapot or cup and freshly boiled water is poured over. The vessel should be covered immediately to avoid the loss of volatile compounds. Allow to steep for 5–10 minutes. The infusion must be strained if loose herbs are used. The drink can be sweetened with honey or rice malt to make it more palatable to the child. Less pleasant tasting herbs may need to be mixed with sweet tasting herbs such as Licorice root, Aniseed or Fennel seed. It generally doesn't make any difference whether the tea is drunk warm or cold. However, certain groups of remedies, such as the diaphoretics used in fever management, should be taken as hot as possible.

Herbal teas made up of flowers, leaves or seeds are normally prepared as infusions.

DECOCTION
A decoction is an extract in water, like the infusion, but prepared by actually boiling the herb. Herbs made up of very hard plant material such as roots and barks are usually decocted (unless they are powdered, for example, Slippery Elm).

To make a decoction, put the measured quantity of herb in a stainless steel saucepan and pour the required amount of cold water over. Cover with a lid, and bring to the boil, then reduce heat and simmer for 5-10 minutes. Strain before serving. As with infusions, decoctions can be sweetened or flavoured with pleasant tasing herbs.

Examples of herbs that are decocted are Licorice root and Dandelion root.

TINCTURE
A tincture is an extract of a herb in a mixture of cold water and alcohol, typically 25, 40, 60 or 90 per cent alcohol depending on the

solubility of the active constituents in the particular herb. Tinctures are concentrated herbal extracts which are convenient to take and they are widely prescribed by professional herbalists and naturopaths. One of the most obvious advantages of tinctures is the very small amount of medicine constituting a dose compared to the infusions and decoctions. The alcohol in the tinctures gives them a strong and warming taste similar to spirits. Many children like the taste of alcohol when it is not too strong and it is recommended to dilute the tincture 4-5 times with water or juice. The amount of alcohol consumed by the child is usually not a source of concern since the dose of the tincture typically will be ½-1 mL. Tinctures are not suitable for children under two years.

The suggested dosage for tinctures will most likely depend upon what your practitioner recommends. If the recommended dosage does not correlate with your practitioner's advice, please follow your practitioner's suggestions as he or she would have made up the mother tincture in the first place and can best tell you how many parts water to tincture is necessary.

Tinctures of single herbs are — with a few exceptions — not available to the public. However, a number of companies produce a range of composite tinctures which are available from health food stores. These products are formulated to treat certain conditions, for example, cough, constipation and headache.

TABLETS
Capsules and tablets containing medicinal herbs are available from health foods stores and chemists. Although some products are of high quality, they are generally not suitable for smaller children.

ESSENTIAL OILS
Essential oils, also known as volatile or aromatic oils, are found in many plants. Plants with a strong aroma will often contain essential oil. Essential oils are unrelated to vegetable oils and animal fats.

Pure essential oils are highly concentrated and potent substances and although they contribute significantly to the therapeutic activity of many medicinal plants, they are all toxic in relatively low doses when taken internally. This applies especially to babies and small children and it is generally recommended not to use pure essential oils internally.

Due to the lipid-solubility of essential oils, they are readily absorbed through the skin.

Thus, applying them to the skin is an indirect form of internal administration. The use of fragrant massage oils (massage oils containing essential oil) on babies should be avoided. You should use a good quality cold pressed vegetable oil such as wheat germ or almond oil instead.

A couple of essential oils can be added to a pure vegetable massage-oil in very low concentration and used therapeutically to relieve colic in babies (see Colic in the A–Z Guide).

Another way of using essential oils is inhalation. This method is employed both in aromatherapy and medical herbalism. The simplest way to administer essential oils this way is to add a few drops of essential oil to hot water, either in a saucepan or in an oilburner. Ceramic oilburners with a small dish for water and essential oil on top and a candle underneath are readily available. Oilburners give the room a pleasant smell and many people have them burning almost constantly, filling the room with evaporated essential oil. This is not a good idea, however, because the constant exposure to essential oil can have a negative effect on the lungs. This especially applies to babies and smaller children. An oilburner with a few drops of eucalyptus oil is ideal when the child has a cold and the airways are congested. Have it burning in the child's bedroom for a couple of hours at night. Do make sure that the burner is out of the child's reach.

Always keep essential oils where children cannot get to them.

Administering Herbal Remedies

Some children absolutely refuse to take anything into their mouths when they feel ill. If your baby or child is like this, there are other ways in which you can administer these herbal remedies.

- A decoction, tincture or infusion may be placed in the bath water at 20 times the recommended dose (for an infant 10–15 times the dose is usually enough).
- A tincture may be rubbed into the skin of your baby's or child's abdomen at three times the normal dose.

These are especially good ways to administer herbs if your baby or child has on-going digestive problems or has a condition that has originated in the digestive system. Because of the delicate nature and porous quality of baby's and young children's skin these two alternative methods of administering herbal preparations work as they allow a good quantity of the preparation to pass through the skin and into the body.

SUGGESTED DOSAGES

Standard dosages are recommended for each particular ailment. In the A–Z Guide to Treating Children's Complaints, however, there are times when the condition may be acute or chronic. In these cases:

- Give one dose three times a day for chronic conditions.
- Give one dose every two to four hours for acute conditions.

There may be times when you may find that your baby or child develops a reaction to a particular herb. It may be that he is allergic or sensitive to it. If this is the case stop the treatment immediately and consult a practitioner for alternative treatments.

Foraging for Herbs

You may be lucky enough to be able to forage for wild herbs where you live. If this is the case many of the herbs suggested in this book are available in backyards and gardens or in the bush near your home if you live in the country or near a national park. Certain precautions should be followed if you are intending to pick your own:

- Make sure that you know what you are picking by consulting a book or a knowledgeable person.
- Do not pick plants that have been sprayed with artificial pesticides or herbicides or which are growing on the side of a busy road.
- Make sure that you take only what is allowed to be picked.
- For certain herbs it is best to pick the leaves and flowers when they have just come up. So, for example, when picking Dandelion leaves, pick them in the beginning of spring when they are small and young and have all the energy of the plant. Later on when the flowers come up, use them for healing or just for eating. After the flowers have died, wait until autumn or winter to pick the root.

Herbal Materia Medica

Aniseed *(Pimpinella anisum)*

The fruits are used medicinally. They contain a volatile oil with a sweet, licorice-like aroma. Aniseed is a relaxing expectorant and a carminative (relieving flatulence). The carmin-

ative action of Aniseed is less profound than that of Caraway and Fennel. The sweet taste of Aniseed makes it an excellent flavouring herb which can be added to other less pleasant tasting herbs.

Parts used: the dried fruit.

Indications: cough (especially dry or spasmodic), croup, flatulence, cough in measles, stomach-ache caused by wind.

Contraindications: none.

CAUTION: do not use Anise Oil for children.

Calendula (Marigold) *(Calendula officinalis)*

A member of the daisy family, this annual plant with its bright orange or yellow flowerheads is familiar to most people. It grows readily from seed and doesn't ask much except a sunny position. Calendula is an excellent first aid plant which should be in any home medicine chest. It is gentle in action and very well suited to children. Calendula has anti-inflammatory, astringent and healing actions.

Parts used: the dried flowerheads.

Indications: bleeding, bumps and bruises, cuts and grazes, chickenpox, conjunctivitis, diarrhoea, eczema (as an ointment), mouth ulcers, mumps, skin irritations, stomach-ache with diarrhoea, thrush, tonsillitis.

Contraindications: none.

NOTE: in American nurseries, members of the genus *Tagetes* (also with orange flowers) are sold under the name Marigold. Make sure you use *Calendula officinalis* for medicinal purposes.

Caraway *(Carum carvi)*

The fruits are used medicinally and make one of the best carminatives. Caraway is suitable for treating colic and may be combined with Fennel for this. It also has gentle expectorant properties.

Parts used: the dried fruit.

Indications: bronchitis, colic, flatulence, stomach-ache caused by wind.

Contraindications: none.

Cascara *(Rhamnus purshiana)*

The bark of this North American tree contains anthraquinones which are a certain type of chemical compounds, most of them with laxative effect. Laxatives of this type can be used *short-term* to relieve constipation when this is caused by bowel atony (over-relaxed musculature) or fever. Cascara and other anthraquinone laxatives (such as Senna, Rhubarb, Aloes and Yellow Dock) should not be used when the constipation is caused by nervousness or muscular tension.

Cascara should always be given with a good carminative such as Fennel, Ginger or Chamomile to prevent cramping pains known as griping.

Parts used: the dried bark.

Indications: constipation associated with colds, flu and fever, constipation caused by over-relaxed bowel musculature.

Contraindications: constipation associated with muscular tension or nervousness.

Catmint *(Nepeta cataria)*

This less-known relative of the Peppermint is an excellent children's remedy which should be kept in the family's medicine chest. Catmint acts as a decongestant in the upper respiratory tract, it is relaxing, reduces fever, stimulates the digestion and relieves flatulence. It is probably the most universal children's herb after Chamomile.

Parts used: the dried herb.

Indications: allergy, colds, earache, fever, headache, sleeping difficulties, stomach-ache (when caused by nervousness or anxiety), teething.

Contraindications: none.

Chamomile *(Matricaria recutica, Anthemis nobilis)*

Chamomile is the children's remedy *par excellence*. Two different species of Chamomile are used medicinally, the Annual Chamomile *(Matricaria recutica)* and the perennial species, Roman Chamomile *(Anthemis nobilis)*. Despite the fact that the two plants belong to different genera their medicinal actions are almost identical. Both can be easily grown in the garden but you will have to grow a lot in order to get enough to make more than a few cups of tea.

Chamomile combines relaxing and anti-inflammatory properties and is a gentle digestive stimulant while at the same time releases any tension in the digestive tract.

It is hard to think of a childhood complaint that will not benefit from Chamomile. Its general soothing effect combined with a pleasant taste (especially if sweetened with a little rice malt syrup or honey) and its more specific actions, makes it the foremost herbal home remedy.

Parts used: the dried flowerheads.

Indications: allergy, colds and flu, colic, diarrhoea, flatulence, headache, sleeping difficulties, stomach-ache, teething, travel sickness, vomiting and nausea. Also any inflammatory and/or feverish condition.

Contraindications: none, except allergy to the herb which is very rare.

Chickweed *(Stellaria media)*

This small, inconspicuous plant is a common garden weed in many temperate parts of the world. It is light green in colour with small white flowers, the five petals being deeply divided, thus looking like ten white petals. What makes it easy to tell Chickweed apart from any other more or less obscure green weed is the single line of fine hairs on the stem of the plant (you must look closely to be able to see this).

Chickweed is anti-inflammatory and has profound skin-healing properties. It is the herb of choice for relieving itchy skin conditions.

Parts used: the whole herb, fresh or dried.

Indications: use topically for cuts and grazes, eczema, skin irritations, all inflamed and/or itchy skin conditions.

Contraindications: none.

Dill *(Anethum graveolens)*

The leaves of this plant are well known as a culinary herb. In herbal medicine, the fruits (usually referred to as seeds) are used. They have carminative properties.

Parts used: the dried fruit.

Indications: colic, flatulence, stomach-ache caused by wind, also given with Cascara to prevent griping.

Contraindications: none.

Echinacea *(Echinacea angustifolia/ purpurea)*

A most attractive member of the daisy family, *Echinacae purpurea* grows happily in most gardens and some gardeners will know it under the name Purple Coneflower.

An old North American Indian remedy, it has become famous in recent years mainly due to its stimulating action on the immune system and is probably the most widely prescribed herb in modern Western herbalism. Useful against all types of infections, whether bacterial, viral or fungal, allergies and auto-immune diseases, it works both locally and systemically. Although the herb is useful in the treatment of acute infections (especially when given in relatively high doses), its real strength is as a preventative.

Parts used: the dried root of *E. angustifolia* or the entire plant of *E. purpurea.*

Indications: allergy, poisonous bites and stings, chickenpox, colds and flu, German measles (rubella), all infections, mouth ulcers, mumps, sore throat, thrush, tonsillitis.

Contraindications: none.

Elderflowers *(Sambucus nigra)*

The Elder was associated with much mysticism in Europe in the olden days and it was considered bad luck to chop the shrub down. Various parts of the plant were used for numerous purposes. The ripe berries make a delicious soup or hot drink while the yellowish-white flowers can be used to make refreshing summer drinks, either in the form of a soft drink or as Elder wine. The flowers are used to reduce fever and they also have anti-catarrhal, anti-inflammatory and expectorant properties.

Parts used: the dried flowers.

Indications: colds and flu, to prevent convulsions caused by high temperature, croup, earache, fever, German measles, measles, sinusitis, sore throat.

Contraindications: none.

Elecampane *(Inula helenium)*

Elecampane is a cough remedy which is especially good for treating bronchial congestion. Although mostly used for more chronic conditions, Elecampane is also useful in some milder cases such as irritating cough in children. Elecampane is also anti-bacterial and a digestive tonic.

It contains volatile compounds so make sure you decoct it under a tightly fitting lid.

Parts used: the dried root.

Indications: asthma, bronchitis, cough (wet, mucus-producing), whooping cough.

Contraindications: none.

Eyebright *(Euphrasia officinalis)*

As the name indicates, this plant is of special value in the treatment of conditions affecting the eye, more specifically conjunctivitis. Eyebright is astringent, anti-catarrhal and anti-inflammatory and is valuable in the treatment of catarrhal conditions of the upper respiratory tract as well as eye complaints.

Parts used: the dried herb.

Indications: allergy, conjunctivitis, sore and watery eyes, croup, earache, sinusitis and rhinitis. Also as a gargle/mouthwash for sore throat and mouth ulcers.

Contraindications: none but best avoided in constipation.

Fennel *(Foeniculum vulgare)*

The swollen leaf bases are used as a vegetable, however, for medicinal purposes, the fruits (usually called seeds) are used. Fennel is a good carminative and one of the best herbs for colic. It is also a mild expectorant, an anti-inflammatory and promoter of milk secretion in lactating mothers. Fennel can be used to flavour other herbal teas as it has a pleasant sweet taste.

Parts used: the dried fruit.

Indications: colic, conjunctivitis, acute diarrhoea, flatulence, stomach-ache caused by wind, vomiting and nausea. Also given with Cascara to prevent griping (sharp cramping).

Contraindications: none.

CAUTION: do not use the essential (volatile) oil of Fennel internally.

Ginger *(Zingiber officinale)*

This well-known spice is an important medicinal plant as well as being indispensable in the kitchen. Ginger stimulates the circulation and digestion, relieves flatulence and provides the best prevention against travel sickness. The herb is pungent so don't give your child Ginger tea which is too strong. Always taste it yourself first and dilute it if the child complains about it being too spicy.

Parts used: the fresh rhizome (underground stem). The dried, powdered rhizome can also be used, but is much more pungent than the fresh so you will need to reduce the dose accordingly. Again, taste it before you give it to the child.

Indications: allergy, colds and flu, flatulence, headache, stomach-ache, travel sickness.

Contraindications: acute stomach upset, diarrhoea.

Golden Rod *(Solidago virgaurea)*

Golden Rod is an anti-inflammatory and anti-catarrhal herb which is very useful for acute as well as more chronic catarrhal (inflammatory) conditions of the upper respiratory tract. It is also an important antiseptic diuretic. The remedy is particularly useful in conditions with an element of nervous tension present.

Parts used: the dried herb.
Indications: allergy, earache, sinusitis, rhinitis, urinary tract infections.
Contraindications: none.

Golden Seal *(Hydrastis canadensis)*

This North American herb is most valuable where there is catarrh (inflammation) of the mucous membranes. It is an astringent and a digestive stimulant with a mild laxative action and it has a beneficial effect on the liver function. It is used as an eye rinse in conjunctivitis.
Parts used: the roots and rhizome.
Indications: allergy, chickenpox (topically), conjunctivitis (topically), diarrhoea, mouth ulcers, stomach-ache caused by poor digestion, thrush, tonsilitis.
Contraindications: hypertension.

Heartsease *(Wild Pansy)* *(Viola tricolor)*

This is the wild ancestor of the great variety of pansies so commonly used for ornamental purposes. It too, can be grown in the garden, and it is readily available from nurseries.

Heartsease has anti-inflammatory and expectorant properties and is widely used in the treatment of eczema and other skin conditions.
Parts used: the dried herb.
Indications: bronchitis, cough (especially wet, mucus-producing), cradle cap, eczema.
Contraindications: none.

Lemon Balm (Balm) *(Melissa officinalis)*

This member of the mint family is easily grown in the garden. As the name indicates, the plant has a strong, lemon-like aroma. Lemon Balm has gentle relaxing and sedative properties and is an excellent children's remedy. It is particularly good for nervous states manifesting themselves as digestive problems and for sleeping difficulties.
Parts used: the fresh or dried leaves.
Indications: headaches and stomach-aches caused by anxiety or tension, nervous bowel, sleeplessness.
Contraindications: none.

Licorice *(Glycyrrhiza glabra)*

Known by every child as a flavouring for sweets (although much modern 'licorice' contains no extract of the plant whatsoever but is flavoured with the essential oil of Anise). This is one of the most widely used medicinal plants in Western herbal medicine as well as in traditional Chinese medicine.

Licorice possesses anti-inflammatory, antispasmodic, soothing and cough-relieving properties and aids the withdrawal from corticosteroid drugs (cortisone). It is said to have a harmonising effect on herbal mixtures and it certainly makes many remedies more palatable than they otherwise would be. Prolonged use of Licorice may lead to water retention and a low salt diet should be followed when taking the herb.
Parts used: the dried roots.
Indications: allergy, asthma, colds, constipation, cough, croup, measles, sore throat, whooping cough.
Contraindications: diarrhoea, oedema, hypertension.

Linden (Lime) *(Tilia europaea et spp.)*

A handsome deciduous tree native to Europe and western Asia. This is not the Lime which produces the green citrus fruits. However, the pale yellow flowers of this tree make one of the most delicate and pleasant tasting of all herbal teas.

Linden is a relaxant, increases peripheral bloodflow and is an important remedy for controlling fevers.
Parts used: the dried flowers.
Indications: to reduce fever, for headache and stomach-ache when a result of anxiety or nervousness, sore throat.
Contraindications: none.

Marshmallow *(Althaea officinalis)*

This attractive plant, the wild ancestor of the Hollyhock, is an excellent demulcent, i.e. it has soothing and mucilaginous properties. The tea which is prepared as a decoction is somewhat viscous. Marshmallow has a soothing effect on inflamed mucous membranes in the gastrointestinal tract and is an important cough remedy.
Parts used: the dried roots or leaves.
Indications: allergy, cough, diarrhoea, measles, sore throat, stomach-ache caused by indigestion with diarrhoea, sunburn, as a drawing poultice for splinters.
Contraindications: none.

Meadowsweet *(Filipendula ulmaria)*

This member of the rose family is a native of Europe and western Asia. It is one of the most important medicinal plants for digestive complaints, especially inflammations and problems associated with too much gastric acid.

Parts used: the dried, above-ground parts of the herb.

Indications: acute stomach upset with or without flatulence, stomach-ache caused by indigestion with diarrhoea, cases of excess gastric acidity.

Contraindications: none.

Mullein *(Verbascum thapsus)*

This stately plant is an important remedy for the respiratory tract. It has soothing properties combined with expectorant action.

Parts used: both the dried leaves and the yellow flowers can be used.

Indications: asthma, bronchitis, coughs, earache, mumps, whooping cough.

Contraindications: none.

Nettle (Stinging Nettle) *(Urtica dioica, U. urens)*

Both the annual and the larger, perennial species of nettle produce an unpleasant stinging sensation which may last several hours. Both are fairly common weeds. The stinging properties disappear completely when the plants are crushed, thoroughly dried or cooked — freshly picked nettle shoots are a most nutritious addition to vegetable soups.

Nettles are high in vitamins and minerals and are part of many traditional herbal teas for breastfeeding women. Nettle is taken internally for skin complaints, especially when the condition has a marked psychological component.

Parts used: the dried leaves and flowers.

Indications: eczema.

Contraindications: none.

Peppermint *(Mentha x piperita)*

Peppermint grows willingly and often profusely in semi-shaded, moist areas of the garden. The plant is a sterile hybrid, and thus does not set seed. It can therefore be propagated only by vegetative means such as cuttings.

Peppermint is an important medicinal plant, especially for a variety of complaints of the digestive tract where it has a calming and relaxing effect, relieves flatulence and increases bile secretion. It also brings down fever. Due to its pleasant taste, it can be used to flavour other less palatable herbs.

Parts used: the leaves (dried or fresh).

Indications: colds and flu, to prevent convulsions caused by high body temperature, fever, flatulence, headache, to manage high fever in German measles, measles, mumps and other infections (best with Yarrow and/or Elderflowers), stomach-ache caused by wind or poor digestion with constipation, travel sickness, vomiting and nausea.

Contraindications: none.

Red Clover *(Trifolium pratense)*

An important fodder plant, the medicinal use of this clover is primarily as a purifying agent in conditions caused by an accumulation of toxins and waste products in the body, for example many skin complaints. The plant also has expectorant properties.

Parts used: the flowerheads.

Indications: eczema and other skin disorders, mumps.

Contraindications: none.

Sage *(Salvia officinalis)*

A well-known culinary herb, Sage is a sun-loving plant which can easily be grown in the garden in rather dry and slightly alkaline soil. Like Thyme and other related plants in the mint family, Sage contains a highly aromatic essential oil. The plant is antiseptic and astringent.

Parts used: the dried (or fresh) leaves.

Indications: topically to stop bleeding, as a gargle or mouthwash for mouth ulcers, sore throat and tonsillitis.

Contraindications: none for topical use or when used as a gargle. However, the herb is not suitable for internal use in small children.

CAUTION: do not use Sage Oil.

Slippery Elm *(Ulmus fulva)*

The inner bark of this North American tree has soothing and protective actions on the mucous membranes in the digestive tract. It has nutritive value and can be used as a bulk laxative when constipation is caused by lack of fibre in the diet.

Due to the fact that the powder swells considerably when it comes in contact with moisture *the dry powder should never be given to children. Always add water first.*

Parts used: the dried, powdered inner bark.

Indications: allergy, diarrhoea, stomach-ache caused by indigestion with diarrhoea, as a drawing poultice for splinters.

Contraindications: none.

Thyme *(Thymus vulgaris)*

Another good example of a familiar kitchen herb which is also an excellent medicinal plant. Thyme is a good anti-bacterial and anti-fungal herb and is one of the most useful, relaxing expectorants. It also helps expel intestinal worms.

Parts used: the dried herb.

Indications: asthma, coughs, croup, measles, mouth ulcers, mumps, sore throat, thrush, tonsillitis, whooping cough, worms.

Contraindications: none.

CAUTION: do not use Thyme Oil.

Valerian *(Valeriana officinalis)*

Valerian is one of the best known herbal sedatives. The dried roots and preparations made from them have a characteristic smell which is stronger than the actual taste of the tea. Valerian can be used in all cases of nervous tension, restlessness and insomnia.

Parts used: the dried roots.

Indications: sleeping difficulties, stomach-ache when a result of anxiety or nervousness, general nervous tension.

Contraindications: none.

NOTE: on very rare occasions, Valerian has a stimulating rather than sedative effect. If this is observed, discontinue the use of this herb.

White Horehound *(Marrubium vulgare)*

A member of the mint family, White Horehound can easily be grown in the garden. It is also a common weed in parts of Australia.

White Horehound is an important stimulating expectorant which has relaxing properties as well. Because of its bitterness it is a digestive stimulant. The bitterness of this herb presents a problem; it actually tastes so bad that it must be flavoured with a sweet-tasting herb such as Licorice or Aniseed.

Parts used: the leaves and/or flowering tops.

Indications: bronchitis, colds with cough, coughs (especially wet, mucus-producing).

Contraindications: none.

Yarrow *(Achillea millefolium)*

Another member of the daisy family which can be grown in the garden. It prefers fairly dry soil and a sunny position. Yarrow possesses a wide range of therapeutic actions and is an ideal plant to have in the home remedies chest. One of the best herbs for controlling high fever, it also has a relaxing and gently stimulating effect on the digestion. It stops bleeding from minor cuts and wounds and acts as a wound healer.

Parts used: leaves and flowers.

Indications: bleeding, colds and flu, to prevent convulsions caused by high body temperature, fever (including high fever in German measles, measles, mumps and other infections), sore throat, stomach-ache caused by poor digestion.

Contraindications: none.

NOTE: rarely, this plant causes allergy in sensitive individuals.

HOME REMEDIES

So many of the solutions to our children's illnesses are to be found, not in laboratories but in the combination of commonsense, the wisdom of our grandparents, parents and friends, and our own kitchen cupboard. I can still hear my mother-in-law describing to me 'Grandma Beck's cure for whatever ailed you. Goose grease, pitch plaster or a good old enema.' If one didn't cure you the others surely would!

My own mother used to hand me a glass of salted water, whenever I complained of a sore throat. 'Gargle, every half hour,' she would say, 'and you'll be right by morning.' Most times it worked!

Home remedies will probably always have a place in the treatment of minor illness and it's just as well as most GPs don't expect you to dash to them with every minor discomfort, injury, ache or pain. It is just as sensible to care for such things at home by simple, safe means.

Home remedies have been handed down from one generation to another through notebooks, cookbooks, in old diaries or just by word of mouth. In the *National Geographic* magazine, it was reported in June 1962, that the early settlers of the Tennessee mountains were 'heavily dependent on homemade remedies'. Some of the plant medicines that were reported were catnip tea (a blood purifier and fever reducer), mustard poultices for colds, honey and alum for sore throats, onion poultices for chest colds, croup and pneumonia, and cobwebs on wounds to stop the bleeding. Many of the medical drugs in use today have been developed on the basis of information and studies derived from plants.

Surely everybody has onions and garlic in their kitchen, and when needed they can provide antibacterial effects for combating the common cold, sore throat or earache. Garlic has been used for centuries to heal all sorts of ailments, including gastro-intestinal problems and respiratory infections. Apple juice can be used when the lymph system needs a good cleansing, or when swollen glands or mumps is the ailment. Combined with cloves which act as a topical pain killer, apple juice will help reduce discomfort when swallowing. Rice, rich in potassium, sulfur, chlorine and phosphorus, is ideal for such conditions as swelling, warts and other skin problems. Bay leaves are another common kitchen cupboard ingredient which make excellent home remedies for bleeding gums, canker sores, and infant thrush. They are highly astringent and contain carminative oils that can soothe upset tummies in infants and digestive problems in children and adults.

Home remedies have been, and will continue to be, non-invasive and successful means for treating many common childhood illnesses.

HOMOEOPATHY

Homoeopathy emerged as a medical science in the late 1700s from the research of the esteemed German physician and chemist, Samuel Hahnemann. He believed that the routine practices of his day such as prescribing poisonous doses of drugs were doing more harm than good. Hahnemann was translating a medical text by the English author, Dr William Cullen but found himself disagreeing with Cullen's explanation that the herb Peruvian Bark, which contains quinine, cured malaria because it was bitter. Hahnemann knew of many bitters and none of the others cured malaria. He decided to experiment on himself and after taking the herb began to experience many of the symptoms associated with malaria. These symptoms recurred each time he took a dose and when he stopped the medicine, his health returned. This was an astonishing revelation to Hahnemann: the opposite to what had been taught: that a drug which cures malaria produces symptoms similar to malaria in a healthy person. Hahnemann carried out further experiments with other drugs and confirmed this principle which was to become the first law or principle of homoeopathy: *like cures like*. This means that a medicinal substance which creates certain symptoms in a healthy person, will cure a sick person manifesting similar symptoms. For example, an onion may cause the eyes and nose to water and sting. If a patient presents to the homoeopath with these symptoms (as in a simple cold) then he may receive the homoeopathic preparation of onion to cure the condition.

Hahnemann found that a single medicine chosen by the homoeopathic method was able to act on the whole person mentally, physically and emotionally. As he found that only one medicine was necessary to cure, he established the second principle of homoeopathy: *only one medicine is to be used at a time*.

In order to prevent all the toxic side-effects of medicines Hahnemann developed a special method of preparation which involved diluting and then shaking (succussing) the substance a number of times. This process is called potentisation and all homoeopathic remedies are prepared in this way. This process not only maintains but even increases the therapeutic value of medicines.

To sum up, the three main principles of homoeopathy are:
1 A substance which creates symptoms in a healthy person will remove similar symptoms in a sick person.
2 Only one remedy is prescribed at a time.
3 Very diluted, and therefore harmless, substances are used.

Homoeopathic Practitioners

Some homoeopaths are first trained in orthodox medicine while others are trained purely in the homoepathic method. A traditional homoeopath (one who uses the essential principles of homoeopathy) will seek to investigate the whole of the presenting complaint and patient history before making a prescription. He or she will only prescribe a single medicine at a time so that clarity and understanding of the process of cure is maintained throughout the treatment.

Acute and Chronic Ailments

Homoeopathic medicine is able to treat the two basic categories of illness, acute and chronic disease. Acute diseases are those which are of limited duration, for example flu, muscle strains or fevers, whereas chronic diseases like asthma or arthritis take hold of the body and do not diminish with time but usually increase their hold. The homoeopathics recommended in this book essentially deal with acute illnesses and first-aid situations. If you are treating your child effectively with homoeopathic medicines but the symptoms keep returning at intervals then your homoeopath may prescribe a chronic (also known as constitutional) medicine to adjust your child's system and prevent further recurrence. Chronic long term diseases and acute illnesses with severe symptoms such as very high fever or persistent or violent vomiting must be treated by a properly trained homoeopathic practitioner.

Tissue Salts

Tissue salts are a limited selection of homoeopathic remedies made from mineral compounds which are natural components of the human body. They were used exclusively by Dr Schussler but have now been incorporated into the broader homoeopathic materia medica. A number of tissue salts are useful in first aid and for treating acute illnesses in the home. These have been included in the Materia Medica section. They are usually available at health food stores.

HOMOEOPATHIC REMEDIES

Homoeopathic medicines act on your child by strengthening and restoring the inherent powers of the body to heal itself. This takes place principally through the 'control' systems of the body, such as the immune system, the nervous system and the hormonal system. Children generally respond quickly to the correctly chosen medicine as their systems are less inhibited by stress, toxins and emotional restraints. Remember, the medicines are very dilute and so do not produce the side-effects that might be experienced with orthodox medicines.

Preparations and Potency

The substances used in homoeopathy are drawn from plant, animal and mineral sources. As mentioned previously the remedies are prepared by dilution and succussion of these substances. There are two main scales of dilution:

- Decimal — which uses a dilution factor of 10 and is notated by an 'X' or 'D' on the bottle.
- Centesimal — which uses a dilution factor of 100 and is notated by a 'C' on the bottle.

If for instance we are looking at a centesimal medicine the first dilution is known as 1C, the second as 2C and so on up to the required strength. If you have the medicine Chamomilla 12C it means that the medicine was diluted by a factor of 100 twelve times. You will see the dilution factor written on the label of each medicine you purchase.

In the Homoeopathic Materia Medica you will find that a number of potencies are suggested for each medicine. These are considered to be most suitable for use in the home and medicines of much higher or lower potency should only be prescribed by the qualified homoeopath. The tissue salts are usually given in the supplied 6X potency.

You should purchase homoeopathic medicines in pillule (small pills) form. These pillules are based on lactose or cane sugar. They can be given dry on the tongue or, if necessary dissolved in a teaspoon of water. They are available from all reputable suppliers of homoeopathics.

How To Select a Remedy

The remedy that is best indicated for your child is the one which is most suitable to the sum total of all symptoms with which he presents. All prominent mental, emotional and physical symptoms which have arisen during the acute illness should be taken into account — proper selection of the remedy must be based on the *whole person*. Homoeopathic remedies stimulate the natural vital forces to encourage a quick return to health.

The following is a guide to the information you will need to correlate the illness to the symptoms of the medicine:

- Possible cause: a fall, shock, grief, exposure to cold wind, chill, an insect sting, etc. For example Aconite has ailments from exposure to cold dry winds.
- Mode of onset: sudden or gradual.
- Location of the symptoms or the pain: for example, head pain may not be located in the whole head but only in the right temple as in Belladonna.
- The type of pain: stitching, burning, tearing, throbbing, etc.
- The modalities (what makes the symptoms better or worse): for example, better for cold, worse for movement, better for pressure, worse for lying down.
- Sides: is it left sided or right sided?
- Discharges: if there is discharge, what is its nature — colour, consistency and colour?
- The general state of the child: is he restless, cold, thirsty, desiring lemonade, wanting

fresh air? (These symptoms are very important, as the whole person is affected.)

- Mental/emotional symptoms: irritability, fearful, weepy, sighing. (Again these symptoms are very important as the whole person is affected.) Homoeopaths have found that where these are prominent, they must be in the symptom picture of the medicine for it to cure.
- Examination and observation: redness, swelling of the affected part, for example, is the child flushed or pale, are the pupils dilated?

When you have noted all the important symptoms, the remedy with similar symptoms, following both the A-Z of Complaints and the descriptions in the Homoeopathic Materia Medica. Only those remedies that are commonly used for many different complaints are covered in the Materia Medica. Referring to both of these sections will help you, especially if more than one remedy seems to be indicated. The remedies are suitable for children from birth to twelve years of age.

How To Administer the Remedies

1 Once the remedy has been chosen on the basis of similar symptoms, one pillule should be dissolved in a teaspoon of water and given to the child in a clean mouth. This is one dose. If the child will not take it in water, the pill may be given dry on the tongue.

To administer homoeopathic remedies in pill form to babies between the ages of six and twelve months it is easier to crush the tablets between two teaspoons until powdery and mix with about a teaspoon of warm or boiled water.

Choose which method works best for you.

2 The child should not drink or eat ten minutes before or after each dose of a homoeopathic remedy (water is an exception).

3 The pillules should not be handled but dispensed into the lid and then into a teaspoon or the mouth as required.

4 If the condition is severe, as in high fever or burns, then the remedy may need to be given every 15-20 minutes (even every 5 minutes for the pain of a burn). When symptoms are of medium intensity, a dose should be given every 2-3 hours and in slight injury, once or twice a day.

5 The most important caution to remember with dosage is to *stop on marked or sudden change for better or for worse.*

If your child is markedly better no further doses should be given. Wait and observe. If he continues to improve, there will be no need of further dosing. If the improvement stops or slows down you can administer doses at longer intervals. In the event that there is no improvement after administering six doses stop the treatment. In this case it is unlikely that you are using the correct remedy. Consult a practitioner of your choice as soon as possible.

If the symptoms get worse, stop the dosing and wait. Occasionally you will find that when the correct remedy has been chosen the symptoms become worse for a short time. This varies from a few minutes in intense conditions (for example high fever) to a few hours in milder conditions (for example sporadic coughing). If there is no improvement after a few hours reassess the prescription. If another medicine is indicated, then it may be given, but if in doubt seek the advice of a homoeopathic practitioner.

6 Any strong aromatic substance (for example eucalyptus oil) used at the same time as a homoeopathic remedy can act as an antidote to the remedy. Use them 30 minutes apart.

Caring for the Medicines

The medicines should be kept away from strong light, heat and strong odours or scents, such as camphor.

Homoeopathic Materia Medica

This section contains the Materia Medica which is simply an alphabetical list of the remedies. Each is discussed in detail to give a complete picture of the remedy, including mental, emotional (fear and anxiety will accompany every ailment however trivial) and physical aspects. The word 'modalities' is a term which means that symptoms are aggravated or ameliorated by certain factors.

Note that the symbol > means better for and < means worse for.

Aconite

A major remedy for shock or for conditions which come on suddenly, after exposure to cold dry winds, such as colds and fevers.

SYMPTOMS CHARACTERISED BY

Suddenness: complaints come on rapidly.

Intensity: symptoms are of a violent nature with intense pain or high fever.

Inflammation: the first stage of inflammation before suppurations (discharge) or mucus sets in.

Pains: violent and sudden, driving the child to distraction.

Over-sensitivity: to pain, smells, touch, etc.

THE CHILD IS

Fearful: of being alone; of crowds; of death. This state may be accompanied by bounding pulse, rapid heart beat or fever.

Restless: tosses, turns, changes position constantly; nervous irritability.

Thirsty: for large amounts.

MODALITIES

Aggravated: after cold dry winds; in the evening; in a warm room; noise; light; tobacco smoke; a shock.

Ameliorated: open air.

THE BODY

Head: sudden violent headache; head full, bursting, worse in a warm room.

Eyes: sudden inflammation with watery discharge only.

Ears: intense earache after exposure to cold dry wind; sensitive to noise.

Nose: water mucus, worse at night; nose bleeds; first signs of a cold.

Face: neuralgia (nerve pain); flushed.

Mouth: gums hot and inflamed; tongue coated white.

Stomach: vomiting due to fear, fright or exposure to cold.

Urine: urine retention after shocks.

Respiration: croup from cold dry wind; throat red, dry, constricted; breathing short and laboured; acute asthma.

Fever: rapid onset; thirsty, restless, fearful; skin hot, dry and red; pulse bounding; photophobia (intolerance of light); intolerance of warmth, throws off the bedclothes.

Recommended potency: 30C

Antimonium Crudum

The sulphide of Antimony is often indicated for children who are inclined to excessive weight gain.

THE CHILD IS

Irritable: and fretful.

Weeps: if looked at.

Symptoms are often accompanied by

Thick milky white coating: on the tongue.

MODALITIES

Aggravated: washing or cold bathing; the heat of the sun or warm room.

Ameliorated: open air and rest.

THE BODY

Head: aches from becoming cold, also from cold bathing and digestive upset from excess fat, acids and fruit.

Digestive tract: thick milky white coating on the tongue; gastric complaints from cold bathing, overheating or overeating; vomiting < for eating or drinking; stomach weak and easily disturbed; stomach is sensitive to pressure; watery diarrhoea mixed with lumps; constant burping and flatulence.

Respiration: whooping cough < for being overheated.

Skin: horny warts; impetigo; scaly, pulsular eruption with burning and < itching night.

Extremities: nails tend to split.

Recommended potency: 12C

Antimonium Tartaricum

Also called Tartar emetic which was traditionally used as an emetic (causing vomiting) but in homoeopathy it is used to cure vomiting. It can be used in cases of near-drowning.

SYMPTOMS CHARACTERISED BY

Drowsiness: great desire or irresistible inclination to sleep after complaints.

Sweat: profuse and cold especially on the face.

THE CHILD IS

Clinging: wants to be carried; cries and whines when touched; will not let you feel the pulse.

Cold: face feels cold and sweat is cold.

MODALITIES

Aggravated: cold and damp; lying down at night; warm room; change of weather in spring; evening.

Ameliorated: sitting upright; cold; open air; belching; expectorating; lying on right side.

THE BODY

Digestive tract: tongue coated thick white with reddened papillae or red edges; craving for apples; vomiting in any position except lying on right side; vomiting until he faints.

Respiration: rattling of mucus in the chest with difficult or no expectoration; cough results in great drowsiness; at birth the child was pale, breathless, asphyxiated from mucus in the larynx.

Skin: cold pale or blue, especially the face; cold sweat; pustular eruptions; pox eruptions: smallpox, chickenpox.

Recommended potency: 12C

Apis Mellifica

For the effects of bites and stings specially where there is swelling. A preparation of the honey bee.

SYMPTOMS CHARACTERISED BY

Swelling: pale waxy swelling due to accumulation of fluid in the tissues, may have rosy red hue and appear in throat, face, about the eyes, joints or abdomen.

Sensitiveness: to touch/pressure.

Pains: burning and especially stinging.

Violence and rapidity of onset: of complaints.

THE CHILD IS

Sad: tearful weeping disposition; weeping day and night; whining.

Irritable: nervous, apprehensive.

Indifferent: to everything that could make them happy.

Clumsy and awkward: drops things.

Thirstless: often associated with scanty urination.

MODALITIES

Aggravated: heat in all forms: warm room, fire, hot drinks; pressure; touch; lying down, especially on the right side.

Ameliorated: cold applications or bath; motion; open air; uncovering; change of position.

THE BODY

Face: puffy swelling of face, eyelids, eyes, mouth.

Throat: tonsils swollen, stinging, rosy red, ulcerated with white secretions.

Respiration: difficult breathing; swelling in the throat or air passages; asthma.

Mumps: swelling soft, rosy, puffy and tender.

Urine: burning and soreness when urinating; scanty urination.

Skin: hives, itchy.

Stings: bee and insect bites — rapid rosy looking swelling, red, itchy and puffy.

Recommended potency: 12C

Arnica

Means 'fall herb'. Important for injuries to soft parts leading to bruising, concussion or haemorrhage or for over exertion.

SYMPTOMS CHARACTERISED BY

Bruised feeling: or lame, sore feeling in the injured part or all over the body as in influenza.

Swelling: of affected part.

Discolouration: blue/black of the affected part.

Restlessness: everything that is rested on feels too hard which necessitates the child to constantly change position.

THE CHILD IS

Fearful of being touched or approached: often because they feel sore and sensitive.

Preferring to be alone: while sick.

Exhausted: from strain, sport or over exertion.

MODALITIES

Aggravated: touch or pressure; motion; over exertion.

THE BODY

Head: hot with body cold; concussion.

Eyes: bloodshot; black eye.

Face: ruddy.

Teeth: to reduce pain and bruising following dental surgery.

Throat: hoarseness from over-use of voice.

Digestive tract: eructations (belches), stool or flatus smelling of rotten eggs.

Extremities: limbs ache as if beaten or bruised; cannot walk or raise arms due to soreness.

Sprains: aching from strains or over-use.

Skin: easy bruising; blue/black discolouration; very sore acne; crops of boils.

Sleep: comatose drowsiness.

Fever: influenza; the body aches and feels bruised.

Recommended potency: 30C

Arsenicum Album

SYMPTOMS CHARACTERISED BY

Burning pains: in any part which is relieved by heat.

Weakness and prostration: exhausted from the slightest exertion; complains of great weakness which is out of proportion to the apparent cause.

Chilliness.

Restlessness: tries to find relief in motion, always moving.

THE CHILD IS

Anxious and fearful: about others; about trifles; of death.

Depressed: thinks he will never recover.

Very restless: in mind and body.

Thirsty: intense thirst, drinks often but only a little at a time.

MODALITIES

Aggravated: cold air, applications, drink or food; after midnight, particularly 1-2 a.m.; lying on the right side.

Ameliorated: warmth and hot applications, except the head; warm food and drinks; open air; sweating; having head elevated.

THE BODY

Head: headache $>$ cold applications.

Nose: colds descend to the chest; thin watery discharge that burns the skin; redness; sneezing.

Throat: burning pain relieved by hot drinks.

Digestive tract: burning pain in stomach; gastric derangement from food poisoning, cold drinks, ice cream, cold fruit, watery fruit, cheese or spicy food; aversion to the sight and smell of food; vomiting with retching and nausea; vomiting of blood, bile, brown, black or frothy mucus. Diarrhoea with painful cramps burning and offensive odour; stools bloody, watery or dark; great weakness afterwards.

Respiration: head colds descend to chest; asthma — unable to lie down; fear of suffocation — must sit or bend forward; burning in chest; cough is worse after midnight.

Skin: cold, blue; cold clammy perspiration.

Extremities: twitching and trembling.

Fever: anxious, restless, burning pains; thirsty for frequent sips.

Influenza: aching; averse to sight and smell of food; tendency to diarrhoea and vomiting.

Recommended potency: 12C

Belladonna

A remedy for fevers and inflammations characterised by sudden onset. Acts mainly on the nervous system.

SYMPTOMS CHARACTERISED BY

Sudden violent onset.

Heat and burning: in all parts, discharges feel hot.

Throbbing: or pulsating of ailments, headaches, abscesses, boils, etc.

Hypersensitivity: ailments worse for light, noise, jarring, touch.

Redness: of the affected part.

Right-sided complaints: symptoms tend to be predominantly right-sided.

THE CHILD IS

Fretful: irritable, nervy, excitable.

Sensitive to cold and draughts: can even get a cold after a haircut.

Restless.

Delirious: in high fevers; may experience hallucinations.

MODALITIES

Aggravated: cold and cold draughts; light; jarring; noise; haircut.

Ameliorated: warmth; sitting still and straight; bending backward.

THE BODY

Head: throbbing headache worse for jarring, light, noise, often on the right side.

Face: pupils dilated; face red, especially the cheeks; eyes glassy.

Throat: red and inflamed, worse on the right side; liquids painful to swallow; glands hot and swollen; tonsillitis.

Digestive tract: tongue strawberry or white coated; desire for lemonade.

Skin: boils, hot and throbbing.

Sleep: moans or screams out in sleep; twitches and jumps; grinds teeth.

Fever: sudden high fever with restlessness, delirium and dilated pupils; skin hot, red and dry; worse for uncovering; head hot but feet cold; influenza; mumps.

Recommended potency: 30C

Bryonia Alba

Has an important action on the pleura which are the membranes covering the lungs, relieving inflammation. It may also act on mucous membranes and reducing excessive secretions.

SYMPTOMS CHARACTERISED BY

Dryness: because of lack of secretion of various glands throughout the entire digestive tract from mouth to rectum; dry cracked lips, mouth, cough and dry hard stools.

Stitching pains: pains sharp, stitch like a needle especially respiratory complaints for example, pneumonia, pleurisy.

Slow onset: most complaints develop slowly.

Hardness: dry hard stools; small hard glands.

THE CHILD IS

Angry: irritable, does not want to be bothered and desires seclusion and quiet.

Thirsty: for large quantities — often or every few hours.

Irritable: cries for something and then refuses it.

MODALITIES

Aggravated: motion, < slightest movement regardless of symptoms; warmth, hot weather; light touch; vexation.

Ameliorated: pressure, keeping the affected part still. > lying on the affected side as it aids in keeping it at rest for example, cough better for keeping completely still or pressing the chest; bandaging; cool open air.

THE BODY

Head: bursting, splitting headache as if everything is pushed out; << motion — even of eyes; stitching tearing pain < cough, sitting up, stooping.

Nose: watery nasal discharge with stuffy nose; dry nose; colds travel to chest.

Face: lips parched; dry, cracked.

Mouth: dry, bitter taste; white coating of tongue.

Digestive tract: nausea and faintness on rising; bitter belching.

Stomach: sensitive to touch; sense of a heaviness or a stone in the stomach; vomiting bile after eating, water, warm drinks, fatty or rich foods; colic < movement and warmth; appendicitis, stools large, dry, hard as if burnt; constipation from poor muscle tone; diarrhoea < in the morning on rising or after cold drinks in warm weather.

Respiration: head colds travel to the chest; presses hand to chest when coughing; dry throat; dry, hard painful cough > pressing chest < warm room; sharp stitching in chest < deep inspiration; pleurisy.

Fever: must lie still; thirst for large drinks.

Injury: injured joint swollen and painful; pain from a fractured rib; twisted knee < slight motion.

Influenza: with painful throat, cough and chest.

Measles: early stages, rash does not properly appear — comes and goes; bronchitis or pneumonia develops instead.

Mumps: hard swelling with tenderness.

Recommended potency: 12C

Calendula Cream (for external use only)

Calendula is a herb with antiseptic and healing properties and is useful for cuts, abrasions or burns (including sunburn) to sooth, heal and prevent infection.

Cantharis

Important for burns and scalds and urinary tract infections associated with burning pains.

SYMPTOMS CHARACTERISED BY

Pains burning: cutting and smarting or as if raw.

Inflammation.

Mucus: stringy.

THE CHILD IS

Irritable: ending in rage.

THE BODY

Throat: as if on fire; great difficulty swallowing liquids.

Digestive tract: burning thirst, but averse to all fluids; burning stools, bloody and shreddy.

Urine: kidney region very sensitive; cystitis; urine burning, scalding with intolerable urging; urine passes only in drops; urine bloody.

Skin: burns and scalds, better for cold water,

just before or just after blisters form; vesicles or blisters full of yellowish fluid.

Recommended potency: 30C

Carbo — Vegetabilis

Charcoal is used for excessive gas and as a toxin remover. In homoeopathy it is known as the 'corpse reviver'.

SYMPTOMS CHARACTERISED BY

Sluggishness/indolence: slow thinking; pains develop slowly; weak digestion; indolent ulcers.

Coldness of surfaces: knees to feet, breath, tongue, sweat, nose, fingertips; associated with blueness of skin.

Putridity: septic states with putrid odour and burning sensation; involuntary putrid stool.

MODALITIES

Aggravated: evening; open air, warm and damp weather; lying down; fatty food; milk; during and after eating.

Ameliorated: burping; fanning; cool air.

THE CHILD IS

Indifferent: dull, indolent.

THE BODY

Face: bluish; cold breath.

Respiration: desire for air — must be fanned; cold breath; asthma after long spasmodic cough with gagging and vomiting < eating, talking; raw, sore chest with difficult breathing < evening.

Digestive tract: averse to meat, milk and fats; burning in stomach/heartburn; belching and gas after eating; simple food causes gas; digestion slow and weak; swelling of upper abdomen or stomach; cramps cause them to bend double.

Collapse: from any cause; lack of air.

Skin: sweat cold clammy and bluish.

Extremities: limbs cold and bluish.

Recommended potency: 12C

Chamomilla

Acts mainly on the nervous system. Used for ailments which come on after anger.

SYMPTOMS CHARACTERISED BY

Over-sensitivity: especially to pain which can be unbearable and drive child to distraction; the child may even scold the pain and everyone else.

Pains: severe and unbearable; < night; associated with numbness of part; faints from pain.

Heat: one cheek hot and red; child hot and thirsty — hot sweaty head.

THE CHILD IS

Restless: with the pain; constantly moving.

Thirsty: excessively, for cold drinks.

Irritable: extremely so — asks for something then throws it aside; cannot return a civil answer; spiteful, snappish and screaming; child fretful, whining and wants to be carried.

Impatient: unreasonable, obstinate.

Moaning: with the pain.

MODALITIES

Aggravated: anger; night; cold; damp; heat.

Ameliorated: being carried; walking; warm wet weather.

THE BODY

Head: hot clammy sweat; throbbing ache on one side; convulsions in child specially during teething.

Ears: ache, swelling and heat drive the child frantic, > heat; sensitive to noise, ear feels stopped.

Eyes: profuse, acrid discharges.

Face: hot and body cold; one cheek red; neuralgia < heat.

Teeth: ache < anything warm in mouth > eating cold things, holding cold drinks in the mouth; hypersensitivity to pain of dental treatment.

Digestive tract: low appetite but desires cold drinks; bitter taste; foul burps; violent vomiting and retching; abdomen distended with gas; colic — child doubles up, screams, kicks, wants to be carried; stool is hot, green, watery, fetid, like chopped eggs and spinach; diarrhoea from a chill, after anger, during teething; excoriation (skin rubbed off) around the anus.

Sleep: sleepless and restless at night; sleepless though tired; moaning, weeping, tossing, and talking in sleep.

Fever: with violent thirst.

Skin: sweats after eating or drinking; night sweats.

Recommended potency: 30C

Coffea Cruda

Made from the raw coffee berries. Symptoms occur after excessive joy and laughter or disappointed love. Used for insomnia, toothache and convulsions in teething children.

SYMPTOMS CHARACTERISED BY

Over-sensitivity: to pain, touch, noise, odours.

Nervous agitation and restlessness.

Despair from pain: which is intolerable.

THE CHILD IS

Irritable and wakeful: sleeplessness associated with an over-active mind.

Weepy: tosses about in anguish.

Moody: cries and laughs easily.

MODALITIES

Aggravated: noise; mental exertion; walking in open air; strong odours; night; touch.

Ameliorated: sleep; warmth; lying down.

THE BODY

Head: convulsions in teething children with grinding teeth and coldness of limbs. Pain as if nail driven into the head.

Eyes: dilated pupils, bright eyes.

Ears: hearing acute.

Nose: smell acute.

Teeth: toothache > holding ice water in mouth < as water warms.

Stomach: eats and drinks hurriedly.

Respiration: dry hacking cough with measles.

Sleep: sleepless from mental activity or excitement.

Extremities: trembling of hands and twitching of limbs.

Skin: painfully sensitive; itchy, scratches until it bleeds.

Recommended potency: 12C

Colocynthis

THE CHILD IS

Angry: may be suffering the effects of anger especially if suppressed; irritable with the pain.

Very restless.

MODALITIES

Aggravated: suppressed emotion; anger; indignation; least amount of food or drink.

Ameliorated: pressure; heat; beinding over; escape of gas; passing stool.

THE BODY

Stomach: nausea and vomiting with pain.

Abdomen: severe cutting or cramping pain, child doubles up from the pain; must press on abdomen; distention of abdomen; sensation of stone; feels like it will burst; sore around navel; cramping diarrhoea; every bite of food followed by a rush of diarrhoea.

Stool: jelly-like.

Extremities: pain and contractions in hips, legs; sciatica which is contractive > pressure, heat, < when still.

Recommended potency: 12C

Ferrum Phos

Indicated where inflammation is present with pain, redness or fever, especially inflammation before the formation of pus.

SYMPTOMS CHARACTERISED BY

Heat: or fever.

Redness.

MODALITIES

Aggravated: motion; night; suppressed sweat.

Ameliorated: cold applications.

THE BODY

Eyes: red, burning, sore; sensation of grains of sand under lid; styes.

Ears: first stage of earache with throbbing and heat.

Nose: bleeding.

Face: flushed.

Throat: first stages of inflamed throat; tonsils red and swollen; pain worse for empty swallowing.

Urine: urine retained in children during fever.

Respiration: beginnings of a cold; bronchitis.

Skin: measles.

Fever: beginning stages of fever before mucus sets in; chill with desire to stretch.

Recommended potency: 6C (The tissue salt preparation of 6X or 12X is also satisfactory)

Gelsemium

This medicine displays two opposite phases:

- Sluggish, relaxed, torpid state. Mental and physical functions are depressed. Muscles respond tardily to the will.
- Hypersensitive, rigid, excitable.

SYMPTOMS CHARACTERISED BY

Weakness: relaxation and prostration of the whole muscular system; lassitude, fatigue; wants to lie down, feels weak.

Functional paralysis: eyelids droop; vision blurred; loss of voice; numbness of the hands.

Heaviness: of body, limbs.

Trembling: of hands, legs, body, tongue; trembling is so severe that it shakes the child like a chill, however no chill is present.

THE CHILD IS

Fearful: problems associated with excitment, anticipation, fear or dread of an event, surgery, social, exams. The effect is diarrhoea, trembling, shivering, chills during first stage of fever.

Apathetic and indifferent: mental faculties dull, cannot think, drowsy with red face; speech becomes thick and slow; eyelids droop; wants to be alone; doesn't want to move.

Thirstless.

MODALITIES

Aggravated: emotions; cold and humid weather; before storms; thinking about ailments; at 10 a.m.; any effort to think.

Ameliorated: profuse urination; sweating; open air; bending forward; continued motion.

THE BODY

Head: headaches from sun, mental stress, anxiety; sensation of band around head above eyes; pain at base of brain > profuse urination; wants head high.

Face: dark and flushed.

Eyes: eyelids heavy, drooping; pain < motion of eyes; pupils dilated; double vision.

Nose: sneezing, running, hot, watery — irritates nose and upper lip; pain at root of nose.

Throat: hoarseness.

Respiration: cough hard and croupy; dry cough.

Digestive tract: diarrhoea green, cream coloured and painless — from emotions, excitement, bad news; involuntary stool.

Extremities: limbs aching and heavy.

Sleep: insomnia from excitement about coming event; exhaustion.

Fever: chill with aching and weakness; chill up and down back; drowsiness and heaviness of limbs and eyelids; great shaking and chattering; no thirst; trembling with long exhausting sweats.

Measles: itching increases when rash appears.

Recommended potency: 30C

Hepar Sulph

An important remedy for suppuration and septic conditions.

SYMPTOMS CHARACTERISED BY

Hypersensitivity: to touch; pain; cold air; specifically dry and cold; faints from pain; slightest thing irritates even to violent behaviour.

Offensiveness: of perspiration, of discharges — often like old rotten cheese.

Suppuration: skin unhealthy — even slightest injuries and scratches become infected.

Splinter sensation: sticking, pricking sore throat; boils and pustules.

Sweating: sweats easily on mental or physical exertion.

THE CHILD IS

Hypersensitive: as above.

Irritable: angry; quarrelsome.

Very sensitive to cold draughts and cold dry winds: cannot bear to have the smallest part uncovered.

MODALITIES

Aggravated: dry cold wind; draught; lying on right side; slight touch; lying on painful side.

Ameliorated: damp weather; wrapping up the head; warmth; after eating.

THE BODY

Ears: throbbing, whizzing; earache very sensitive to touch > wrapping up; pustules in the ear; infection extends from throat.

Nose: sneezes in cold wind; hayfever; discharges first watery then thick and offensive; yellow discharge from one nostril.

Throat: sensation as though plug or splinter is lodged when swallowing; suppuration (formation or discharge of pus) of tonsils; hoarse.

Respiration: dry hoarse cough < cold food; rattling loose cough; expectoration thick and yellow; suffocating choking cough; difficult breathing and wheezing.

Skin: unhealthy skin — every little injury suppurates or ulcerates; sensitive ulcers or abscesses; offensive perspiration.

Injury: red, swollen, painful/suppurates.

Recommended potency: 12C

Hypericum

A primary remedy for injury to sensory nerves or for injury to parts rich in nerves, such as fingers, toes, spine, brain and tail bone. It is also used as a preventative against tetanus.

SYMPTOMS CHARACTERISED BY

Shooting pains: darting, stitching, along the nerves.

Radiating pain: pain at the site of injury radiates towards the centre of the body.

Excessive painfulness of the part: pain is disproportionately severe indicating involvement of the nerves.

THE CHILD IS

Suffering nervous depression: following wounds or surgical operations.

Sensitive to cold.

MODALITIES

Aggravated: touch; damp; cold; foggy weather.

Ameliorated: lying on the affected side.

THE BODY

Face: lockjaw.

Teeth: toothache > for lying on the painful side; dental surgery, to reduce the pain of the drill.

Neck and back: consequences of spinal concussion; tail bone painful, pain radiating up the spine and down the limbs after a fall; painfully sensitive spine.

Extremities: crushed fingers, nail torn or injured; phantom pains of an amputated limb.

Skin: puncture wounds, standing on a nail, animal bite; preventative for tetanus.

Recommended potency: 30C

Ignatia

A remedy to calm the emotions, especially when ailments come on after grief, bad news, fright, disappointed love or anger.

SYMPTOMS CHARACTERISED BY

Sensation of a ball in inner parts: for example lump in the throat, abdomen or rectum.

Spasm: twitching, jerking, hiccups.

Contradictions: for example parts better for hard pressure, upset stomach better for indigestible foods.

THE CHILD IS

Moody: from laughter to tears, joy to grief.

Weeping: sobbing, weeps in solitude, worse for consolation, silent grieving.

Sighing.

Grieving: regret, remorse.

Giggling: laughing over serious matters.

Desires: sour foods, acid foods.

MODALITIES

Aggravated: emotions; grief; anger. Coffee; sweets.

Ameliorated: lying on the painful side; hard pressure; warmth; urination.

THE BODY

Head: pain like nail sticking into the head, better for lying on the painful side.

Mouth: easily bites the inside of cheeks.

Face: twitching of muscles and eyelids.

Throat: lump in the throat, cannot be swallowed; sore when not swallowing or when swallowing liquids but better for swallowing solids.

Digestive tract: empty, all gone sensation in the stomach not better by eating; vomiting better for indigestible foods such as cabbage and onions but worse for bland foods; sweets aggravate; sharp stitching pain shoots up the rectum.

Respiration: coughing increases the desire to cough; anxiety felt in the chest; breathing is difficult.

Extremities: twitching spasms after emotions.

Sleep: sleepless from grief; many troubled dreams; twitching as goes off to sleep.

Recommended potency: 30C

Ipecacuanha

SYMPTOMS CHARACTERISED BY

Nausea: persistent and accompanies most complaints, is not relieved by vomiting.

Haemorrhage: from any orifice of the body.

THE CHILD IS

Irritable.

Uncertain: full of desires but does not know what for.

Thirstless.

MODALITIES

Aggravated: warmth; damp; lying down.

Ameliorated: open air; cold drinks.

THE BODY

Face: deathly pale with blue rings around the eyes.

Nose: bleed (see Haemorrhage below).

Digestive tract: tongue is clean; constant nausea and vomiting but vomiting does not relieve; vomits jelly-like mucus; nausea and vomiting after over indulgence in food, cakes, pastry or ice cream; profuse salivation; griping pain in the intestines; greenish diarrhoea, frothy.

Respiration: sudden onset of ailments; must sit up to breathe; violent suffocative cough; asthma returning periodically; coughs with each breath; feels full of mucus but nothing comes up; whooping cough; rattling cough; sense of weight on chest.

Haemorrhage: profuse, active, bright red blood with nausea; blood does not coagulate.

Pulse: weak.

Skin: cold sweat.

Recommended potency: 12C

Ledum Palustre

SYMPTOMS CHARACTERISED BY

Upward movement of complaints: pains move upward.

Coldness: affected parts cold to touch but > for cold applications.

Parts puffy: about puncture wounds or swollen joints.

MODALITIES

Aggravated: warmth of any kind, heat of the bed; covering; night.

Ameliorated: cold; cold bathing, even use of ice; uncovering the part.

THE BODY

Eyes: bloodshot; black eye from injury with blunt object.

Extremities: unnaturally cold but ameliorated by cold; easy spraining of ankles; puncture wounds — puffy and cold > cold; joints swollen and hot but not red in acute conditions.

Skin: bruises which do not respond fully to Arnica specially if part is cold and numb.

Stings: effects of bites and stings from animals or insects: bee, hornet or wasp; pains extend up; part cold or numb; sensitive to touch.

Wounds: puncture — puffy and cold, > cold.

Teeth: pain from injection.

Recommended potency: 12C

Mag Phos

This medicine acts on muscles and nerves. Chiefly a pain remedy especially in cramping and spasmodic pains.

SYMPTOMS CHARACTERISED BY

Cramping or spasm.

Pains relieved by heat.

Pains relieved by pressure.

MODALITIES

Aggravated: cold, draughts.

Ameliorated: warmth; pressure and doubling up; rubbing.

THE BODY

Head: pain or neuralgia relieved by warm applications.

Ears: earache from cold air.

Teeth: toothache, shooting pains relieved by warmth.

Digestive tract: hiccup day and night. Flatulent colic better for bending double, warmth and pressure, or drawing the legs up; abdominal cramps.

Urine: bed-wetting from nervous irritation.

Extremities: cramping, writer's cramp, muscle tension.

Recommended potency: 6C (the tissue salt preparation at 12X is satisfactory)

Mercurius Sol

SYMPTOMS CHARACTERISED BY

Suppuration: tendency to pus formation which is offensive — abscesses, quinsy (abscess around the tonsils), boils.

Ulcers: which burn, sting or suppurate.

Offensive odours: of body sweat, discharges and saliva.

THE CHILD IS

Angry or irritable.

Salivating or sweating: profusely; these do not relieve the complaint.

Weak and trembling.

MODALITIES

Aggravated: night (sunset to sunrise); lying on the right side; heat or cold; wet weather; perspiration; warm room or bed.

Ameliorated: rest.

THE BODY

Ears: stitching pains < night; middle ear infection; abcesses.

Nose: much sneezing; thick green or profuse

watery nasal discharge making upper nose and lip sore.

Throat: smarting, raw and sore throat; tonsillitis — deep redness of tonsillar area; difficulty swallowing; ulcers on tonsils; glands of the neck swollen, tender, inflamed; stitching pains extend to ear on swallowing; fluids return through the nose because of tonsillar swelling.

Mouth: profuse salivation, drooling; metal taste of saliva; bad odour; thickly coated tongue, yellow or white; teeth leave imprint on the edge of the tongue.

Digestive tract: green, bloody, slimy stools; thirst for cold drinks; painful diarrhoea with 'never gets done' feeling.

Skin: pustular infection, boils; profuse sweat.

Urine: persistent urging to urinate with intense burning.

Recommended potency: 12C

Natrum Muriaticum

SYMPTOMS CHARACTERISED BY

Periodicity: often < 10.00–11.00 a.m. — fevers and other ailments; annual hayfever.

Dryness: of mucous membranes — mouth, lips, tongue, vagina, skin and anus which fissures.

THE CHILD IS

Suffers ailments from grief: loss, anger < consolation; will often seek solitude to cry.

Thirsty: for cool drinks.

Desires: salty food.

Irritable: hates fuss and often refuses consolation.

MODALITIES

Aggravated: lying down; seaside; music; noise; warm room; mental exertion; heat; at 10-11 a.m.

Ameliorated: open air; cold bathing; lying on right side; going without regular meals.

THE BODY

Head: anaemic headache in young girls; headache throbbing, bursting, like hammers, with visual disturbances < daytime, sun, study.

Eyes: watery from the wind; coughing or laughing; sore eyes from over study.

Nose: watery or white nasal discharge; sneezing from annual hayfever; stopped passages.

Face: herpes on lips or other parts of the face.

Digestive tract: desires salt; tongue mapped with red islands; thirst for cold water; constipation with dry or crumbly stool; watery diarrhoea.

Skin: herpes or vesicles on lips, chin or nose.

Sleep: sleepless from grief.

Recommended potency: 6C

Nux Vomica

Suited for ailments from over indulgence, excesses of stimulants or from food poisoning.

SYMPTOMS CHARACTERISED BY

Spasm: of voluntary and involuntary muscles, i.e. stomach, bladder, rectum; this spasm involves constant urging but little satisfaction, for example, upset stomach with much straining and retching before vomiting.

Oversensitiveness: to external impressions such as noise, light; trifling ailments are unbearable.

Drawing pains.

THE CHILD IS

Irritable: very irritable because of their oversensitiveness; everyone displeases or annoys; they answer curtly and rudely; dissatisfied, wanting to tear things; many have a violent temper.

Critical and fault finding: perfectionists.

Impatient.

Desire to be left alone.

Cold: dislikes draughts and open air.

Desire: stimulants, alcohol, spicy foods, fats.

MODALITIES

Aggravated: over use of stimulants, alcohol, tea, coffee and tobacco; overeating especially fatty, rich foods; anger; excessive mental labour.

Ameliorated: moist humid atmospheres; by strong pressure; evening.

THE BODY

Head: morning headache < moving the eyes, < light or noise; headache from over indulgence, from the sun; pain better for pressure and quiet.

Nose: colds after exposure to cold dry wind; stuffed up indoors but flows freely outdoors; sneezing with itchiness inside nose.

Digestive tract: weight and pain like a stone in the stomach 1-3 hours after eating; nausea, vomiting with much retching, difficult to vomit; food poisoning; indigestion; constipation with frequent ineffectual urging, then only a small amount passes; diarrhoea with straining, after bad food.

Urine: must strain to urinate.

Sleep: sleep in the afternoon but awake at night; cannot sleep after 3.00 a.m. wakes irritable.

Fever: great heat but chills on the least moving or uncovering.

Recommended potency: 30C

Phosphorus

SYMPTOMS CHARACTERISED BY

Haemorrhage: great tendency to; profuse nosebleed; small wounds bleed profusely.

Hypersensitivity: to all external impressions.
Weakness and trembling: from nervous debility or loss of vital fluids for example, diarrhoea, bleeding.

THE CHILD IS

Anxious/fearful: of dark, death, thunder.
Excitable: easily; produces heat all over.
Over-sensitive: to light, touch, sound, odours.
Restless.
Weakness: is great.
Thirst: is great for cold or iced drinks.
Chilly.

MODALITIES

Aggravated: lying on left; left side generally; touch; physical and mental exertion; change of weather; evening; twilight; warm food and drink.
Ameliorated: lying on right; open air; sleep; rubbing; washing in cold water; cold food and drink.

THE BODY

Head: ache from odours.
Nose: profuse bleeding; bleeding from nose blowing.
Throat: hoarseness; painless loss of voice; painful laryngitis.
Respiration: cough — croupy, hard, dry, tickling, rasping < for breathing cold air or speaking; violent tickling when speaking; racking cough when trembling; painful throat on coughing; colds descend to chest.
Digestive tract: desires salt; great thirst for cold drinks which may be vomited once warm in the stomach; burning pains in stomach or intestines; weak empty sensation in stomach; vomiting blood and undigested food; sour taste and belching.
Colds: travel to the chest.
Fever: thirst for cold drinks; appears well despite temperature.
Haemorrhage: profuse bleeding anywhere.
Teeth: Excessive bleeding after dental work.
Recommended potency: 12C

Pulsatilla Nigricans

SYMPTOMS CHARACTERISED BY

Changeability: of symptoms for example, weepy then laughing; no two stools alike.
Pains wander: often accompanied by chilliness; the greater the pain the greater the chill.
Discharge: thick, bland, yellow/green for example, eyes, nose, expectoration.

THE CHILD IS

Mild: gentle, yielding, timid, fears the dark and crowds.

Moody: easily moved from laughter to tears; indecisive.
Weepy: cries easily, cries when telling their symptoms.
Consolation: ameliorates, wants sympathy; desires to be carried.
Craves open air: asks for windows to be open.
Thirstless: even with dry mouth.

MODALITIES

Aggravated: twilight; heat; warm room; rich fatty food; too many clothes.
Ameliorated: open air; slow movement; cold applications; cold food and drink.

THE BODY

Head: wandering pains > open air.
Ears: difficult hearing as if ears stuffed; earache; sensation as if something forced out; throbbing < at night; red swollen external ear; thick yellow bland discharge.
Nose: thick yellow mucus abundant in the morning, stoppage in evening and indoors; nose runs freely in open air.
Teeth: ache > cold water < warm things and warm room.
Eyes: styes — especially on upper lid or from eating fat, greasy or rich food; conjunctivitis.
Digestive tract: desires something but doesn't know what; desires butter; dry mouth with lack of thirst; bitter taste; nausea in the morning; vomits clear yellow liquid in morning; weight as if a stone in the stomach especially on waking; stomach pain one hour after eating; wants clothes loose around abdomen; diarrhoea — watery, green, yellow, changeable stools.
Respiration: dry cough in the evening — loose in the morning; dry or rattling cough evening and night; paroxysms of cough with gagging or choking; thick yellow expectoration; must sit up to relieve cough; sense of weight on chest.
Fever: with no thirst.
Sleep: on back with arms above head; sleepless from recurring thoughts.
Skin: fever goes down after measles rash appears; chickenpox.
Mumps: moves to reproductive parts.
Recommended potency: 12C

Rheum

Prepared from Rhubarb and is especially useful during teething.

SYMPTOMS CHARACTERISED BY

Sourness: in odour of stool, odour of sweat and in disposition.

THE CHILD IS

Screaming: especially while urging and passing stool.

Impatient, irritable: restless and wanting many different things.

MODALITIES

Aggravated: from teething and eating.

Ameliorated: warmth and wrapping up.

THE BODY

Head: sweat of scalp is constant and profuse; the hair is always wet and may smell sour.

Teeth: difficult teething with restlessness, irritability, pale face and sour smell.

Digestive tract: colic with very sour stool < uncovering, even of a limb; < standing > doubling up; stool is sour, fermented, slimy or acrid.

Recommended potency: 12C

Rhus Toxicodendron

For complaints after exposure to cold and damp, catching chill, getting wet, lying on damp ground. 'Also used for over exertion, straining or over stretching.

SYMPTOMS CHARACTERISED BY

Better for continued motion.

Worse for rest: worse for the first movement.

Restlessness: constantly changes position.

Pains tearing: bruised, better for heat.

THE CHILD IS

Restless.

Sensitive to cold.

Desires cold drinks: which aggravate; cold milk or sweets.

MODALITIES

Aggravated: night; cold; becoming cold; change of weather; rest.

Ameliorated: warmth; pressure; rubbing and moving about.

THE BODY

Head: tearing pains.

Eyes: swollen, inflamed after exposure to cold and damp.

Nose: sneezing after getting wet, colds.

Face: cold sores around the mouth; glands swollen and painful; mumps.

Digestive tract: tongue coated white with a triangular red tip; great thirst with dry mouth; diarrhoea copious and bloody.

Respiration: hoarseness from over using the voice > speaking; dry teasing cough worse at night or when chilled.

Extremities: stiffness after rest and on beginning to move but better with continued gentle motion; weakness of lower limbs; strains; sprains; restlessness of lower limbs at night; swollen knees; hot, painful, swollen joints.

Skin: itchy with blisters, red, swollen, like chickenpox or effects of poison ivy; eruptions moist.

Fever: easily chilled, < least uncovering with pain in the limbs; chill preceeded by cough, alternating with heat, with desire to stretch.

Recommended potency: 12C

Ruta Graveolens

Acts on cartilage, flexor tendons, eye muscles, which are largely tendinous, joints and wrists. Chief remedy for injured or bruised bones.

SYMPTOMS CHARACTERISED BY

Bruised or lame sensation: all over especially limbs and joints; often attended by restlessness.

Deposits of hardening: formation of deposits in bones periosteum (the membrane which covers the bones), tendons and about joints; nodules left after bruising.

Weakness: legs give out on rising from chair, ascending or descending steps; paralytic stiffness in wrist; lassitude and heaviness in limbs.

Sensation of pressure: on the bladder as if continually full, at root of nose, deep in eye sockets.

THE CHILD IS

Sensitive to cold: ailments from cold and damp weather or after becoming cold.

Restless: turns and changes position frequently.

Thirsty: violent thirst for cold water.

MODALITIES

Aggravated: cold wet weather; cold applications; lying on painful side; ascending or descending steps; over exertion.

Ameliorated: scratching; rubbing; motion; lying on back.

THE BODY

Head and Eyes: headaches, soreness or blurred vision after eye strain; redness and heat in eyes as if burning; pain at root of nose.

Digestive tract: burning, gnawing pain; tension in abdomen > milk.

Neck and Back: ache > lying on it — feels bruised and sore.

Extremities: tendency to boney deposits in periosteum, bones and tendons; repetitive strain injury; legs weak, heavy and restless — cannot support the child; injury to bones — bruised, periosteum and tendons with formation of hard swellings which are tender and slow to heal; straining and over exertion — especially of wrists and ankles; dislocations; pain after osteopathic or chiropractic manipulations; tendonitis.

Teeth: deep aching.

Recommended potency: 12C

Staphysagria

SYMPTOMS CHARACTERISED BY

Irritation and hypersensitivity: specially of nervous system; easily offended; tips of fingers sensitive, scars sensitive, vagina very sensitive to touch.

Pain: stinging, cutting like a knife; stitching especially where the pain is after an operation.

THE CHILD IS

Sensitive: to slightest impressions, easily offended.

Easily offended: great indignation about things done or said by others, ailments after insult; can't confront.

Anger: ailments from suppressed anger; resentment — violent outbursts; throws things

Trembles: from nervous excitement or suppressed feelings.

MODALITIES

Aggravated: least touch; pressure; anger; grief; insults.

THE BODY

Head: aches from anger or suppressed feelings.

Eyes: recurrent styes.

Digestive tract: colic after anger; severe pain after abdominal operation.

Urine: painful urination, frequency.

Skin: pain of an incised wound; neuralgia after surgery.

Recommended potency: 30C

Sulphur

SYMPTOMS CHARACTERISED BY

Burning and heat: heat on crown of head, soles, eyes, skin and diarrhoea burns.

Itching: of skin, throat, anus.

Redness: especially in orifices — lips, urethra, anus, eyes.

Offensiveness: stool, sweat, breath, mucus, etc.

THE CHILD IS

Critical/irritable.

Thirsty: but eats little.

MODALITIES

Aggravated: 11.00 a.m.; bathing; washing;

standing; warmth of bed; scratching;

Ameliorated: lying on right side; dry warm weather.

THE BODY

Digestive tract: very thirsty, eats little; sinking feeling or hungry one hour before lunch or 11.00 a.m.; burning and itching of anus; ineffective urging alternating with diarrhoea; constipation as if 'something left behind'; diarrhoea sudden, changeable, yellow, watery, slimy, undigested; painless morning diarrhoea drives him out of bed; stool hard, dry, dark, held back from pain.

Skin: rough, hard, dry, scaly, itching and burning < heat.

Extremities: burning heat especially in soles.

Chickenpox: intense itching of pox.

Fever: flushes of heat, sweating of single parts — sulphurous odour; feet cold.

Recommended potency: 12C

Veratrum Album

SYMPTOMS CHARACTERISED BY

Rapid loss of energy: faintness and collapse.

Cold sweat: specially on the forehead.

Cramping: pain in the chest, abdomen, fingers or toes.

General icy coldness: of face, nose, feet, hands or arms.

Great unquenchable thirst: specially for icy or cold drinks.

THE CHILD IS

Delirious: this may be accompanied by the desire to cut and tear, praying, cursing or howling.

Craving: iced water or cold drinks.

MODALITIES

Aggravated: exertion; drinking.

Ameliorated: hot drinks and walking about.

THE BODY

Digestive tract: violent vomiting and nausea aggravated by drinking and the least motion; vomiting after bad food; cutting colic; profuse diarrhoea which is gushing, watery or green; painful constipation of infants where the stool is large, hard and in round black balls.

Respiration: continuous violent cough with retching < cold drinks.

Fever: with coldness, thirst, collapse, paleness and sweat on the forehead.

Recommended potency: 30C

CHINESE MEDICINE

If you are unfamiliar with Oriental culture beyond your favourite Chinese restaurant, the principles of Chinese medicine may seem strange and far-fetched. However, if you decide to delve a bit deeper into the world of traditional Chinese medicine, you will find a highly refined yet fundamentally simple theory. Chinese medicine uses natural products and herbs with an emphasis on preventing illness. Ch'i Po, Chief Minister to the Yellow Emperor had this to say about healing: 'To take medicine only when you are sick is like digging a well only when you are thirsty — is it not already too late?'

Philosophy

One of the fundamental principles of Chinese medicine is to treat the whole person. It is based upon the study of people in relationship with themselves — in body, mind and spirit — and with the universe. In Imperial times the court physician did not receive payment if the emperor fell ill, since this was believed to be a sign that the physician was not performing his job properly. A single symptom or part of the body is never treated, because it is not believed that a symptom can be considered all by itself; the whole must be viewed and the patient must be acknowledged as an individual.

Chinese remedies do not have undesirable side effects and they generally take longer to restore harmony to the individual than Western treatments. It is believed that to maintain health and well-being we need fresh air, clean water, the right mental attitudes, exercise and most important, good food. Food is essential for life because it is transformed into fuel for the body, and it is also a great source of pleasure. It forms the focus of nearly every social gathering.

A Difference in Syntax

Perhaps the biggest obstacle in understanding Chinese medicine is the way that words are used in describing health and sickness. The Chinese doctor believes that we are greatly influenced and affected by natural phenomena. He may describe someone as suffering from cold air in the lungs which causes their cough.

Classification of Body Types

The Chinese believe that children can be classified into two types relating to their strengths or weaknesses of body and character. These types I will refer to as 'Sun' and 'Moon' (traditionally known as Yin and Yang). During illness, the characteristics of each particular type become more pronounced.

SUN	MOON
usually strong and sturdy	thin, empty-looking
boundless energy	tires easily
not bothered by minor complaints	upsets easily
usually have a positive outlook	negative outlook
when they become ill their body battles the disease quickly	recovers slowly
prone to high temperatures	low prolonged fever
doesn't need much sleep	sleeps a lot
heals quickly	takes a long time
often has good colour in face	pale and often puffy

HOT	COLD
reddish complexion	pale complexion
feels hot most of the time	feels cold most of the time
doesn't like to wear clothes	likes to wear lots of clothes
sweats often	hardly ever sweats
bad breath	no strong breath odour
great appetite	poor appetite
drinks a lot	not thirsty most of the time
body of tongue red, may have yellow coating	body of tongue pale, sometimes with a white coating
likes cold foods	likes hot or warm foods
urine is scanty and strong	urine is clear and copious
aggressive, strong-willed	submissive
doesn't like blankets	likes lots of blankets
needs little sleep	needs lots of sleep

Sun and Moon Patterns

The sun child is like a bull charging at his enemy. He has a strong immune system, but his energy still needs to be directed to override the illness.

The moon child does not have the same strength and even though his symptoms appear milder it is important to build up his immune system by giving him strengthening tonics to increase his vital energy.

Classification of the Nature of Illness

Illness can also be classified into two types: hot and cold. These descriptions relate to the physical symptoms of the illness. With a hot condition the child has a clammy and sweaty body with a flushed face and high fever.

With a cold condition, the child has a pale complexion, urinates a lot, can't get warm no matter how many clothes he puts on and is not at all hungry.

Chinese Herbs

The most fundamental type of treatment within the realm of Chinese medicine is Chinese herbs. The traditional way of taking these herbs is by bringing them to the boil in water and then simmering to extract their essence. Then the liquid is strained, decanted, and taken at specific times. There are over 5000 ingredients listed in Chinese herbal medicine but only about 500 are commonly used today. They are blended together in exact amounts and precise ratios — a formula may contain from six to thirty ingredients.

Chinese herbs are classified into drug properties which include the five flavours, four

The Effects of Food Preparation on Body Heat

TYPE OF PREPARATION	EFFECT
raw foods	lowers body heat
pickling (brine)	lowers body heat
steaming	slightly cooling
boiling	slightly cooling
pan-frying	raises body heat
deep-frying	raises body heat considerably
grilling	raises body heat considerably
baking	raises body heat greatly
roasting	raises body heat greatly

essences and four directions of actions.

The four directions: floating, sinking, ascending and descending. Ascending and floating refer to herbs that have an upward and outward effect and can induce sweating. Sinking and descending herbs possess a downward and inward effect — they cause contraction thus relieving coughs for example. The four directions also relate to different sites of disease in the body.

The four essences: cold, hot, warm and cool indicate their therapeutic effects and the body's reaction.

The five flavours: generally speaking salty-tasting herbs have purging and softening effects; sour-tasting herbs have astringent effects which prevent or reverse abnormal leakage of fluids or energy; bitter-tasting ones, like bitter melon have purging and fortifying effects, and rhubarb (also bitter) regulates the bowels as well as getting rid of excess heat in the body; sweet-tasting ones like Licorice and Ginseng, have tonifying and regulating effects; and pungent-tasting herbs such as fresh Ginger have promoting and dispelling effects.

A practitioner of Chinese medicine will rarely use one single flavour to treat an illness but will combine two or more flavours.

It is difficult to get children to take Chinese herbal teas because they have to drink so much and the teas are unpalatable no matter how much honey or sugar you may mix with them. So it is best to use desiccated extracts made from the classical formulas, or Chinese paediatric patent medicines which are made into tiny pills, syrups or powders. The Chinese medicines recommended for the complaints covered in this book are patent medicines or desiccated extract formulas. They can be purchased in Chinese pharmacies in the Chinatown areas of most large cities. For those people who do not have easy access to these shops I have included a list of Chinese pharmacies who are willing to mail order.

Causes of Disease

The Chinese classify the causes of disease as:
- external — environmental
- internal — emotional
- miscellaneous — all those which are neither external or internal

Diseases which are caused by other than external factors should always be referred to a professional practitioner. In this book, therefore, only external causes will be dealt with.

External

Environmental causes are classified under the following headings and describe how people are affected by climatic and seasonal changes.
- cold
- heat
- damp
- dry
- wind

So someone who has hay fever will dread spring flowers, the rheumatism sufferer can predict rain by the aching in his bones, thundery weather will often set off a migraine headache. If you observe children's behaviour, you may notice that it often reflects the outside elements. We are as much part of nature as the ocean and the sky and therefore must be affected by natural seasonal and climatic changes in the same way.

Chinese medicine diagnoses disease according to nature using these elements. If your child is suffering from a cold or the flu, for example, he would be described in Chinese terms as suffering from an attack of wind-cold or wind-heat. Children naturally suffer from many illnesses each year and some are necessary to help them build up their immune system. However, you can protect your child against unnecessary bouts of illness, by dressing him in warm clothes in cold weather, and by keeping the back of his neck covered as the so called 'wind-gate' of the body is located just at the base of the neck.

Wind

Wind is said to be the trigger of illness. It is capable of rampaging through the defensive energy of the body and taking the other elements (hot, cold, damp and dry) for a ride. Wind has the ability to penetrate and can make the illness move more quickly. We may become restless as cats do, or irritated, or affected by what the wind carries, such as pollen, viruses, bacteria, germs, dust and pollution. The most unpleasant wind is that from the East, associated with spring, which brings about flu, headaches, aches and pains, colds and diarrhoea. Wind is associated with severe conditions which rise quickly and fall just as quickly leaving a change behind them. Typical wind conditions are allergies, muscle cramps, convulsions, itching skin and strokes.

Cold

Children are particularly vulnerable to cold because their organs and immune system are not yet fully developed and are therefore more susceptible to environmental changes. In addition, external factors such as stress or lack of touch can predispose them to frequent bouts of cold-related symptoms. The obvious signs of extreme cold are cold hands and feet, lowered temperature, slow circulation of the blood, aches and pains in the body, pale face, inability to sweat, slow pulse and numbness in the toes and fingers. When the whole circulatory system is slowed down our body cells do not receive their required amount of oxygen and blood and so the *Chi* or energy is blocked. Some of the symptoms may be nausea, indigestion, burping, hiccupping, diarrhoea, flu and aches and pains in the whole body and head.

If the condition is aggravated by wind (wind-cold), your child may have a sudden attack of diarrhoea with contracting abdominal pains, thin, watery, clear phlegm, lots of body aches, itchy, watery eyes and nose, sneezing, chills and fever, together with cold hands and feet. If you do not treat the condition and the wind is not dispersed from the body, then it can invade the lungs (indicated by a cough or, more seriously, bronchitis or pneumonia) or the stomach which would produce some symptoms as nausea, vomiting, diarrhoea or constipation, loss of appetite and fatigue.

When the symptoms are a stuffed nose, possibly a sore throat or an uncomfortableness around the glands, chills and fever, and thick, yellow phlegm, it is more likely to be a wind-heat condition.

To make matters a bit more complicated, a cold condition can reverse itself into a wind heat one as the body fights the pathogen. In this case it is better to see a practitioner who can assist you in making a clearer diagnosis and prescribe the appropriate medication.

Wind cold and wind heat patterns largely correspond to such conditions as flu, colds, upper respiratory tract infection and sometimes tonsillitis and pneumonia too.

Heat

In children, illness resulting from heat is more serious than from cold conditions. It can develop from being in hot places, eating hot, spicy foods, or spending too much time in the sun without proper protection. Symptoms are rough, chapped skin or dry lips, a dry cough, thirst, dry mouth, desire for cold drinks, constipation, sweating, red skin, irritability, bleeding from the nose and gums and red eyes.

Children with these symptoms may also exhibit an 'over heated temper' manifesting as hysteria and possible neurosis, and children who eat a lot of animal fat or sugar may find that their bodies will try to cope with this heat excess by producing skin eruptions such as acne, pimples and boils. It is usually quite a sudden manifestation, and it is quite commonly experienced during dry, hot summers and cold, dry winters and especially in centrally heated environments.

Swimming and hot steamy baths are recommended, along with cheese, asparagus, soymilk, eggs and tofu. These will help moisten the body. Avoid foods such as nuts, fried foods, chocolate and oranges.

Dampness

Dampness in the body can produce changes in behaviour, mood and well-being, vomiting, shortness of breath and tightness in the chest, dull aches and pains, excess mucus, a variety of skin problems and chronic diarrhoea. Excess humidity upsets the fluid balance and causes fluid retention in the body. Children who have had broken bones or the makings of arthritis can often tell if it is going to rain because the humidity that precedes the rain causes blockages in the body chi or energy and manifests as pain.

Dryness

This condition is brought on by dry weather and usually comes about before heat arises in the body. The symptoms are a dry mouth and lips, thirst, dry skin, a dry cough, constipation, little urine, itchy skin and dry eyes. It causes feelings of irritability and restlessness.

Children Are Not just Miniature Adults

Babies are physiologically, emotionally and anatomically different from adults. Up until the age of six, their digestion is considered to be inherently weak. Practitioners of Chinese medicine believe that almost all the diseases of children under six years of age begin as a form of indigestion, and that the best medicine for children is a well-balanced and regulated diet.

For example according to Chinese paediatrics, there is an internal pathway or channel connecting the intestines and stomach to the inner ear. When food is not digested and just sits in the stomach and intestines it transforms into a heat-like quality and rises up this internal pathway to the inner ear where it fulminates. Pain arises and perhaps there may even be a discharge of some sort from the ear. This is an indication that there is dampness as well as heat. The traditional Chinese medical treatment of earache in children is geared towards clearing the heat from the digestive tract, cleaning out the stomach and intestines of the stagnant food, getting rid of the dampness and strengthening the whole digestive system. This will lower the fever and get rid of the pain.

Eating the Wrong Food

Perhaps the most often neglected cause of sickness is eating the wrong food. Eating and drinking indiscriminately injures the stomach and spleen and changes the metabolism, predisposing one to disease. For example, if we give our children too much fatty food it can cause an accumulation of phlegm in the chest. There are certain guidelines that would be beneficial to follow:
- Stop eating when your stomach is 75 per cent full so that the digestive system is not overworked.
- Avoid taking too much salt as it has an addictive effect and is a known stimulant particularly affecting the kidneys.
- Do not eat too much sugar as it creates mucus throughout the system.

Chinese Herbal Materia Medica

This Materia Medica of selected Chinese herbal formulas has been simplified and abridged for the purposes of this book. There are other indications and applications for most of the formulas listed here, however these are more applicable to adults than to children.

Bai Shao Gan Cao Tang (Shao Yao Gan Cao Tang)

Action: nourishes blood, calms the liver and alleviates spasms, harmonises liver and stomach.
Indications: weakness in the legs, painful muscle spasms, pale face, pale lips.
Tongue: pale with thin white coating.
Application: colic, muscle spasms or cramping.

Ban Xia Xie Xin Tang

Action: harmonises stomach and intestines, dispels pathogenic 'Cold' and 'Heat' factors.
Indications: hardness of epigastric region, nausea, vomiting, loss of appetite, oral ulceration, abdominal pain, diarrhoea, coughing or vomiting frothy mucus.
Tongue: the coating is yellow and greasy.
Application: acute gastroenteritis, mouth ulcers, motion sickness.

Bao He Wan

Action: reduces food stagnation, harmonises the stomach.
Indications: abdominal distention and fullness, occasional abdominal pain, belching, acid regurgitation, nausea and/or vomiting, aversion to food, symptoms aggravated by eating, may also be diarrhoea.
Tongue: a thick greasy coating which may be yellow.
Application: indigestion due to overindulgence, acute gastroenteritis.

Bu Fei Tang

Action: tonifies the Qi (vital energy), stops sweating.
Indications: shortness of breath, spontaneous sweating, occasional chills and feverishness, coughing, wheezing.
Tongue: pale
Application: asthma, bronchitis.

Chuan Pei Mo

Action: moistens lungs, clears 'Heat', promotes circulation of Qi, transforms 'Phlegm'.
Indications: cough with thick yellow sputum which is difficult to expectorate, dry and sore throat, loss of appetite, sensation of constriction in the chest.
Tongue: red and dry with little coating.
Application: bronchitis, laryngitis, pharyngitis.

Da Cheng Qi Tang

Action: purges 'Heat' accumulation from the intestines.
Indications: fever, severe constipation and flatulence, localised distention and fullness of abdomen, abdominal pain which increases on pressure (or touch), abdomen is tense and firm.
Tongue: red with a dry yellow or yellow-brown coating.
Application: constipation, uncomplicated intestinal obstruction, acute uncomplicated appendicitis.

Contraindications: not for those with a weak constitution, seek professional help in cases with appendicitis.

Er Chen Tang

Action: eliminates 'Phlegm' and 'Dampness', harmonises spleen and stomach.
Indications: profuse watery sputum or mucus which is white in colour, abdominal fullness, nausea and/or vomiting, coughing.
Tongue: pale with white greasy or oily coating.
Application: nausea, vomiting, headache, cough, bronchitis.

Fu Ling Ze Xie Tang

Action: eliminates 'Dampness', harmonises stomach, promotes urination.
Indications: gastric regurgitation, thirst, abdominal distention, abdominal pain.
Tongue: coating is white and may be thick.
Application: regurgitation of milk in infants.

Gan Mai Da Zao Tang

Action: nourishes the heart, calms mind and emotions, harmonises stomach and spleen.
Indications: anxiety, depression, crying spells, easily startled, over-excitement, insomnia, frequent waking, poor appetite, yawning excessively.
Tongue: pale with very little coating.
Application: insomnia, bed wetting, night fears, night crying, anxiety.

Ge Gen Tang

Action: dispel 'Exterior' attack by 'Wind'-'Cold' factors, relieve muscle ache of the neck.
Indications: fever, intolerance of cold drafts, absence of perspiration, muscle ache of neck.
Tongue: no abnormalities.
Application: common cold, influenza, headache.

Gui Pi Tang

Action: replenish Qi (vital energy) and blood, strengthen heart and spleen.
Indications: insomnia, forgetfulness, nightmares, fatigue, decreased intake of food, complexion is sallow or pale.
Tongue: pale, thin white coating.
Application: poor sleeping habits, weakness, fatigue.

Gui Zhi Tang

Action: dispels 'Exterior' attack by 'Wind'-'Cold' factors, strengthens the 'Defensive' energy, (i.e. resistance).

Indications: chills and fever, sweating, decreased body resistance, increased sensitivity to cold drafts, nasal congestion, headache.
Tongue: no abnormalities.
Application: common cold, influenza, hives.

Huang Lian Jie Du Tang

Action: dispels 'Heat' and 'Toxins'.
Indications: high fever, irritability, dryness of mouth and throat, nose bleeds, boils, suppurative infections.
Tongue: red with a yellow coating.
Application: boils, nose bleeds, dysentery.
Contraindications: do not use if there is absence of coating on the tongue.

Huang Qi Jian Zhong Tang

Action: replenishes Qi (vital energy), warms the stomach and spleen.
Indications: low energy, fatigue, perspires easily, gets out of breath easily, abdominal pain, frequent urination, cold hands and feet.
Tongue: pale with thin coating.
Application: abdominal pains, bed wetting, anaemia, constitutional weakness.

Huo Xiang Zheng Qi Tang

Action: dispels 'Wind' and 'Cold', eliminates 'Dampness', harmonises stomach and spleen.
Indications: Diarrhoea, nausea and/or vomiting, loss of appetite, chills and fever, abdominal pain, abdominal distention, flatulence.
Tongue: Coating is thick, white and greasy.
Application: acute gastroenteritis, common cold, diarrhoea.

Jin Fang Bai Du San

Action: Dispels external attack by 'Wind', 'Cold' and 'Dampness', alleviates pain.
Indications: fever and chills, absence of sweating, headache, pain and stiffness of the neck, generalised body aches.
Tongue: thick white coating.
Application: common cold, influenza, conjunctivitis, epidemic parotitis.

Jin Gui Shen Qi Wan

Action: warms and tonifies the kidneys, warms the lower half of the body.
Indications: cold sensation in lower half of body, weakness of legs, low back pain, tenseness in lower abdomen, frequent urination, bed wetting, cough, asthma, diarrhoea.
Tongue: pale and swollen with a thin white moist coating.

Application: bed wetting, chronic bronchitis, asthma.

Jin Ling Zi San

Action: promotes circulation of Qi, drains 'Heat', alleviates pain.
Indications: abdominal pain that is aggravated by heat and pressure, irritability.
Tongue: normal or red with a yellow coating.
Application: abdominal pain.

Li Zhong Wan

Action: warms and strengthens the spleen and stomach.
Indications: diarrhoea with watery stool, nausea and/or vomiting, loss of appetite, abdominal pain which is relieved by heat and pressure, absence of thirst.
Tongue: pale with a thin white coating.
Application: gastroenteritis, irritable bowel syndrome, chronic bronchitis, cold sores.

Liang Fu Wan

Action: warms the stomach and spleen, dispels 'Cold', promotes the circulation of Qi, relieves abdominal pain.
Indications: abdominal pain that is relieved by warmth, absence of thirst, preference for warm beverages.
Tongue: coating is white.
Application: abdominal pain.

Ling Gui Zhu Gan Tang

Action: warms and strengthens the spleen, resolves 'Phlegm' and 'Dampness'.
Indications: cough with copious amounts of clear and watery sputum, cold hands, feet and possibly also abdomen, nausea and/or vomiting, stools are loose or watery.
Tongue: pale with a white, oily coating.
Application: cough, bronchitis, vomiting, diarrhoea.

Liu Jun Zi Tang

Action: strengthens the spleen, resolves 'Phlegm', stops vomiting.
Indications: loss of appetite, nausea and/or vomiting, abdominal distention or sensations of bloating, fatigue, weight loss, cold hands and feet, cough with copious amounts of thin, clear or white sputum.
Tongue: pale with a distinct white greasy or oily coating.
Application: indigestion, poor appetite, vomiting, inability to gain weight, anaemia, cough, bronchitis, chronic asthma (take between attacks).
Contraindications: do not give with fever.

Liu Mo Tang

Action: promotes movement of Qi, directs 'rebellious' Qi downwards, moves the bowels.
Indications: abdominal distention and pain, constipation, belching, irritability, symptoms aggravated by emotional upsets.
Application: emotionally related — abdominal pain, bloating, constipation, and belching.

Liu Wei Di Huang Wan

Action: enriches the 'Yin', nourishes the kidneys.
Indications: delayed closure of anterior fontanel, low energy, bed wetting, delayed development (i.e. standing up, walking, head hair growth, teething, speaking), sleep disturbances, sweating at night.
Tongue: red with little or no coating.
Application: delayed development (physical or mental), fatigue and low energy, disturbed sleep, asthma, bed-wetting.

Long Dan Xie Gan Tang

Action: drains 'Fire' from liver and gall bladder, clears and drains 'Heat' and 'Dampness' from the lower part of the body.
Indications: pain in the hypochondrial area, headache, dizziness, red and sore eyes, earache, swelling in the ear canal, bitter taste in the mouth, irritability, painful urination, burning sensation in the urethra, swelling, heat, redness, and itching of the external genitalia, vaginal discharge.
Tongue: red with a yellow coating which may be greasy.
Application: acute conjunctivitis, acute otitis media, suppurating infections of the external auditary canal, acute cystitis, urethritis, eczema of the external genitalia, migraine headaches, herpes zoster, orchitis, epididymitis.
Contraindications: not to be taken long term. Not to be taken in cases with spleen deficiency or deficiency of body fluids.

Ma Zi Ren Wan

Action: moistens the intestines, drains 'Heat', promotes movement of Qi, unblocks the bowels.
Indications: constipation with hard stool, frequent urination.
Tongue: dry yellow coating.
Application: constipation, haemorrhoids.

Mai Men Dong Tang

Action: replenish body fluids in the stomach, directs 'rebellious' Qi downwards.
Indications: coughing, spitting of saliva, wheezing, dry and uncomfortable sensation in the throat, dry mouth, thirst.
Tongue: dry and red with little or no coating.
Application: gastritis, bronchitis, pharyngitis.
Contraindications: cough due to external 'Wind'-'Heat' or 'Wind'-'Cold'.

Mu Xiang Shun Qi San

Action: promotes smooth circulation of Qi, clears 'Heat', nourishes blood, tonifies spleen, eliminates 'Phlegm' and 'Dampness'.
Indications: irregular bowel motions, belching, abdominal distention, abdominal pain, indigestion.
Tongue: yellow and greasy coating.
Application: stomach ache due to improper eating, constipation, indigestion.

Qian Jin Nei Tuo San

Action: clears 'Heat', dispels 'Toxins', tonifies Qi, nourishes blood.
Indications: red, swollen, painful, suppurating lesions, weak constitution.
Tongue: either pale or red, with yellow coating.
Application: carbuncle, furuncle, suppurative otitis media.

Qian Shi Bai Zhu Tang

Action: tonifies Qi, eliminates 'Dampness', promotes circulation of Qi.
Indications: poor appetite, abdominal pain and distention, nausea and/or vomiting, diarrhoea, poor digestion, low energy, tires easily.
Tongue: pale with a thick white coating.
Application: child with weak constitution and poor digestion with diarrhoea.

Qing Fei Yi Huo Tang

Action: clears 'Heat' from lungs and liver, eliminates 'Phlegm' and 'Toxins', moistens lungs and throat.
Indications: raspy cough with yellow sputum, dry and sore throat, fever, dark scanty urine, constipation, may also be mouth sores and bleeding gums.
Application: bronchitis, aphthous ulcers, laryngitis.

Qing Wei San

Action: clears 'Heat' from the stomach, cools the blood, nourishes Yin.

Indications: gums sore, red and swollen, mouth ulcers, facial swelling, fever, bad breath, dry mouth, pain and swelling of tongue and/or lips.
Tongue: red with little or absent coating.
Application: stomatitis, gingivitis, glossitis, halitosis.

Qing Xin Cha

Action: clears 'Heat' from the heart, nourishes Yin, replenishes body fluids.
Indications: dream disturbed sleep, anxiety, irritability, thirst.
Tongue: may have a red tip.
Application: insomnia, emotional instability.

Ren Shen Bai Du San

Action: disperses external 'Wind' and 'Cold', dispels 'Dampness', tonifies the Qi.
Indications: high fever and severe chills, shivering, absence of sweating, pain and stiffness of the head and neck, aches and pains in the limbs, nasal congestion, productive cough.
Tongue: pale with a thick greasy coating.
Application: common cold, influenza, early stage dysentery, early stage measles; for child with delicate constitution.

Ren Shen Jian Pi Wan

Action: strengthens the spleen, reduces food stagnation, stops diarrhoea.
Indications: reduced appetite with difficulty in digestion, bloating of abdomen, watery diarrhoea, weak constitution (pale face, low energy, quiet, etc.).
Tongue: pale with a thick greasy coating.
Application: gastroenteritis, dysentery, ulcerative colitis, nervous dysfunction of the gastrointestinal tract.

San Huang Xie Xin Tang

Action: drains 'Fire', relieves toxicity, dries 'Dampness'.
Indications: fever, irritability, restlessness, flushed face, red eyes, dark urine, constipation or diarrhoea, there may also be jaundice, localised distention in the upper abdomen, ulcers on tongue and/or in mouth.
Tongue: red with a greasy yellow coating.
Application: acute gastroenteritis, dysentery, mouth ulcers.

San Zi Yang Qing Tang

Action: directs the Qi downwards, transforms 'Phlegm', reduces food stagnation, relaxes the diaphragm.

Indications: coughing and wheezing, copious sputum, loss of appetite, digestive difficulties.
Tongue: white greasy coating.
Application: bronchitis, asthma, spasms of the diaphragm.

Sang Ju Yin

Action: disperses external 'Wind' and 'Heat', stops coughing.
Indications: slight fever, cough, slight thirst.
Tongue: normal.
Application: common cold, influenza, bronchitis, acute tonsillitis, acute conjunctivitis.

Sha Shen Mai Men Dong Tang

Action: clears 'Heat' from lungs and stomach, moistens lungs and stomach, generates body fluids, nourishes lungs and stomach.
Indications: Hacking cough with scanty sputum, dry throat, thirst.
Tongue: red with little coating.
Application: common cold, influenza, bronchitis, whooping cough.

Shao Yao Tang

Action: clears 'Heat', relieves 'Toxicity', promotes circulation of Qi and blood.
Indications: abdominal pain, tenesmus, diarrhoea with pus and blood, dark scanty urine, burning pain around anus.
Tongue: red with a yellow greasy coating.
Application: dysentery, acute enteritis, ulcerative colitis.

Shen Ling Bai Zhu San

Action: tonifies Qi, strengthens spleen and stomach, resolves internal 'Dampness'.
Indications: muscular weakness, fatigue, poor appetite, pale complexion, abdominal distention, indigestion, nausea and/or vomiting, diarrhoea.
Tongue: pale with a white greasy coating.
Application: chronic gastroenteritis, malabsorption.

Sheng Ma Ge Gen Tang

Action: disperses external 'Wind' and 'Heat', causes rashes to surface.
Indications: fever and chills, headache, generalised body aches, sneezing, coughing, red eyes, tearing, thirst.
Tongue: red and dry.
Application: early stage of measles.

Si Jun Zi Tang

Action: strengthens the spleen, tonifies the Qi.

Indications: pale or yellowish complexion, low and soft voice, speaks little, poor appetite, may have dull abdominal pains or discomfort, loose stools, weakness and fatigue, eyes lack brightness, may sleep with eyes slightly open, may have blue vein or blue tint between the eyebrows, may be a yellow hue in the area between the eye lids and eye brows and also the whites of the eyes.
Tongue: pale and may be swollen with tooth marks on the edges.
Application: for child with poor digestion and weak constitution.

Si Ni San

Action: promotes circulation of Qi, regulates the spleen, harmonises liver and stomach.
Indications: abdominal pain, belching, reduced appetite, pain or discomfort below the ribs, bitter taste in the mouth, nausea and/or vomiting, irritability, depression, cold fingers and toes.
Tongue: red and may have a yellow coating.
Application: emotionally related — abdominal pains, discomfort, indigestion.

Teng Hua Bai Du San

Action: clears 'Heat', drains 'Dampness', eliminates 'Toxins'.
Indications: itching skin rash, fever, cough, nasal congestion.
Application: measles — second stage (skin eruptions just beginning to appear).

Tian Wang Bu Xin Dan

Action: enriches Yin, nourishes blood, tonifies the heart, calms the mind and emotions.
Indications: irritability, fatigue, insomnia with restless sleep, poor concentration ability, mental confusion; forgetfulness, dry hard stools, there may also be ulcers in the mouth and on the tongue, low fever and night sweats.
Tongue: red with little or no coating.
Application: poor sleeping habits, night crying, oral ulcers, personality disorders.

Tuo Li Xiao Du Yin

Action: clears 'Heat', pushes 'Toxins' outward, expels pus, tonifies Qi, nourishes blood.
Indications: red, painful, hot swellings without discharge of pus.
Application: carbuncles, furuncles, middle ear infection.

Wu Ling San

Action: promotes urination, drains 'Dampness', strengthens spleen.

Indications: nausea and/or vomiting, diarrhoea, generalised sensation of heaviness, difficulty in urinating.

Tongue: white coating which may be moist or greasy.

Application: acute gastroenteritis.

Wu Wei Xiao Du Yin

Action: clears 'Heat', relieves 'Toxicity', cools the blood, reduces swelling.

Indications: localised swellings on the skin which are red, hot and painful, fever, chills.

Tongue: red with a yellow coating.

Application: carbuncles, furuncles, erysipelas, conjunctivitis, urinary tract infection.

Xiang Ru San

Action: disperses external attack by 'Cold' and 'Dampness' in the summer season, harmonises stomach and spleen, transforms 'Dampness'.

Indications: aversion to cold temperatures, skin is warm to the touch, absence of sweating, sensation of heaviness in the head, headache, abdominal pain, nausea and/or vomiting, diarrhoea, stifling sensation in the chest, easily tired.

Tongue: white greasy coating.

Application: common cold, gastroenteritis.

Xiang Sha Liu Jun Zi Tang

Action: strengthens the spleen, harmonises the stomach, promotes the circulation of Qi, alleviates pain.

Indications: poor appetite, feeling full after eating very little, belching, abdominal distention and/or pain, nausea and/or vomiting, loose stools or diarrhoea.

Tongue: pale with a thick greasy white coating.

Application: chronic gastroenteritis, poor digestion.

Xiang Sha Yang Wei Tang

Action: strengthens the spleen, resolves internal 'Dampness', dispels 'Phlegm', promotes circulation of Qi, harmonises stomach and spleen.

Indications: poor appetite, loss of taste, inability to eat more than a little at a time, bloating after eating, nausea, flatulence, localised distention in the abdomen, abdominal pain or discomfort, general weakness and fatigue, loose stools or diarrhoea.

Application: chronic gastroenteritis, poor digestion.

Xiang Su San

Action: promotes free circulation of Qi, dispels external attack by 'Wind' and 'Cold'.

Indications: fever and chills without sweating, headache, stifling sensation in the chest, poor appetite, belching, localised sensation of swelling in the upper abdomen.

Tongue: normal.

Application: Common cold, stomach flu.

Xiao Chai Hu Tang

Action: dispels external attack by 'Wind' and 'Cold' that has begun to penetrate into the interior of the body, tonifies Qi.

Indications: alternating fever and chills, dry throat, bitter or sour taste in the mouth, dizziness, irritability, sensation of fullness in the chest and below the ribs, difficulty in taking a deep breath, heartburn, nausea and/or vomiting, reduced appetite, may also be diarrhoea.

Tongue: normal.

Application: common cold, influenza, bronchitis, epidemic parotitis.

Xiao Jian Zhong Tang

Action: warms and strengthens the stomach and spleen, alleviates spasmodic abdominal pain.

Indications: intermittent spasmodic abdominal pain, pain is relieved by heat and pressure, pale lustreless complexion, frequent urination, poor appetite, cold hands and feet, low energy, easily fatigued, may also have low fever.

Tongue: pale with a thin white coating.

Application: abdominal pains, bed-wetting, anaemia, fever of unknown origin.

Xiao Qing Long Tang

Action: dispels external attack by 'Wind' and 'Cold', resolves fluid congestion, warms the lungs, directs 'rebellious' Qi downwards.

Indications: fever and chills (chills predominating), absence of sweating, productive cough with sputum that is copious, white, sticky and difficult to expectorate, wheeze, stifling sensation in the chest, generalised body aching with sensations of heaviness, absence of thirst.

Tongue: moist coating.

Application: acute bronchitis, acute episode of chronic bronchitis, bronchial asthma, influenza.

Contraindications: not to be used long term.

Xiao Yao San

Action: promotes circulation in liver Qi, strengthens the spleen, nourishes the blood, harmonises liver and spleen.
Indications: pain and sensation of distention below the ribs, headache, dizziness, bitter taste in the mouth, dry mouth and throat, fatigue, reduced appetite, abdominal bloating and sensation of fullness, hiccup, depression, irritability, symptoms aggravated by emotional upsets, may also have diarrhoea or constipation or alternating.
Tongue: pale.
Application: emotionally related gastro-intestinal disorders.

Xie Bai San

Action: drains 'Heat' from the lungs, stops wheezing.
Indications: cough, wheeze, fever, symptoms tend to worsen in the late afternoon, sputum which is scanty and difficult to expectorate, dry mouth.
Tongue: red with yellow coating.
Application: bronchitis, whooping cough, pneumonitis from measles.
Contraindications: conditions due to external attack by 'Wind' and 'Cold' or 'Wind' and 'Heat', conditions due to 'Phlegm' and 'Dampness'.

Xing Su San

Action: dispels external attack by 'Cold' and 'Dryness', promotes free circulation of lung Qi, resolves fluid congestion.
Indications: mild headache, chills, absence of sweating, productive cough with watery sputum, nasal congestion, dry throat, dry mouth.
Tongue: a dry white coating.
Application: bronchitis.

Xuan Du Fa Biao Tang

Action: clears 'Heat', eliminates 'Toxins' dispels external attack by 'Wind', 'Cold' and 'Heat', promotes free circulation of lung Qi, resolves 'Phlegm'.
Indications: fever, mild chills, nasal congestion, cough, sore and swollen throat, may also be diarrhoea.
Tongue: normal.
Application: early stage measles (before skin eruptions appear).

Yin Qiao San

Action: dispels external attack by 'Wind' and 'Heat', clears 'Heat', relieves 'Toxicity'.
Indications: fever, mild or absent chills, headache, thirst, cough, sore throat, nasal congestion.
Tongue: may have a red tip and the coating is thin and white or thin and yellow.
Application: common cold, influenza, acute bronchitis, measles, epidemic parotitis.

Yue Ju Wan

Action: promotes movement of Qi, releases stagnation.
Indications: abdominal pain, fullness and distention, flatulence, acid regurgitation, belching, nausea and/or vomiting, reduced appetite, indigestion, stifling sensation in the chest, mild cough with copious sputum.
Application: functional gastro-intestinal disorders.

CHINESE REMEDIES IN THE A-Z GUIDE TO CHILDREN'S COMPLAINTS

'External' refers to diseases that occur in the more superficial parts of the body (e.g. common cold).

'Internal' refers to diseases that occur in the deeper parts of the body, affecting the internal organs (e.g. when a cold or flu goes to the chest and the infection reaches the lungs).

'Deficiency' refers to a lowering or reduction in the functioning of an organ or bodily system.

'Excess' refers to an overactivity of an organ or bodily system. It also refers to an accumulation or build-up of pathological substances in the body (e.g. 'Heat', and 'Toxins' which refers to the painful inflammation due to a bacterial infection which usually produces pus.)

'Dampness', 'Heat', 'Cold', 'Dryness', 'Phlegm' and 'Wind' all refer to pathogenic factors which may invade the body from the outside or be generated on the inside of the body due to imbalances of various kinds.

'Stagnation' refers to a blockage in the normal circulation of various substances in the body (e.g. Qi, blood and food are commonly involved in this pathological process).

Zhi Gan Cao Tang

Action: tonifies Qi, nourishes blood, enriches Yin.

Indications: irritability, insomnia, shortness of breath on mild exertion, constipation, dry mouth and throat, easily startled.

Tongue: pale and shiny without coating.

Application: poor sleeping habits, night crying, constipation, nosebleeds.

Zhi Tou Chuang Yi Fang

Action: clears 'Heat', eliminates 'Toxins', dispels 'Wind' from the skin.

Indications: skin lesions which are itchy and have a yellow or pus-like exudate, may also have hard stool or constipation.

Tongue: red with a yellow coating.

Application: eczema, dermatitis.

Contraindications: not to be used for 'Deficiency' conditions.

Zhu Ye Shi Gao Tang

Action: clears 'Heat', generates body fluids, tonifies the Qi, harmonises the stomach.

Indications: prolonged low fever (from a febrile illness), sweating, complexion is red, vomiting, irritability, thirst, dry mouth, lips and throat, cough, stifling sensation in the chest, may also have restlessness and insomnia.

Tongue: red with little coating.

Application: pharyngitis, bed-wetting.

MASSAGE

The Importance of Touching

It doesn't matter how old or young you are, most of us love to be touched. It is the sense upon which all others are based and is probably the earliest to develop in the human embryo. Even though everyone is different in how often, by whom, when and where they like to be touched (and these differences are often class or culture based), it is one of the most important forms of communication in our lives.

For centuries, both in the East and West, parents and grandparents have used their hands and sometimes even their feet to gently massage the bodies of their newborn infants. It played a major role in strengthening the relationship between parent and child and resulted in happy, calmer, healthy babies.

A long line of scientific studies from around the world confirm that touching is almost as nourishing for baby as mother's milk. The research suggests that babies who get plenty of extra holding and caressing, especially in the first few months of life, smile more, have more satisfying relationships with their parents and cry less. Research indicates that infants that aren't touched enough simply don't grow properly at all.

In 1915, Dr Henry Chapin, a New York paediatrician, reported that in ten cities, in every institution except one, every infant under two years of age died. The realisation that this was caused by being deprived of touch immediately resulted in boarding out babies instead of leaving them in the institutions. After World War II, studies were done to establish the cause of a disease called marasmus (wasting away) responsible for infant mortality not only in institutions, but the best homes and hospitals as well. As a result of the study, hospitals introduced new guidelines that included picking up, carrying and mothering infants at least several times daily. Another very early study found that the earlier a baby's skin is stimulated the greater the influence upon the development of the immunological system. This has important consequences for a child's future resistance to infections and disease.

People now understood that in order for children to grow and develop to their peak, they need to be handled, carried, cuddled, caressed, stroked, kissed and cooed to, as often as possible.

More recent studies have proved these early results. Dr Saul Schanberg of Duke University Medical Centre in North Carolina and Dr T. Fields of the University of Miami Medical School gave massages to ten out of twenty premature infants in intensive care for ten days in a row. They compared the growth and development of these babies with the ten who weren't massaged. The massaged infants gained 47 per cent more weight each day, appeared more active and alert, showed more mature infant behaviour and were discharged from the hospital on an average of six days earlier.

The slowed growth of infants deprived of mother's touch is a kind of survival mechanism, according to Dr Schanberg. The absence of touch indicates the absence of a mother, which is a life-threatening situation. The energy normally directed to growing, therefore, shifts to maintaining the body. It is now considered impossible to spoil a baby with too much affection and touching.

Unfortunately, with the passing of the extended family in our society, the tactile stimulation of babies is left solely to the mother who is often too busy to give the attention she'd like. However, the ancient art of infant massage is undergoing a renaissance in the West, and bodywork therapists, holistic health practitioners, childbirth educators, and even paediatricians are praising the practice as its emotional, physical and psychological benefits become more and more evident. And, not only can the positive effects be seen in the infant, but the person giving the massage also reaps benefits.

The Benefits of Massage

When the foetus is floating around in the amniotic fluid it is continuously exposed to a soothing massage. Most of its first prenatal sensory experience is tactile, so it virtually goes without saying that the importance of being lovingly touched will be vital to a baby's well-being. This factor is crucial to their survival and emotional well-being in the first few months of their lives.

During the first few months and years of an infant's growth, regular massage can help to ensure successful development. It can facilitate positive long-term emotional and psychological growth and relieve and prevent certain physical, emotional and psychological ailments common to children.

Massage not only tones the skin and muscles, but also has the capacity to stimulate the internal organs, which helps to maintain and promote their healthy functioning. It can regulate involuntary activities, such as digestion and circulation, and has successfully been used in the East for thousands of years to support health and prevent illness.

One of the most common findings from parents who regularly massage their children is that the children become more and more relaxed and overcome stress better because the massage gives them a very good form of release. At the same time as these more visible results, massage stimulates the infants' circulatory, respiratory and gastro-intestinal functions. Common ailments such as colic and wind are often quickly relieved.

Best of all, massage enhances bonding between parents and child because it contains all of the vital ingredients: smiling, skin-to-skin contact, eye-to-eye contact, soothing sounds, peaceful environment, cuddling, interaction and nurturing. And not only is it good for the child and the parent-child relationship, but massage is good for you, the parent, as well. Knowing that you are able to contribute to your child's well-being and pleasure is very rewarding.

If a mother and her child are not able to make the important physical, primal bond immediately after birth (this may be due to premature birth, caesarean section or perhaps an infant has been adopted and has experienced separation from the mother at delivery or shortly thereafter), massage can be an important tool in re-establishing that bond. In these instances it would be vital for the massage to begin within two months of the birth.

Not only is massage vital for healthy infants, but massage specialists have found that it can also be quite a useful and effective tool in growth and recovery from illness for the deaf, blind, and hospitalised infants.

How To Massage Your Child

When To Massage

You can begin massaging your child as soon after birth as the navel is healed. At this early stage you should only use a gentle all-over stroking massage. When your baby is over four months of age, then you may wish to concentrate on more specific areas like the hands, feet, back, ear, etc. However, there will be occasions when stroking alone is most appropriate and soothing. You are the best judge of your child's moods and needs so don't be afraid to trust your own intuition about the type of massage necessary.

As soon as your child becomes ill you should begin treating him with massage. You should, however, always choose a time when you can feel relaxed and your child will be receptive. For babies, after a bath is a lovely time to massage for colic. For older children, in the evenings at bedtime is a good time for chronic conditions such as bed-wetting or asthma. If, for example, you are rushing out the door to an appointment or are feeling anxious, this may not be the time to try and fit in a massage treatment for abdominal pain.

Where To Massage

Be sure when you are doing any massage that your child is warm and the room temperature is comfortable. This is especially important for babies. Placing a warm (that is, comfortable to your wrist) water bottle on your child's back or abdomen, can add to his relaxation.

When using the trigger points or reflex points for the feet, you can be carrying your child in your arms. When giving your child a massage, he should ideally be lying down on a bed or a mat or blanket on the floor. You should be comfortable too. If you are sitting on the floor, prop yourself up with cushions or lean against a wall, sitting cross-legged or with your legs spread apart with the child lying between them. Your spine should be straight, with most of your movement coming from the centre of your body through your arms and hands. Babies will need to be propped up on a pillow to feel a sense of security and closeness to you. A changing table can also be used for babies.

What To Use

Ohashi, a practitioner and teacher of Shiatsu (Japanese massage), gives some techniques that can be used with infants in his book, *Touch For Love*. He suggests stroking or rubbing your baby with a soft brush, such as an infant's hairbrush, a pad of cheesecloth or a folded cotton handkerchief, a warm teaspoon, one or two fingers, or your whole hand covered with warm oil.

When using the pressure points, you don't need oil or lotion. However, using a light natural vegetable oil or lotion when doing the massage strokes makes the movement easier as well as more soothing on your child's skin. Oils are better than lotions because they soak into the skin more easily and most lotions dry more quickly. What you put on your child's skin is important because the skin absorbs easily. Babies can be highly sensitive and allergic to some oils and as they are fond of tasting everything they come into contact with, use an oil that is safe for their digestive system.

Mineral 'baby oils', are non-organic oils made from a non-food petroleum base. These oils are known to dry the skin and clog the pores, and may also deplete the system of vitamins.

The best oils to use are almond oil, apricot kernel oil, sunflower oil, vitamin E oil, avocado oil and olive oil. These can be bought at either health food stores or grocery stores. Unscented oil is also better for infants. If you want to use lotions, look for ones with natural ingredients such as safflower oil, aloe vera, cucumber, lanolin, glycerin, and jojoba oil. Remember that the first ingredient listed on the pack will be the major one in the product. If the first ingredient listed is water, choose something else as water will dry out the skin.

Watch the child's skin for any reaction. Children can be more reactive to the nut oils so you might have to switch to safflower or apricot oil. Wipe off any excess oil with a towel or wash cloth to keep child's skin clear and prevent clogging of pores or rashes.

Analgesic products such as tiger balm, oil of olbas, and eucalyptus ointment can be used during massage on children older than twelve months of age to help open up the bronchial tubes.

Massage and Touching

When you are massaging your child you are also teaching them about their bodies and touch. Through your touch they will learn what feels good, safe and healthy and when they want to be touched. As parents we are responsible for our children's bodies until they are old enough to care for them themselves. It is important, therefore, that even with an infant you ask their permission to touch their body and do so with love and respect. This is one way you can start teaching your child about what constitutes safe and healthy touching, and that they do have the right to say no.

SECTION 2

Preventative Care

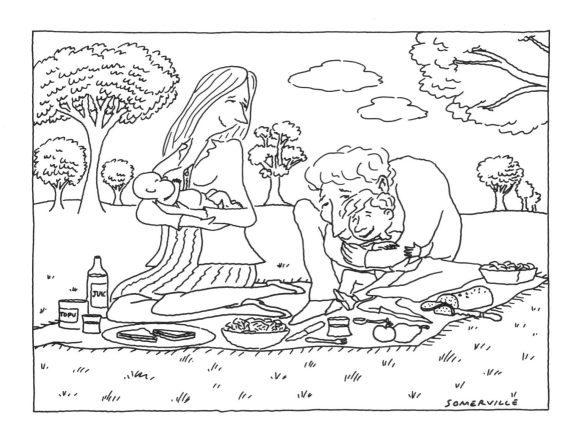

CHILDHOOD ILLNESSES

The speed at which illness progresses in children can be quite alarming. Temperatures can soar, chest complaints can rapidly develop into pneumonia and diarrhoea can quickly become severe. Fortunately children respond very quickly to treatment.

Just before the onset of an illness, you may notice that your child's stools begin to change in colour — they may become greenish and will probably be loose. Shortly thereafter, he may develop a runny nose and a change in temperament will be evident. If you don't catch it in time an earache may develop, and later it could find its way down into the lungs and a cough could arise.

Digestion and Illness

Digestive disturbances are often the cause of illness, particularly in children under six years of age. Even whooping cough, asthma and eczema can sometimes be caused by disturbances in the digestive system.

Common Causes of Digestive Disturbances

Demand feeding: most infants' digestion is weak and inefficient and needs a certain amount of time to perform at optimum level. If your baby is fed too much too often his digestion becomes impaired.
Irregular feeding: maintain a schedule for small regular meals, every 2–3 hours except in times of sickness. This will support the digestive system without taxing it too much.
Cold and excessive fluids: drinking with a meal or drinking too much before or after a meal dilutes the stomach acids and digestive juices causing poor digestion. Cold drinks also prevent the stomach from functioning properly.
Over-feeding: many children are fed too much food. Never force food onto your child.
Indigestible food: because of the delicate nature of infants' digestive systems, easily digested foods such as rice milk or puréed cooked vegetables and fruits should be the first solid foods you give your child.

Repeating Patterns

If a child with a healthy immune system develops an infection or illness, he usually recovers in a matter of days or weeks. However sometimes one or two of the original symptoms remains and never seems to clear. This pattern has been linked to recurring problems such as earaches, sore throats, chest infections and tonsillitis.

These are the likely symptoms for a child who hasn't completely shaken an illness:
- low energy
- energy drops each day at the same time
- prone to catching infections quite easily
- constant cough or runny nose
- unhappy most of the time
- exhibiting some symptoms of the original illness, for example, in mumps there is irritability, and swollen glands, in whooping cough there is a chronic malingering cough.

Why Is My Child Ill so Often?

It's not unusual for children to have several bouts of colds and coughs during the winter. Young children have few antibodies, so when they first come into contact with viruses or bacteria, they have very little protection. Once they become infected, however, they will develop antibodies. The problem is that viral infections like the flu have many different strains, so that even if your child had the flu last year, he will only have built up antibodies to that strain. If there is a different one this year, those antibodies will have no effect.

Children are particularly prone to illness when they start school or playschool and are in touch with a lot of other children. *This is normal. They are building up their immune system*. A normal, healthy child will have many infections, particularly in the first six years.

FOOD AND NUTRITION

Breast Feeding

Colostrum, a yellowish liquid, is present in the breasts before the baby is born and lasts for about three days afterwards. It is rich in protein, and also contains antibodies to protect the baby against a wide range of diseases, 'including polio, influenza, the Coxsacki group of viruses and salmonella' says Shiela Kitzinger in her book, *The experience of breastfeeding.* According to Paul Buisseret, in 'Common manifestations of cow's milk allergy in children', 'The newborn baby's gut is immunologically very vulnerable and colostrum has an extremely important function in providing a kind of primer of protective paint with this immunoglobulin-rich fluid in concentrations much higher than those of the mother's blood.' Without such protection, the newborn is exposed to respiratory, bacterial and intestinal viral infections.

Over a period of several days, the colostrum changes into thin milk and then by about the end of the second week it finally evolves into mature milk. Breast milk contains anti-stapholococcus factors, vitamins, minerals and live enzymes. It is constantly changing and adapting itself to the baby's needs. As your baby grows the protein and fat content of the milk decreases.

How Long To Breast Feed

The World Health Organisation recommends breast feeding for at least the first four to six months of baby's life. Only a nursing mother can make the best decision for herself and her baby. But it should be continued for as long as both mother and baby are happy with it.

Drugs and Breast Milk

You should consult a health care practitioner if you are taking any drugs while breast feeding. They can enter your milk supply and may pose a risk to your baby.

There are far too many variables involved to be able to cover the problems in detail,

however, the following guidelines will be helpful.

- Drugs that enter the bloodstream directly are more concentrated and are therefore likely to be more concentrated in the breast milk.
- Some drugs bind to proteins in the mother's blood system and some don't. The protein-binding capacity of a drug limits to some degree the concentration that the baby receives.
- Highly alkaline drugs (those with high pH levels) pass into the milk at higher concentrations than do more acidic drugs (lower pH).
- Every drug has a certain 'peak effect' which is a point at which its action and its passage into the breast milk, is maximised. Beyond this point, the level of concentration in the

---

CAFFEINE LINK WITH SMALL BABIES

Women who consumed at least 4½ oz of caffeine a day doubled their risk of delivering a baby weighing less than 5½ lbs, compared with those who gave up caffeine during pregnancy.

Moderate caffeine consumers also doubled their risk of delivering a baby showing intra-uterine growth retardation. Heavy consumers quadrupled their risk of growth retardation. Both low birth weight and intra-uterine growth retardation are associated with increased risks of infant illness and mortality.

A study done by Pennsylvania State University has found that drinking coffee, tea or cola in moderation, say two to three cups a day, should not pose a threat to the baby through his mother's milk.

However, some babies may be affected by the smallest amount. They may become restless and may cry continuously. Especially in the first three weeks after birth, too much coffee can make both mother and baby nervous and upset.

breast milk decreases. If you know when the peak effect is, you can co-ordinate feeding times with non-peak periods of drug activity.

- Premature babies may have too few liver enzymes and other detoxifying agents to be able to successfully break down and move drugs out from the body.
- Whether or not a drug is fat soluble or not can determine its effect on the baby. The fat content of mother's milk increases from morning to midday, and then drops off toward evening and it also increases as the feeding goes on. So by rescheduling or reducing the feeding times fat-soluble drugs can be decreased in the milk given to the baby. Water soluble drugs appear in the beginning of the breast milk, so expressing first will help to alleviate the drugs in this case.
- Caffeine is found in many foods as well as over-the-counter medications such as cold remedies, weight-control aids, pain relievers and stimulants. Only about one per cent of the caffeine ingested by a mother appears in her breast milk, but the amount can accumulate in the baby's system. Some of the more common responses are hyperactivity and wakefulness which can sometimes be misinterpreted as colic or other minor ailments.

Time that is spent breast feeding can be a rich and rewarding experience for both you and the baby. The non-verbal communication of touching, feeling, seeing and smelling all enhance a baby's first experiences. However, bottle feeding can also be rewarding when it is done with love. Shiela Kitzinger sums it up well when she says, 'The quality of the relationship is more significant than whether the milk comes in breast or bottle.'

Weaning

All babies and children need to suckle and be comforted, and if they don't have access to prolonged nursing, they will have to find it in other ways. If your child is not ready to give up the breast, try introducing a bottle, pacifier or blanket and see if this can help to make the transition smoother. However, it's important to recognise that this object will need to be used for *as long as the child needs it*, not when you think it is time for him to give it up.

Gradual weaning is usually the most successful — slowly dropping one feed at a time, leaving until last the one, at night, just before

sleep. However, how you wean is ultimately up to you and your baby. Follow your instincts, no one can know better than you on this matter. Despite old beliefs, responsible long-term breast feeding cannot 'spoil' children, and in fact it can provide much of what little children really need, eventually producing more secure and independent people.

The Joy of Eating

First Foods

At the age of six months or thereabouts, most babies indicate a desire for solid food. Start your baby off with puréed vegetables and cereals, such as rice cream, porridge and barley. It is best not to introduce wheat until the baby is at least ten months old as it's often linked to allergies and coeliac disease (a malabsorption condition). Some foods such as grains are digested better when cooked, because the starch in the plant fibres expands, causing the cell walls to rupture and yield their nutrients more easily. Once your baby starts to get teeth, try bite-sized pieces of cooked vegetables and fruit to exercise his gums.

Introduce foods one at a time and wait three to five days before introducing the next one. This way you can see if there is any allergic reaction. Rotate foods as much as possible and don't use any seasoning. If your baby develops either a nasal mucous discharge or loose stools from the food, then it should be stopped for a while until the digestive system is strong enough to handle it. Because of the immaturity of the intestines, meat is not considered a beneficial choice.

HOW MUCH IS ENOUGH?

A few tablespoons at a time is all that is usually required in the beginning. Your baby will let you know when he wants more. If you notice that in the baby's stools certain foods are going out the same way as they went in, don't worry, it's only that some foods are not being fully absorbed. Gradually, as the digestive system becomes more fully-developed, digestion improves.

It is best to leave cabbage family vegetables (broccoli, cauliflower, Chinese greens, lettuce, brussel sprouts, etc.) until at least nine months as they are often difficult to digest.

Taste Sensations

As infants develop, so too do their preferences for different tastes. Towards the end of an infant's first year of life, his ability to know what he needs is so well developed that he can actually select a diet that is nutritious and wholesome according to his needs. C. Davis, in a study done called 'Self selection of diet by newly weaned infants', in the *American Journal of Diseases of Children,* Vol. 36 'found that babies did not choose the 'proper' diet of cereals and milk, supplemented by small amounts of fruit, eggs and meat. If a foodstuff contained a nutrient that the babies need, their physiology caused it to taste good — even cod liver oil'. Until infants are two or three years old, their sensation of flavour is not completely developed. However too much sweet food will weaken the digestive system and can produce mucus, whereas a little bit will warm and support the stomach and even help a child grow.

Is Milk Necessary?

In many respects dairy food is neither traditional nor healthy. It was only in the 1930s that we started to consume them in large quantities at all, and 90 per cent of the world's population up until the middle ages hardly ever drank milk. Cow's milk has been shown to be implicated in 74 per cent of allergic skin reactions, and in 89 per cent of asthma and hay fever cases according to John Button, author of *How to be Green.* Many children find it difficult to digest the lactose (milk sugar) in dairy products, and if they continue to consume them, can often develop allergies. Asians and black Africans do not drink milk after they are weaned, and their bones develop normally. (Their skeletons are also resistant to osteoporisis because of their low consumption of animal protein.)

Although milk is touted to be a high-calcium, high-protein food, it contains only 3.3 per cent protein, and 3.8 per cent is saturated fat, supplying 40 per cent of our saturated fat intake and 30 per cent of our total fat intake. There is lots of calcium in milk but there is also plenty in dried fruit, sesame seeds, potatoes, green vegetables, peas and mushrooms. It is probably wiser and healthier to use dairy products as embellishments rather than daily, staple foods.

From Three Onwards

By three years of age, a child will be eating the same food as the rest of the family. Balance is the key to good health.

A well-balanced diet should be ideally based on seasonal, fresh, organically grown produce and wholefoods, free range, chemical free chickens and eggs and organic and/or biodynamically raised meat (if desired). (*Fresh* meaning the best quality seasonal or dried produce; *whole* meaning, unrefined, unadulterated, as complete in structure and nutrient composition as possible.) These include nuts, fruits, whole grains (rice, barley, oats), pulses and beans, fish, vegetables, free-range and organic eggs, organically reared meat and fowl. So-called health foods are not necessarily wholefoods. They can be just as refined and processed and more expensive than their competition. Organically grown and biodynamic produce is produced without the use of chemical pesticides, artificial fertilisers or growth hormones, and make use of manure, bones, and natural compost. Meat and fowl that are free range and organic and/or biodynamically raised are free to roam about and are fed whole grains and preferably allowed to eat grass that has not been chemically treated.

Eating seasonally is one of the best ways to ensure that the produce you buy is fresh. All highly refined and processed foods and those containing additives or preservatives should be avoided as the original nutritional balance, so essential for well-being, is upset during refining and processing. Even a refined product, fortified with a selection of the vital nutrients stripped off in refining, is still only a partial food.

Sharing Foods

The sharing of food is one of the most important ways that we socialise. If the food that we provide at home isolates our children socially they will not want to invite their friends home to enjoy it. What is needed is a little of both worlds; something that they want to eat and something that you want them to eat. Providing that they get one meal a day that is nutritionally sound, you probably don't have to concern yourself too much with their other meals. They will inevitably share their lunches as all kids do! If we want our children's friends to share our food we must allow our children to share their friend's food once in a while, no matter what it's like.

Basic Guidelines for Food Selection

- avoid fatty foods
- avoid refined sugar
- eat more complex carbohydrates
- eat fewer refined and processed foods
- avoid food colouring and preservatives
- eat seasonally

- eat organically-grown produce when available
- eat meat sparingly
- decrease mucus-forming foods
- eat wholesome breakfasts, not sugar-laden cereals

Cooking Techniques

- steaming, pressure cooking, boiling or baking for the first year
- baking, grilling or roasting can be incorporated after one year and then
- light sauteeing after two years
- shallow frying after three years

Mucus-forming Foods

- cream
- butter
- cheese
- roasted peanuts
- too much orange juice or oranges (more than one orange a week)
- bananas
- excessive sugar
- too much fatty food
- too much meat
- too much salt

Foods that Reduce Mucus

- onions
- watercress
- garlic
- mustard
- salt-pickled plums (Japanese or Chinese)
- parsley
- saltwater pickles
- celery
- green tea
- bancha tea (Japanese)
- jasmine tea
- lemon

Food Guide

4-6 MONTHS

Texture: semi-liquid purées; no added seasoning and no lumps.
Preparation: peel fruits and vegetables; remove seeds, pips and strings; boil or, preferably, steam (save water and use for purée or soup); purée or sieve.
Suggested foods: pumpkin; rice cream; apple sauce; pear sauce; cooked fruits in season.

6-8 MONTHS

Texture: lumpy foods, but soft; the texture of

> Stainless steel, glass corningware or enamel are the best materials for cooking. Avoid aluminium at all costs. Food should be prepared just before eating if possible, and discarded after 24 hours if not eaten.

cottage cheese. Add liquid where necessary. Finger foods such as carrot and celery sticks can be given now, especially if your baby is teething.
Preparation: peel fruits and vegetables; remove pits and seeds; mash.
Suggested foods: as above together with (add one at a time): sweet potato; carrots; peas; wholegrain cereals; soups; fruit or vegetable jellies; cooked fruit wedges; steamed and mashed banana; rice cream cereal (see box below).

RICE CREAM CEREAL

1 cup brown or white organic rice
6-8 cups purified water
1 tablespoon roasted sesame seeds (hulled)
Wash rice the night before.

If using brown rice, bake on a baking sheet in a pre-heated oven 180°C (350°F) until a nutty brown colour.

Grind if possible along with sesame seeds or leave whole or use freshly ground brown or white rice flour.

Combine the cereal and water in a saucepan and gradually stir to prevent lumps forming until it begins to boil. Simmer covered, over low heat for 40-60 minutes. Add more water if too thick.

In order to retain the nutritive properties in brown rice and other whole grain cereals they should be cooked immediately after grinding; when exposed to air, grains begin to oxidize and lose some of their nutritive qualities.

Any cereal can substituted for rice.

8-10 MONTHS

Texture: chunky with lots of finger foods.
Preparation: peel fruits and vegetables; remove seeds, pips and strings; serve raw or cooked, cut into slices or sticks, or chopped or grated.
Preparation of fish: trim off fat, bones and skin; steam or poach; mince finely to ensure all the bones have been removed.
Suggested foods: as above as well as toast;

ALL ABOUT SUGAR (SUCROSE)

Sucrose, also commonly known as sugar, is a refined carbohydrate and is made up of two sugars, fructose (fruit sugar) and glucose. Sucrose can be found in sugar cane, dates, figs, maple syrup and beetroot. Most of the sucrose that we consume comes from sugar cane.

For the last fifty years or so, there has been a significant rise in sucrose consumption. About 50 kilograms per person is consumed each year, with the highest consumption among teenagers.

It is likely that the following conditions are strongly associated with, or can be caused by, a high intake of sucrose. It is advisable therefore to consider reducing sucrose consumption in all cases.

Adverse effects of sucrose consumption
- tooth decay
- increased susceptibility to infection (weakens the immune system)
- obesity
- gastrointestinal ailments such as indigestion and diarrhoea
- hypertension (in some individuals a high sucrose intake produces an increase in blood pressure)
- hyperactivity in children
- anxiety
- depression
- acne
- dandruff
- eczema
- dermatitis
- allergies
- increased losses in the urine of the essential trace mineral, chromium, (associated with atherosclerosis, elevated blood cholesterol levels, and diabetes)

Beneficial effects of sucrose consumption
- Hiccups — these very often respond well to drinking a water and sugar solution.
- Intravenous feeding — when people are unable to take food by mouth they can benefit greatly from a salt, sugar and water solution.
- Wound healing — if wounds are unable to heal by themselves, the local application of sugar or honey can greatly assist the healing process.

Ways to reduce sugar intake
- Don't give your child excessively sweet foods until he demands it: babies often develop more savoury tastes if they are not exposed to sweet-tasting foods.
- Never give your child a bottle of milk, juice, soft drink or cordial to put him to sleep. Sugar stays in the mouth while the baby sleeps, allowing tooth decay to start.
- Never dip a pacifier in sugar or honey.
- Never add flavour or sweetener to a bottle; if a baby refuses to drink water he cannot be thirsty.
- Use fruit for desserts.
- Look into what is available at the school canteen and try to persuade your child to spend his pocket money on healthy foods.
- Offer water and diluted fruit juice for drinks. Remember that the effect of artificial sweeteners in young children is not known, so their consumption should be limited.
- Never send your child to school with sticky sweet foods when he is not able to clean his teeth afterwards.
- Look for alternative rewards — dried fruit, a book or a game.
- Limit sweet foods, lollies, chocolates, sweet biscuits and rich cakes to special occasions, or once each week.
- Check ingredient lists for glucose, maltose, honey, maltodextrins, golden syrup, molasses, fructose, lactose, dextrose, corn syrup solids, treacle and concentrated fruit juice. Although all have different names, they all become glucose in the body, and all have the same effect on teeth.

mashed potato; fish or chicken broth; unsalted rice or rye crackers; noodles.

10-12 MONTHS

Texture: depends on teeth, finely chopped, grated, chunky.

Preparation: peel fruits and vegetables; remove seeds, pips and strings; steam or boil.

Suggested foods: to all the above foods, add soft rice; green vegetables; fish; noodles; bread; all seasonal fruits and vegetables; fish or chicken broths; rice or mung bean noodles; green beans; unsalted crackers; citrus fruits.

FOOD IS MEDICINE

In the 4th and 5th centuries BC, Hippocrates, a Greek physician spoke of allowing food to be our medicine. He taught that the effects of climate, temperature, occupation and food were the things to look at when deciding upon the cause and cure of illness.

Modern science and medicine has recently begun to reassess some of its findings and to agree with this ancient wisdom. People are starting to look more and more at their diet and see the direct connection between health and well-being. What we eat, what it is made from, how we eat is vitally important.

ONE YEAR OLD

Texture: as above.

Preparation: as above, plus baking, grilling or roasting.

Suggested foods: as above with dried beans; fresh and dried peas; very small amounts of mashed, cooked tofu; yoghurt; eggs (introduce the yolk first); fresh herbs.

TWO YEARS AND OLDER

If your child is lacking strength and vitality, it may be necessary to introduce more broths of fish, chicken, beef and lamb into the diet.

Texture: any.

Preparation: as above.

Suggested foods: as above, along with nuts; seeds; white meat; more herbs; miso soup; a little more salt; custards.

Teaching Children about Nutrition

Many young children don't actually know how food is grown and many of them think that it comes in boxes or cans. 'Instant' foods have led to a widespread ignorance of where food actually comes from.

More than ever, children today have a dynamic relationship to the package and T.V. commercials rather than the actual food. Name, colour, and design of the package identify the food, not the contents or point of origin. In the past, how and what to cook was passed on by mum or grandma, and they learned by helping out in the kitchen. Today with demanding school, work and leisure schedules, microwave ovens and the increasing abundance of fast food restaurants, many meals are eaten on-the-run

or away from home, leaving little time in the kitchen for the children to learn about cooking.

We must teach our children about nutrition if we want them to be strong and healthy. Begin to involve your child more in the kitchen as well as with the shopping. Smell a melon, tap a watermelon, test to see if a pineapple is ripe (does the leaf come out easily when it is gently pulled?). Read labels and discuss what the different ingredients are. Look for foods that are additive- and preservative-free, organically grown, and explain why you are doing so and how they differ.

Vitamin and Mineral Supplements

In this day and age it shouldn't be difficult to provide a healthy, balanced nutritious diet for your child, which will provide them with all the vitamins and minerals they need. However, the huge number of vitamin and mineral supplements available today are enough to make any parent feel that her child might need them because he is not getting all that is required from his daily food intake. And even if you give your child what you consider to be a good balanced diet, he doesn't necessarily eat everything put in front of him. So how can you be sure that your child does get an adequate intake of his daily vitamin and mineral requirements?

Paediatrician, Dr Kathy Christofell who practices at the Children's Memorial Hospital in Chicago, feels that most supplementary vitamins are a 'waste of money' unless they are given for specific problems such as when a child refuses to eat, when drugs interfere with the body's ability to absorb vitamins and minerals or when a child has been diagnosed with a vitamin deficiency disease.

Some people have claimed that vitamins can be used to counteract pollution stemming from the environment. Dr Christofell says that 'there is little evidence to support the claims that megavitamin therapies are helpful or that vitamins are useful in combating environmental pollutants.'

There are two sides to the story as Dr Dunn, an Oak Park, Illinois paediatrician states: 'when a child has been on a diet low in nutrients and high in sugar and so-called junk foods, he may require high doses of certain vitamins, minerals and/or enzymes to restore biochemical balance.

Subsequently, biochemical balance may be maintained through an appropriate diet and a multiple vitamin/mineral supplement designed for the child's needs.' He also believes that a good, natural hypoallergic diet is one of the most important ways of supporting children's well-being. However, there are times when vitamin, mineral and amino acid supplementation is necessary to provide all of a child's needs.

According to Sherry Hardy, paediatric dietitian at Primary Children's Hospital in Salt Lake City, there is very little possibility of vitamin deficiency in healthy babies and children in America, as most get adequate intake of all the vitamins they need providing they eat a sound and balanced diet.

Many parents believe that if they are taking vitamin and mineral supplements, it must be fine for their children to take them. This is not necessarily the case. Giving vitamin and mineral supplements to children without even investigating what their needs are can be detrimental and large doses of certain vitamins can even be poisonous. There is very little evidence to prove that vitamins are helpful during illness either.

Your children will no doubt experiment with food that does not provide adequate nutrition, but there is nothing wrong with the odd packet of chips or a lolly or two, providing that they don't take the place of more nourishing food on a regular basis. Introduce healthy snacks such as muesli, wholemeal cookies sweetened with fruit juice instead of sugar, 100 per cent fruit juices, candy without colouring and sugar, and breads made from organically grown wholegrains. These will not compromise your child's vitamin and mineral requirements.

Don't overcook your food, serve lots of raw fruits and vegetables when appropriate and serve lots of fish and homemade desserts. Good eating habits are the best way of making sure that your children get all their vitamin and mineral needs to grow and stay healthy. Some foods are richer in vitamins and minerals than others but as long as a wide variety of foods are eaten there is no need for concern.

How to Prevent Weight Problems

Obesity is now 'the leading nutrition problem of all children' according to William Dietz, Ph.D., director of clinical nutrition at the New England Medical Center in Boston. A study, conducted in 1987 and reported in the *American Journal of Diseases of Children*, showed that since the 1960s, obesity has increased by 54 per cent among children between the ages of 6 and 11 and by 39 per cent in the 12 to 17 age bracket.

There are many things that parents can do to prevent weight problems in their children. One of the most important is not to force children to eat when they are not hungry. They should be allowed to follow their own needs. They will naturally know what their body needs and regulate their eating accordingly, unless they are lacking certain vitamins and minerals. The best way to handle children's idiosyncrasies around food is to let them make their own decisions about when and what to eat. Provide healthy foods that your children like and leave the rest up to them. Bake your own pies and cakes and have the children help; give them the ingredients and let them try it on their own. Do not supply non-nutritious foods (anything processed, fried, salty, oily, or full of sugar like lollies and sugar desserts). If you find your child overeating or undereating, change the volume of food consumed. Change the quality first, especially if your child is eating junk food, and even if the volume remains the same for a while, eventually overeating or undereating will cease to be a problem and excessive cravings for junk foods will disappear.

Set a good example yourself and encourage your children to do more exercise like walking, bicycle riding, or playing outdoor sports. Enroll them in after-school athletic activities and invite children over to play a game of soccer, baseball or basketball. Hand out little rewards (incentive devices) for all the players so no hard feelings evolve. Get into the game yourself and invite other parents to do the same.

Vegetarianism — A Way To Go?

Bringing up children at the best of times is complex and difficult enough, so those people who choose to give their children a vegetarian diet are really very brave. Mention the possibility of serving a meatless or, even worse, a dairyless, diet for children, and you will immediately provoke fear about 'getting enough'. Protein and calcium are usually the big issues, with friends and relatives pushing for the cheese and milk diet for strong bones and teeth!

If you decide to raise your children as

vegetarians, there are a number of issues to be considered. For example, when and what kinds of foods should be introduced and what kinds of social pressures will the children face because of such a 'weird' diet? Dr Christine Northrup, an obstetrician-gynaecologist in Maine, feels that the best way to raise a healthy child *is* without meat. She believes that vegetarian diets generally provide more vitamins and trace minerals than the more common diet. Of course you need to know how to provide a balanced diet, and learning how to feed a child any type of balanced diet is challenging.

How Do I Give My Child Enough Protein?

One of the first questions that I am asked is how to give a child enough extra protein for healthy growth. It's important to realise that children do not need that much extra protein. For the first year breast milk is enough. From 12–14 months your child should get his protein from soyfood, grain and bean combinations, and vegetables. Children who eat eggs and dairy products will receive lots of protein and even diets without dairy and eggs will still be adequate enough. The Farm, a well-known vegetarian community in the U.S., which has published numerous books on soyfoods and nutrition, suggest that about two-thirds of a child's protein requirements can come from soy products, such as soybeans, tofu, soymilk and soy yoghurt (½ cup of tofu provides 10 grams of protein; 1 cup of soymilk provides 7 grams). Between the ages of one and three, 24 grams of protein is all that is required. The remaining one-third of the protein can come from rice and bean combinations, nuts and vegetables. Children who have an intolerance to soy products will do well enough from just these foods and peanut butter and high-protein baby cereal. It is virtually impossible to get too little protein from a diet that contains a wide variety of whole-foods. Too many of today's health problems such as kidney stones and calcium loss stem from just the opposite problem — too *much* protein in the diet.

Children and Low Fat Diets

Another common concern is that a low fat, high fibre diet is good for adults, but dangerous for children. It is true that children under the age of two need more fat in their diet than adults do, because the essential fatty acids and energy supplied by the fat are extremely vital. That's why breast milk is so important — it is high in fat. After the age of two, a child's digestive system can obtain all fatty acids necessary for growth and vitamin absorption from seeds, beans, peas, nuts, cooking oils and avocados. As yet, not one case of fat-soluble vitamin deficiency has been reported among children on a vegetarian diet.

Martha C. Cottrell, M.D., a New York based family doctor, feels that a fat intake of between 20–30 per cent of total calories is safe for most active children, and believes that by adopting a grain and vegetable based diet, children will automatically receive lower, but adequate levels of fat.

Calcium

Calcium is another sticky point that comes up when discussing vegetarianism. Breast milk is the best source of calcium. It is two to three times more absorbable than the calcium in cow's milk. According to Judy Krizmanic, in an article in *Vegetarian Times*, January 1990, 'studies have suggested that milk's high protein content causes its calcium to be washed right out of the body. Rather than drinking cow's milk, a growing child may do better to get calcium from the same place the cow does: plants. Especially good calcium sources are dark leafy greens (broccoli, collards, kale, mustard greens), tofu and chickpeas. Sesame seeds, almonds, filberts, cashews and the butters from these seeds and nuts are also excellent.'

If dairy products are being eliminated from your child's diet, make sure that he gets plenty of sunshine. The best source of vitamin D is sunlight which reacts with the skin's oils to form vitamin D.

What About Iron?

Dried fruits such as raisins, sultanas, figs, apricots and prunes, silverbeet, mushrooms, winter squash, sea vegetables (arame), and algaes (spirulina), tofu, grains such as cornmeal, millet, brown rice and cracked wheat (bulghur) and blackstrap molasses all contain more than adequate amounts of iron. To help increase absorption, add foods rich in vitamin C such as lemon juice and cook in iron pots.

The B12 Issue

Vitamin B12 is a controversial subject among vegetarians. It is one vitamin that you can't always get from a healthy, vegetable-based diet. But B12 deficiency can show up even if you eat meat because certain factors in the digestive tract can keep the vitamin from ever reaching the cells, according to Nathaniel Mead, medical researcher and journalist who specialises in health and environmental topics.

B12 deficiency can lead to all sorts of ailments from severe degeneration of the spinal cord and brain, to depression, mental illness, epileptic-like seizures and hallucinations. However, it is not enough to think that a low B12 diet is the only cause of B12 deficiency. According to Mead: 'At least 97 per cent of B12 absorption takes place in the final section of the small intestine, and the amount absorbed increases as the amount in the diet decreases. Saliva, gastric juices, intestinal proteins, pancreatic enzymes and calcium ions all collaborate to ensure the optimum uptake of B12 by the bloodstream via the intestine.'

High intake of animal food can actually work against B12 absorption as the body's need for B12 increases in proportion to the amount of fat and protein in the daily diet. Other factors also come into play. Certain aspects of a diet may somehow interfere with the body's ability to absorb B12. Pregnant women and nursing mothers, for example, need twice the amount of B12 and if they are deficient their bodies will produce B12 deficient milk. If their digestive abilities or diet are poor, however, they may not be able to provide the amount of B12 necessary.

Vegetarianism, therefore, does not necessarily lead to B12 deficiency and is certainly not the only cause. We may just have over-consumed vitamin B12 rich foods (US diets provides 5-7 times more B12 than recommended by nutritionists) in the past from animal sources and now it will take several generations before we can adapt to low B12 diets.

AN OUNCE OF PREVENTION
- avoid over-eating
- avoid too many flour products
- avoid too many oily foods
- minimise under-cooked soy products
- include more fermented foods such as miso, tempeh, sauerkraut, pickles
- include small amounts of animal foods occasionally, if appropriate

A Challenge

In-laws, grandparents and your children's friends may make it difficult for you and your child, especially if he is being teased and is

FUN WITH FOOD

Help your child squeeze some orange juice into a glass. Then make some juice from a can of frozen orange juice concentrate. Have your child taste each from a separate glass. Talk about the differences. Which one tastes better, sweeter, more bitter, etc? Explain the difference between a juice and a juice drink. (Drink is mostly water, sugar and flavouring, even though it may contain some percentage of actual juice which is usually written on the label.)

Involve your child in making biscuits. Use wholemeal flour for one kind and white for another. Look at the difference and discuss it from a nutritional aspect.

Teach children to pack their own lunch boxes with foods they can share as well as sandwiches. Try carrot and celery stick with dip, or slices of fruits or tangerine wedges, nuts, biscuits or dried fruits.

feeling rejected. Talk to your son and listen to what he has to say. Share food with other vegetarian families and, if your child is not coping well with the pressure, ask him what he would like to do. If changing his diet to conform to the other children at school is necessary, *do it!* He can eat vegetarian foods at home. No doubt he will reject certain foods anyway, as all children do. One day it may be tofu for breakfast, lunch and dinner and the next week he won't look at it at all.

Here are some suggestions that may help:
- Make foods attractive and palate-pleasing to your children.
- Encourage your child to help prepare meals (they like to eat what they cook).
- Stick to foods that are comforting and familiar like pancakes, noodles, pizza, vegetable burgers, pies, and potato pancakes.
- Make sure that your child tries each new food and if he rejects it don't make a big deal out of it.
- Further reading: *Vegetarian Baby*, Sharon Yntema, Ithaca, N.Y., McBooks Press, 1984; *Vegetarian Children*, Sharon Yntema, Ithaca, N.Y., McBooks Press, 1987; *The Complete Guide and Cookbook for Raising Your Child As a Vegetarian*, Michael and Nina Shandler, N.Y., Ballantine Books, 1986.

SLEEP PATTERNS

It's true when they say no two peas in the pod are ever the same. My first child was an excellent sleeper from the word go and the second one was just the opposite. He napped three hours at a time till the age of three, she 45 minutes till the age of 2½. So when the question arises as to how much sleep your child needs, the answer is simple: nobody knows! Each child has different needs and no two are the same. Some sleep 16 hours straight, others wake in the night three or four times and only require 12 hours sleep. Usually children under the age of one year of age need 14-16 hours a day, but mine didn't. From the age of one up until four, 12-14 hours seemed to be the rule of thumb in my household; from four until seven, 10-12 hours.

Some children will nap until the age of three or four, others only till two years of age. What your child does during the day will determine how much sleep is needed. So does his mood and nervous system. If he gets up without any difficulty then his sleeping habits are fine for him.

Getting children to go to bed is another kettle of fish. Most children rebel, and will tell you that they are not tired. I have found the best way to get them ready is to dim the lights and even light a candle, preferably no loud or strenuous activities before bedtime; and if he is feeling scared or anxious about something, taking the time to give him a special story, song or cuddle before going to sleep.

Too much food before sleep can cause restlessness and possibly bad dreams. Hot baths can be calming and relaxing, but some children might in fact be envigorated by them.

If your child seems frightened, try leaving a light on in the room and if something is frightening him, remove it. Lay with him until he falls asleep (if possible), holding him close so he can feel your heartbeat. Make bedtime special by putting on special pillowcases, sheets and blanket covers that he will want to snuggle up with. Leave a window open so that there is adequate fresh air, and if sleep is still a problem, try making a herbal sleeping pillow. These have been used for centuries to cure insomnia, depression and nightmares.

Herbal Pillow

250 g (8 oz) dried rosemary
250 g (8 oz) dried thyme
250 g (8 oz) dried lavender
125 g (4 oz) dried hops
250 g (8 oz) dried rose buds

Mix all the herbs together in a bowl. Stuff them into a pillowcase and cut it to the right size. Sew up the ends. Then place it inside another pillowcase and cut it to the right size. Finish off the edges and give it to your child to hold, not to sleep directly on. You can even make it in the shape of any stuffed animal that your child likes. In this case, you will need to change the volume of herbs to suit the size of the animal.

HUGGING, ROCKING AND LAUGHING

A child first learns about tactile sensation from the contact he has with his mother. Even though a healthy child will grow up exhibiting a sense of independence, touch is still intrinsic to his feelings of well-being and self-esteem.

According to Jim Kehoe, professor of psychology at the University of NSW, 'touch is very important in establishing bonding and a sense of trust in the first two years of a child's life.'

In today's society many children and adults suffer from 'skin hunger', a need to be touched. Men particularly are uncomfortable with hugging children after they reach a certain age or because they are of the same sex. Parents may often stop being affectionate with a child of the opposite sex because they begin to associate touching with sexuality. But hugs and other forms of touching help to establish intimacy and trust and are one of the ways you can help your child develop into a secure adult.

Rocking

A gentle rocking motion while feeding, singing to or just holding your baby has a calming effect on both of you. After all he became used to motion while in the womb. A whimpering or crying baby can often be soothed by a slight rocking of the cradle.

Benefits of the Rocking Motion

In both babies and adults, rocking improves circulation. It promotes respiration, discourages lung congestion and stimulates muscle tone. There is scientific evidence that rocking has the ability to stimulate the balance mechanism in the inner ear, which promotes the baby's ability to be more attentive and alert.

When baby is too cold, rocking helps to warm him. Conversely when the baby is too warm, rocking has a cooling effect and is soothing to the baby's nervous system as well.

Physical Benefits of Rocking

Ashley Montagu, in his book, *Touching, the human significance of the skin*, further suggests

that, 'A baby, especially, that is rocked, knows that it is not alone. A general cellular and visceral stimulation results from the rocking. Again, especially in babies, the rocking motion helps to develop the efficient functioning of the baby's gastrointestinal tract. The intestine is loosely attached by folds of peritoneum to the back wall of the abdominal cavity. The rocking assists the movements of the intestine like a pendulum and thus serves to improve its tone. The intestine always contains liquid chyle and gas. The rocking movement causes the chyle to move backward and forward over the intestinal mucosa. The general distribution of chyle over the whole of the intestine undoubtedly aids digestion and probably absorption.'

Rocking and Premature Infants

Many studies have been done about the possible benefits of rocking on two-and three-month old premature babies. It was found that weight gain, crawling, muscle tone, head lifting, and strength of grasping were significantly better in those infants that were rocked.

Laughter

Laughter may have a far more important role in healing than we think. The notion that laughter can reverse the course of sickness, or keep healthy children healthy, is itself laughed at. But it is an absolutely essential ingredient of human nature and it is even possible that we cannot live without it. In his book, *Philosophical Foundations of Health Education*, Ronald S. Laura argues that contrary to the traditional medical view, 'humour is a powerful antidote to some illnesses and can assist in preventing others.'

Dr Alice M. Isen, at Cornell University compared the mental behaviour of people who had just seen a funny film with individuals who had not. She showed that the comedy induced creative mental energy and positive feelings for problem solving in those who saw it.

How Laughter Heals

When we laugh, it is as if we are giving ourselves an internal massage, as all the organs are moved, stroked and manipulated. Circulation is definitely improved as more blood travels to the vital organs of the body. Children love to laugh. They like comics, cartoons, playing jokes on one another, tickling, and telling funny stories. They should always be encouraged to do so.

Why Children Laugh

REASON FOR LAUGHING	AGE OF CHILD
A happy atmosphere; children will not laugh unless they are comfortable in their surroundings.	People of all ages will laugh when they are happy.
Jokes, funny stories and funny faces.	Jokes will usually make older children laugh, and funny faces are great for the younger set.
Expectation. If a familiar person plays with the child, by tickling him for example, he will usually laugh.	Usually an infant's first smile is because of the recognition of his mother or father.
Release of tension. Children often laugh to hide nervousness, for example when they have have been naughty.	This is most common among 3-6 year olds.
Mistakes. Children often laugh at their own deliberate word mistakes, and those of others.	From about 18 months to 2½ years, depending on the situation.
Messages. A laugh can mean 'Don't worry, I'm all right' or 'It was only a joke'.	This is most common among older children (over three), who can communicate in more complex ways.
Silly language. Often children laugh a 'nonsense talk', when they are able to talk and make up words by themselves.	This is most amusing to 3-5 year olds.
Infectious laughter. Children often laugh in response to the laughter of others, or to feel accepted.	Applies to all ages, although 4-6 year olds are more likely to laugh because they feel they should, even if they appreciate the humour.
Ridiculous situations.	Children from the age of two will laugh at something silly, or laugh when others laugh.
To create a rapport. A child will often laugh as a request for friendship.	Applies to all ages.
Surprise.	Children under 2½ prefer familiarity to surprise. They love you saying 'boo', but only if they are prepared for it.

Adapted from 'What Makes Your Child Laugh', Clare Shaw, *Practical Parenting*, July 1991.

VACCINATIONS

Most orthodox doctors are in favour of children being immunised. They usually suggest the following immunisation schedule:

At two months: triple antigen (DPT) and Sabin oral (pertussis (whooping cough), diptheria, tetanus and polio).

At four months: as above.

At six months: as above.

At fifteen months: measles/mumps/rubella (MMR).

At eighteen months: triple antigen.

At approximately four-five years: CDT, i.e., combined diptheria and tetanus; and Sabin oral. This is recommended before pre-school entry, i.e., before the child is exposed to the risk of infection from his peers.

However, there are many doctors and health care practitioners who are opposed to immunisation. In this chapter we present both sides of the debate, so that you can make your own decisions. There is a legal aspect to this too, some schools will not accept unimmunised children.

The Case Against Immunisation

Vaccinations have been developed to deal with the infectious diseases of childhood such as measles, mumps, German measles, whooping cough and diptheria. Vaccinations are designed to give a person a mild form of a disease via the use of immunisating agents made up of dead bacteria or viruses. This is done to produce specific antibodies that are thought to protect the organism when the real thing comes along.

However, some of these so called 'miracles' can actually produce a variety of illnesses which can in some instances be more serious than the disease for which they were intended. Walene James in her book *Immunization — the reality behind the myth*, points out that, 'Injection of foreign substances — viruses, toxins, and foreign proteins — into the bloodstream, i.e., vaccinations, have been associated with diseases and disorders of the blood, brain, nervous system, and skin. Rare diseases such as a typical measles and monkey fever as well as such well-known disorders as premature ageing and allergies have been associated with vaccinations. Also linked to immunisations are such well-known diseases as cancer, leukemia, paralysis, AIDS, multiple sclerosis, arthritis, and SIDS (Sudden Infant Death Syndrome).

Long Term Effects

Although vaccines have been in use for most of this century, there has been little research done on any possible long-term side-effects. There is a growing suspicion that immunisation may be partly responsible for the dramatic increase in auto-immune diseases. These are diseases whereby the body's own defence mechanism cannot distinguish between foreign invaders and ordinary body tissue, resulting in the body destroying itself.

John Gamble in *Vaccination — exploring some myths*, has this to say, 'Most of the infectious diseases are either inhaled or swallowed through the mucous membranes of the lungs or stomach. Here the antigen meets IgA, a particular antibody which lines the mucous membranes. This is the first line of defence. The disease then enters an incubation period of 1-2 weeks before symptoms show, when a vaccine is given, it is injected straight into the bloodstream, avoiding the antibody which lines the mucous membranes. These large amounts of viral genetic tissue and nucleic acid (produced in animal, not human, culture) can, when thus injected, unite with the DNA of human cells. The transformed cells are then recognized by the host's immune system as foreign ... These transformed cells, containing latent viruses, may become the focus for the body's own immune system — i.e., the body starts to attack itself ...'

A Child's Immune System

According to Dr Richard Moskowitz, 'childhood diseases are decisive experiences in the physiologic maturation of the immune system which prepares the child to respond promptly and effectively to any infections he may acquire in the future. The ability to mount a vigorous, acute response to infectious organisms is a fundamental requirement of health and well-being.'

Common Immunisations

MEASLES
Only rarely does a case of measles result in complications. According to the publication 'Morbidity and mortality weekly report', February 5, 1988, published by the Center for Disease Control, more than half of the reported cases of measles in the U.S. in the first half of 1987 were in children who had been fully vaccinated. The live virus vaccine was introduced in America in 1963, although the measles mortality rate had already dropped radically from 13.3/100,000 cases to 0.3/100,000 by 1955. Five to fifteen per cent of vaccine recipients react with mild rash or fever, and some doctors believe that the measles vaccine can result in mental retardation, meningitis, paralysis, seizure disorders and muscle disorders.

MUMPS
Mumps, usually experienced in childhood, does not normally require medical treatment. Most children are immunised against mumps along with measles and rubella at about 15 months of age. Vaccination is recommended because if the disease is contracted by a male adult, he may contract *orchitis*, a condition which affects the testicles. In rare instances, this can cause sterility. Dr Robert Mendelsohn, a paediatrician for more than thirty years who was Associate Professor of Preventative Medicine and Community Health at the School of Medicine of the University of Illinois, believed that the vaccine can affect the central nervous system, and cause encephalopathy (a brain disease) and deafness as well as bruising, itching and a rash, although these reactions are extremely rare. The vaccination is not guaranteed to provide lifetime immunity.

GERMAN MEASLES (RUBELLA)
The only risk involved with German measles is when women contract the disease during their first trimester of pregnancy, thus endangering their foetus. This fear is used to justify the immunisation of all children, boys as well as girls. There is virtually no need to protect children from this disease. According to Dr Robert Mendelsohn, 'the greater danger of the rubella vaccination is that it may deny expectant mothers the protection of natural immunity from the disease. By preventing German measles in childhood, immunisation may actually increase the threat that women will contract rubella during their childbearing years … Study after study has demonstrated that many women immunised against rubella as children lack evidence of immunity in blood tests given during their adolescent years. Other tests have shown a high vaccine failure rate in children given rubella, measles, and mumps shots, either separately or in combined form.'

Side effects of rubella vaccination can include various nerve disorders, painful joints, arthritis and numbness, pain or tingling in the peripheral nerves. These symptoms are often temporary and may not occur immediately after immunisation.

DIPHTHERIA
Most cases of diphtheria have disappeared and it is questionable whether the disease's disappearance was due to the immunisation programs or to natural decline. There is ample evidence that the incidence of diphtheria was already declining before immunisation started. During a 1969 outbreak of diphtheria in Chicago, the city Board of Health reported that four of the sixteen victims had been fully immunised and five others had received one or more doses of the vaccine. Only two retained full immunity. Of those who contract diphtheria, on the average, more than half are fully

---

CHILDREN'S ILLNESSES

When children first start preschool or playgroup, it may seem as if they are never without a cold, cough or sniffle. Some doctors recommend antibiotics for minor infections, but even though children aren't born with all the antibodies their immune systems need to combat illnesses throughout life; the way to build them up is through small doses of the appropriate infections.

By the time a normal, healthy child reaches the age of six he will probably have had thirty-seven infections. Of these seventeen are minor colds, seven are serious colds, three are ear infections, six respiratory infections perhaps including one bout of croup and one of bronchitis, two are diarrhoea and two skin infections.

immunised. There seem to be no significant harmful effects from the vaccine, however no research has ever been conducted to determine what the long-term effects might be.

CHICKEN POX

No vaccine available.

PERTUSSIS (WHOOPING COUGH)

The vaccination for whooping cough is one of the most controversial and is given along with vaccines for tetanus and diphtheria in the DPT or triple antigen vaccination. Evidence shows that the number of whooping cough cases rises with decreased vaccinations but that it has become an increasingly mild disease, particularly in developed countries where nutrition and sanitation have improved. In several European countries, where the number of whooping cough cases has risen since compulsory vaccination was abandoned, the number of deaths attributed to the disease has dropped.

Vaccination does not guarantee that children immunised against whooping cough will not contract the illness. Dr Gordon T. Stewart, head of the Department of Community Medicine at the University of Glasgow, Scotland, noted that there were outbreaks of whooping cough in children who had been vaccinated. Now, he says, '30 per cent of our whooping cough cases are occurring in vaccinated patients. This leads me to believe that the vaccine is not all that protective'.

TETANUS

This is technically not a childhood disease, but a potentially dangerous, sometimes fatal, bacterial infection. One to five tetanus inoculations are recommended beginning at the age of two months.

Common Side-effects

The common side-effects of vaccinations are crying bouts, local skin conditions such as pain, redness and swelling, and a shock-like state.

When you are considering whether to give your infant the DPT vaccine (triple antigen), be sure to consider his medical history. Here are some well-accepted contraindications.

- Convulsions or seizures with or without fever occurring within three days of receiving the DPT vaccine.
- Evidence of allergic hypersensitivity to the vaccine.
- A high fever within 48 hours of receiving the vaccination.
- Collapse or shock-like state within forty-eight hours of receiving the vaccination.

- History of severe allergies. Barbara Fisher, author of *DPT: a shot in the dark*, reported that about 10 per cent of children who react violently to the pertussis vaccine have a history of milk allergies. She believes that many of the babies who do not survive after the vaccine may have had a predisposition to histamine production and go into some sort of shock.
- Persistent crying, lasting three or more hours, or an unusual, high pitched cry occurring within forty-eight hours of receiving the DPT vaccine.
- Personality changes that occur within one week of receiving vaccination. Changes in behavior, forgetfulness, disorientation and prolonged episodes of staring. These can be symptoms of brain damage.
- Delay the vaccination if the infant was premature or low in birth weight or if he has a viral infection or cold. Fisher has reported that there is evidence that children older than seven are especially reactive to the DPT vaccine and should avoid it if possible.

The Chinese Approach to Childhood Illness

Practitioners of Chinese medicine divide infections into two categories: harmful and beneficial.
Harmful: these do not strengthen the body
polio
diptheria
whooping cough
Beneficial: the Chinese believe that these childhood diseases help to rid the body of harmful poisons.
measles
mumps
chicken pox
German measles

The Case for Immunisation

It is said that the development and availability of vaccination is one of the major advances in medicine in the 20th century (the other two being the development of anaesthesia and the discovery of antibiotics). We all know that many people in the earlier years of this century died of illnesses which were endemic or epidemic, such as pertussis (whooping cough), diptheria and measles. We now rarely see cases of these infections, excepting for sporadic outbreaks in unimmunised populations. From an epidemiological point of view, it is generally agreed that mass vaccination is responsible for this enormous change. We have seen an enormous reduction in mortality and morbidity from most contagious illnesses.

PERTUSSIS (WHOOPING COUGH)

This is a highly infectious disease. It is said that 90 per cent of non-immune household contacts will become infected. There is no evidence that passive protection is conferred transplacentally. Many cases are sub-clinical and are therefore undiagnosed. Infection results in immunity, but second cases do occur.

The currently recommended vaccine is a suspension of killed bacteria, which is combined with diptheria and tetanus toxoid, and is injected intramuscularly.

New acellular pertussis vaccines are being tested and they appear to be associated with a good antibody response and fewer adverse reactions. It is probable that in the future, this will become the vaccine of choice for Pertussis immunisation. All infants should proceed through the course of immunisation unless there is a specific contraindication. Each time a child is vaccinated, the parents should be asked to observe the child for adverse reactions and report these to the practitioner. It is recommended that parents give their child Paracetamol, which helps to minimise the possibility of an adverse reaction.

Adverse reactions may be local or systemic. Local reactions at the site of the injection, which include redness, swelling, tenderness and apparent pain are common. Rarely bacterial or sterile abscesses form at the site of the injection. Systemic reactions include fever, drowsiness, irritability, persistent crying, decreased appetite and vomiting. These are not uncommon in the first few hours following injection, but generally resolve rapidly. Mild reactions do not preclude further vaccination. Very severe adverse reactions are uncommon; these include high fever, convulsions, persistent (three or more hours) or unusual cry, colds with a shock-like state and encephalopathy. Other attributed associations, for example infantile spasm and sudden infant death syndrome appear not to be etiologically associated. It appears that the risk of catastrophy from disease is far greater than that from the vaccine.

Pertussis vaccine is said to be contraindicated in children who have neurological disorders, for example uncontrolled epilepsy.

TETANUS

Tetanus and pertussis vaccine are combined. Tetanus vaccine is known to cause very mild local and systemic reaction, such as redness and swelling and myalgia. However, these things are transient and in no way dangerous. The only contraindication to the administration of tetanus vaccine is a history of systemic hypersensitivity to the vaccine. Tetanus is now a very rare illness.

DIPTHERIA

Cases of diptheria are now rarely seen. The vaccine is administered along with the pertussis and tetanus vaccine. It is important to note that the passive protection which children have, which is conferred transplacentally, is lost within the first six months of life. The only absolute contraindication to the administration of this vaccine, is a previous systemic hypersensitivity. Adverse reactions, such as irritability and fever are not uncommon, but very transient.

POLIO

This is administered by Sabin oral preparation, along with the vaccines mentioned above.

MEASLES

Mortality and morbidity from measles has been dramatically reduced throughout the latter part of this century. Measles vaccine has only been available recently. Currently, it is presented with mumps and rubella vaccine in the MMR II preparation. The most common side effect of this vaccine is a modified measles-like illness, which occurs ten days to two weeks after the vaccination. It takes the form of a high fever, irritability, a rash and lymphadenopathy. Rarely, one sees a mild form of measles encephalopathy, secondary to the vaccine. The above mentioned side-effects settle spontaneously.

MUMPS

Mumps vaccine is presented with the measles and rubella vaccines. Side-effects which include fever and local irritation, are transient and very mild. This vaccine does not seem to produce any problems.

RUBELLA

Rubella vaccine is given with measles and mumps vaccine. Side-effects of the vaccine include a low-grade fever, irritability and possibly a mild rash; there are also documented cases of arthralgia, secondary to the vaccine. The side-effects of this vaccine do not seem to be a great problem.

BOOSTING YOUR CHILD'S IMMUNE SYSTEM

Immunity is the body's ability to resist harmful substances such as bacteria, viruses and poisons. If one of these substances does enter the body, antibodies are produced to get rid of it as soon as possible. But a strong immune system depends upon a healthy outlook as much as a healthy body. For this, your child needs to feel loved, happy and secure.

The more physical contact you have with your baby, the more likely he will be to thrive socially, physically and emotionally. Most important, playing with your baby and making him feel good, makes him happy, and helps to develop better performances on standard perceptual and cognitive tests. As the late Pulitzer Prize-winning biologist René Dubos witnessed in his work, happiness may be less trivial for the future of humankind than we've recognised. 'Happiness is contagious. For this reason its expression is a social service and almost a duty. The Buddhists have a saying about this commendable virtue: *only happy people can make a happy world*. Since optimism and cheerful spirits are indispensable to the mental health of technological societies, the most valuable people may turn out to be not those with the greatest ability to produce material goods but those who, through empathy and happiness, have the gift of spreading a spirit of good will.'

How To Ensure a Healthy Immune System

Breast feeding your baby will protect him from a number of infections. Lactoferrin and lysozyme, two chemicals found in breast milk, are said to protect the infant from infection by inhibiting or destroying the growth of bacteria (Goldman et al., 1982). There are also many other resistance factors in breast milk, including interferon which can assist the child's developing immune system function. (Chandra, 1978).

A healthy digestive system is essential for a strong and vital immune system. In under-developed countries where there is widespread malnutrition and poor sanitation, there is low resistance to disease and infection. In developed countries, where sanitation is good, the pervasiveness of processed, sweet and refined foods, and the overuse of preservatives and pesticides, has lowered our resistance, depressed our immune system and may cause epidemics such as measles.

To ensure a healthy digestive system, avoid chemically treated, processed and refined foods. Don't use sugar or salt in excessive amounts. Don't serve your children too many fatty foods, and limit the amount of animal products you give. Encourage your children not to overeat.

Processed and refined foods place unusual and unnecessary stress on our body's metabolic system which in the short term is hardly noticeable, but as time goes by the damage that it causes may be irreparable.

Contributing Factors Affecting Health

THE OZONE LAYER

CFCs (Chlorofluorocarbons) are gases that are used in a wide variety of processes. When they reach the upper atmosphere they break down the ozone layer, which absorbs up to 99 per cent of the sun's damaging ultraviolet rays. Skin cancer and damage to marine life and plants can be some of the possible results.

NUCLEAR POWER AND RADIATION

Nuclear accidents have clearly shown how radiation can wipe out whole communities and cause irreversible damage. The Irish sea is now the most radioactive-contaminated place in the world.

DIOXIN CONTAMINATION

Dioxins are artificially produced, extremely toxic by-products of various chemical reactions and are generally agreed to be the most dangerous chemical known. They are a by-product of the chlorine-bleaching process of the paper industry, and are also caused by car exhaust fumes, some pesticides, herbicides and industrial and municipal waste incinerators. Once they get into the environment, dioxins build-up through the food chain until they contaminate women's breast milk. In the long term they are thought to affect the immune system and the reproductive system, causing birth defects.

SMOG

The sun's rays on smog can cause:
- nose, throat and eye irritation
- respiratory ailments like asthma
Long-term effects:
- nausea
- skin rashes
- lead poisoning
- headaches
- reduced resistance to infection
- bronchitis
- conjunctivitis
- lung cancer

WATER

Believe it or not, our bodies are mostly water — about 70 per cent water by volume in fact. Many essential body functions need water. Cleansing is one of the most important of these functions, with the water needed to flush toxins out of our bodies. That is why it is vital that the water we drink is as pure as possible.

Increasing population has led to urban encroachment into water catchment areas and, therefore, the contamination of our water supplies by septic tank drainage, sewage and agricultural pesticides and fertilizers. Urban run-off is one of the greatest pollution problems facing water quality in and around population centres, while agricultural chemicals, especially fertilizers, present the greatest hazard to water quality in country areas.

Phosphorous, which is contained in both agricultural and sewage fertilisers, stimulates the growth of algae and other aquatic plants. Water supply authorities are forced to add chemicals to our water to control these. The decay of the dead plants, however, releases nutrients back into the water and this causes the growth of bacteria and other undesirable organisms. These are often too small to be effectively filtered out of the water and so the addition of other chemicals to disinfect the water is necessary. This disinfection is normally done by adding chlorine to the water. However, it is known that the high chlorine concentrations needed to treat heavily contaminated water can produce potentially carcinogenic by-products called trihalomethanes.

'Chemicals such as tranquillisers and contraceptive hormones which have passed through the human body have also been detected in "cleaned" water. Little is known about the effects of the 1,200 or so other micropollutants which have been discovered in drinking water … In 1981 the Water Research Council [London] reported that "most" of the 343 organic compounds it had identified in drinking water "have never been evaluated in terms of safety".'

From *The Green Alternative* by Peter Bunyard and Fern Morgan-Grenville.

NITRATES

'High levels of nitrates can also increase the risk of a very rare blood disease, methaemoglobinaemia (where the blood's ability to carry oxygen is diminished). This occurs in bottle fed babies whose feeds are made up with tap water'.

Radio Times, 3-9 June, 1989.

HOME POLLUTANTS

If you have a child who has been feeling depressed, tired, or has had recurring throat and chest infections, he could be a victim of his own environment. Chemicals that have been introduced into our daily lives to beautify, make cleaning easier or help control insects remain in our homes and can accumulate in our bodies and remain there for years. Many of the common household products we use regularly have not been tested for potential long-term health effects on humans. Further, products that are fairly safe when used as directed can cause serious harm in the hands of a curious child. Typical hazardous products include:
- household cleaners
- pesticides
- paint products
- swimming pool chemicals
- pet care products
- personal hygiene products
- automotive fluids
- disinfectants

Indoor air pollution is much the same. Stoves and gas heaters that are unflued can pose dangerous situations as they produce waste gases, nitrogen oxides and carbon monoxide, which become more and more concentrated if the rooms are not properly ventilated. These can be a contributing factor to respiratory problems such as asthma.

A great number of homes are not properly ventilated and are damp. These factors may lead to a build-up of moulds and fungal spores which may also start an asthmatic attack.

LOVING RELATIONSHIPS

A secure, loving and emotionally stable home environment can be just the remedy for some children with frequent minor aches and pains, colds, headaches, thumb sucking, nail biting, bed-wetting and erratic sleeping habits. There are lots and lots of folk remedies for these common complaints, some of which work for some children but not for all. You can usually deal most successfully with these problems if you are aware of your child's emotional needs, and if you constantly reassure him of your love.

STRESS

Stress also plays an important part in the functioning of the immune system. It has been shown that poor mental and emotional health and well-being cause lower resistance and allows for more severe forms of infection. This should be taken into consideration when determining the cause of your child's illness. Stress is just as likely to occur in a child as in an adult.

Loving and Touching

Children thrive when they receive positive reinforcement and praise for what they do and who they are. They like to succeed and be acknowledged. Giving your child attention, encouragement, and love is one of the best ways to ensure his immune system is working at its fullest capacity.

It is also important that children are physically touched. It doesn't matter whether it is on the hand, shoulder, head, back or bottom; these are non-verbal messages of love. Research done at U.C.L.A. has shown that 'hugging relieves many physical and emotional problems and can help people live longer, maintain health, relieve stress and promote sleep'.

Psychologists have shown that the effects of love on the body can be seen and in fact even measured. Bernie S. Siegel, M.D. sums it up beautifully in his book, *Peace, Love and Healing*. 'An unloved infant will have retarded bone growth and may even die; a stroked infant grows faster. The effects of peace of mind are measurable too: people who meditated, as well as those who confided traumatic experiences to diaries rather than repressing them, were shown to have enhanced immune function ...'

Children and Meditation

Meditation reduces the physical symptoms of stress. It slows the breathing and heart rate and lowers the blood pressure. The main advantage in teaching children to meditate is that they can use the technique later to deal with the stresses of adolescence and adulthood. People who have been brought up to meditate are unlikely to use drugs or alcohol for stress relief.

When you are meditating, let your child sit with you. Explain to him that the word 'meditation' means to consider thoughtfully and reflect upon, and that any situation can be meditative. Silently washing the dishes, the car, going on a bushwalk together, or putting away the toys together, doing it as slowly and attentively as possible, will demonstrate how to bring a meditative quality into everyday activities.

No Instant Results

Don't look for instant changes or results. Be patient, consistent and loving and be clear about your own motivations and expectations. Do not force him into meditating.

Techniques

- Gather a group of children together, play some dance music and let them run wild — jumping, screaming or dancing. Let them do this for five to ten minutes. Join in if you like.
- Then put on another piece of music that is slower and dreamier and let them move around again to their own rhythm for five to ten minutes. Dim the lights for more atmosphere. You can also tell them a story to encourage them to relax a bit more, and perhaps get them to act out the story as you tell it.

Then choose one of the following techniques:
- Gather a group of children together and pair them off. Give them a candle to share and let them sit opposite each other and focus their attention on the centre of the flame for the count of ten. Get them to close their eyes briefly (a minute or so) and then repeat five times. A flower may be used instead of a candle.

- Sit them opposite each other, get them to hold hands and look into the centre of each other's eyes for the count of twenty. Get them to see how long they can keep the eye contact without moving.
- Have all the children lie on their backs in a circle with their heads facing into the circle. Get them to close their eyes and focus on their breathing or some soft music.

Apart from lessening or eliminating symptoms such as irritability, hyperactivity, tense or stiff shoulders, headaches, tiredness, lack of concentration or poor sleeping habits, meditation can help children to be more attentive, happier, livelier and more content.

A QUICK REFERENCE TO A VITAL IMMUNE SYSTEM

- Breast feeding lays the foundation for healthy emotional and physical well-being and breast milk is the best nutrient for babies.
- A healthy diet should consist of about 80 per cent fruits, vegetables and whole grains. The balance can be made up of either animal or vegetable protein.
- Foods should be as whole, natural and as unrefined as possible.
- Fruits, vegetables and grains should be fresh, seasonal and organically grown wherever possible.
- Do not overcook foods especially those containing water-soluble vitamins.
- Make sure that your child gets plenty of foods containing protein, essential fatty acids, vitamins A, E, B2, B5, B6, folic acid, vitamin B12 and vitamin C. The most important minerals required for proper functioning of the immune system include copper, zinc, iron, manganese, magnesium, and the trace elements germanium and selenium.
- Encourage your child to sit down, chew well and eat slowly.
- Avoid refined sugar as studies have shown that its consumption weakens the immune system.
- Make sure that your child gets plenty of fresh air, adequate exercise and pure water.
- Give your child plenty of tickles, hugs, kisses and cuddles daily!!! Set aside five minutes each day, perhaps before bedtime. Sit or lie together for five minutes, either breathing with each other and quietly reflecting, telling stories, just cuddling or tickling each other. You will be amazed at how nurturing this is for *both* of you!

SECTION 3

A-Z Guide to Children's Complaints

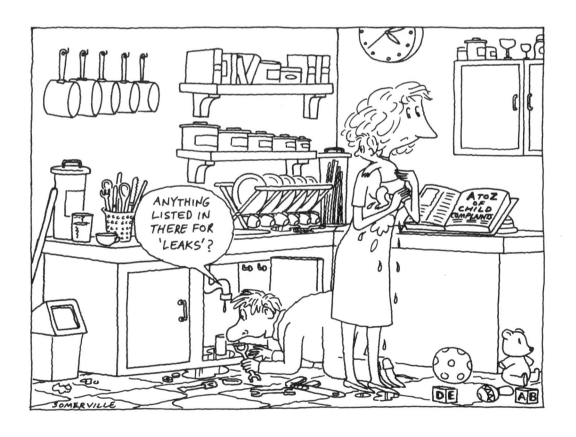

ABDOMINAL PAIN

Sometimes when your child complains of a tummy ache it's difficult to locate the exact place of discomfort. It's even possible that the pain is actually moving around. Paediatricians talk about these non-specific pains as 'non-organic recurrent abdominal pain'. These are pains that are considered to have no particular cause, are located around the umbilicus and can be quite severe.

They can be related to a number of different problems, including food allergies (see Allergies, Food Intolerance and Chemical Sensitivity); improper intestinal flora, when bacteria or fungi in the intestine are of the wrong proportions or in excessive quantities; or a toxic digestive system, when the bacteria or fungi in the intestine is poisonous to the whole body.

In some cases the pain can be caused by an infection, overeating, a virus, tension of the abdominal area due to nervousness, fear or other types of stress, wind, change of environment, etc. Abdominal pain can also be a side-effect of many conventional medicines, for example antibiotics which can cause abnormal bowel flora to develop. Weak digestion which is the result of unhealthy eating habits or a weak constitution, can also encourage the formation of unhealthy flora. It can also be a problem in babies who have not been breastfed. Breast milk helps to establish the bifidus bacteria in the child's stomach. These bacteria are responsible for controlling other pathological bacteria and fungi in the bowel.

CAUTION

Seek medical attention as soon as possible if:
- **Your child exhibits severe pain that persists for more than 2-3 hours.**
- **The pain is accompanied by severe vomiting or diarrhoea.**
- **There are headaches that persist for more than 24 hours.**

It's helpful to initially treat abdominal pains with herbal teas and some simple massage. This will be enough to ease the pain if the problem was just some stubborn 'wind' that refused to move.

General Treatment

- If your child complains of a sore tummy suggest that she goes to the toilet, preferably squatting, to try to clear away air or stagnant matter from the bowel.
- Teach your child to relax the abdomen using abdominal breathing, so that the abdomen expands out on the 'in' breath.

Floppy doll tummy balloons

- Ask your child to lie down on her side.
- Tell her to breathe in through the nose and make her tummy go out like a balloon.
- Tell her to breathe out slowly and then go limp like a rag doll.

Home Remedies

Pour boiling water over 1 teaspoon of chamomile flower heads, cover and let steep 5-10 minutes. Strain. Tea bags can also be used. Dilute with warm water for infants and young children (under the age of two). Do not use a sweetener. Chamomile tea is good for reducing inflammation or relieving spasm.
- Pour 1 cup boiling water over ½ teaspoon fennel or dill seeds and set aside for 5 minutes, then strain.
- Combine 1 cup water with ½ stick of cinnamon, and simmer 5-10 minutes, then strain. This is good for relieving pain related to wind and bloating.
- Grate enough ginger to make ¼ teaspoon. Mix with 1 cup boiling water, ½ teaspoon lemon juice and ½ teaspoon honey. This is good for reducing inflammation in the digestive tract.
- Pour 1 cup boiling water over a peppermint

tea bag. Peppermint tea relieves spasm in the digestive tract.

All teas may be taken three times per day.

Naturopathic Diet for Bowel Cleansing

This ten day diet can be used every few months if your child has abdominal pain or any sign of bowel disturbance such as constipation, loose odorous stools or flatulence. It is a diet high in fibre, particularly soluble fibre, and low in meat protein. It is a balanced diet and can be followed for long periods of time or even indefinitely with no danger to the child.

This diet encourages the correct type and quantity of bacteria to develop in the bowel.

Use an abundance of:

- WHOLE GRAINS, which should be eaten at least at two out of three meals per day, for example, oats, barley, brown rice, millet, polenta.
- LEGUMES, which should be eaten at one meal per day, with a whole grain for best protein utilisation, for example, lentils, haricot beans, berlotti beans, adzuki beans, lima beans, mung beans (if no flatulence occurs).
  To prepare: soak beans overnight in water. Throw away water, cover with fresh water, and cook till tender.
- VEGETABLES should be included in two meals per day, using at least two different varieties.
- NUTS AND SEEDS. A small quantity, about 15 g (½ oz) daily, of unroasted nuts and seeds may be used, e.g. sunflower seeds, almonds, cashews, pine nuts.
- FRUIT, including dried fruit, may be eaten freely as long as it does not suppress the appetite for grains, legumes and vegetables.
- YOGHURT, unsweetened, add your own fresh fruit, about ½-1 cup daily.
- MISO SOUP
- MEAT AND FISH. As fish is the most easily digested meat this can be eaten two or three times per week. All other meat is best kept to a maximum of once per week.
- No eggs.
- No cheese except ricotta or cottage.
- AVOID ALL PROCESSED FOOD, particularly processed grains such as white flour or white rice. Avoid sugar and foods containing sugar.

Processed breakfast cereals that contain sugar and are not made from whole grains, including bran, should not be used. Food that contains artificial additives, colourings and preservatives should not be eaten.

SUPPLEMENTS are part of the bowel cleansing program but are not essential to this diet. However, they will speed up the effects of this diet and amplify its effectiveness.

- Oat bran — 4 teaspoons per day
- Linseed (ground) — 4 teaspoons per day
- Lactobacillis acidophilus powder — see Appendix 6: Friendly Bacteria
- Lactobacillis bifidus — see Appendix 6: Friendly Bacteria

Homoeopathic Remedies

See Colic, Constipation, Diarrhoea, Nausea.

Chinese Remedies

1 'External Cold' (Attacks Spleen and Stomach)

Sudden onset of pain. Aggravated by pressure or touch and eating. May also have nausea and vomiting. Limbs are cold. Likes warmth. May have fever. Complexion is darker than normal. Fingernails are red. Red vein at 'San Guan' (see app. 8). Loose stools. Pale urine. May have a runny nose with clear watery mucus.

LIANG FU WAN

XIANG SU SAN (if child also has a cold)

QIAN SHI BAI ZHU TANG (if child also has diarrhoea)

LING GUI ZHU GAN TANG (body is cold, pain relieved by warmth, no fever, tongue is pale, clear watery vomit, pale or white complexion)

2 'Deficiency' (of Spleen and Stomach)

Pain is dull and continuous. Relieved by pressure or touch and warmth. Eating causes discomfort. No appetite. Abdomen is cold and distended. Loose stools. Tiredness especially after eating. Tongue is pale and swollen with scalloped edges (i.e. tooth marks). Pale or yellowish complexion. Pale lips. Hair may be brittle with split ends. Eyes are dull. Speaks little. May sleep with eyes slightly open. May have a blue vein or bluish tint between the eyebrows. There may be a yellowish hue in the area between the eyelids and eyebrows and also the whites of the eyes.

XIANG SHA LIU JUN ZI TANG
HUANG QI JIAN ZHONG TANG (with cold hands and feet)

3 'Heat' (in the Stomach and Intestines)

Strong colicky pain. Abdomen may appear or feel swollen. Pain aggravated by warmth, pressure or touch. Prefers cold food and drinks. Prefers light clothing or coverings. Red complexion. Red lips and tip of nose. Purple fingernails. Purple vein at 'San Guan' (see app. 8). May grind teeth when sleeping. Thirst. Constipation. Dark and scanty urine. Bad breath. May have sores in mouth and gums or bleeding gums. Tongue is redder than normal, may be a crack down the middle. Tongue coating is thick and yellow. Pulse is more rapid than normal.

HUANG LIAN JIE DU TANG

4 'Phlegm-Damp Accumulation'

Abdomen feels and appears swollen. Pain aggravated by pressure or touch and eating. Loss of appetite. Head and body feel heavy. Coughing or vomiting frothy mucus. Tiredness and depression. Complexion is yellowish. The white part of the eyes (sclera) may also have a yellow hue. Loose stools. Tongue coat is thick and appears greasy.

BAN XIA XIE XIN TANG

5 'Food Retention'

Pain is persistent and colicky, and aggravated by pressure or touch and eating. Abdomen feels and may also look full and swollen. May also have belching (foul tasting and smelling) and vomiting. May be constipated at first, then foul smelling flatulence and diarrhoea which brings relief. Tongue has a thick coating and appears greasy. The area between the upper lip and nose may have a yellow or dark hue.

BAO HE WAN
REN SHEN JIAN PI WAN (weak constitution, chronic problem, chronic loose stools or diarrhoea, pale complexion, pale lips, dull eyes, pale tongue body, speaks little, poor appetite).

6 'Qi Stagnation'

Pain is spasmodic and changes location. Aggravated by pressure or touch and emotional upsets. Abdomen feels and may also appear to be full and swollen. Pain is temporarily relieved by belching and flatulence. Alternating constipation and diarrhoea. Tongue has a thin coating.

SI NI SAN (cold fingers and toes, rest of body warm, tongue red — not pale).
XIAO YAO SAN (pale complexion, pale lips, weakness, tiredness, tongue pale).
JIN LING ZI SAN (pain aggravated by hot food and drinks, tongue red).

Massage

1 First, relax the muscles with a warm hot-water bottle at the base of the child's lower back or abdomen.

2 With your child lying down on her back, in front of you, lift her legs and bend them at the knees, placing her feet back on the floor. Massage in downward strokes from below the rib cage to the pelvis, hand over hand. Your hands should conform to the child's abdomen and be relaxed but firm. Do this six times.

3 Massage in a clockwise motion making half circles one hand over the other, around the abdomen. Feeling for any tight or restricted areas. If you discover a tight area hold your hand over this spot for three to five minutes and direct your own warm, loving energy into it, waiting for a softening of the tissue. Feel your child relax as you breathe together.

If your child won't lie down, you can carry her or hold her and massage the bottom of both feet. To do this, use your thumbs to make tiny thumb prints from the heel to the middle of the foot, pressing in as deeply as is comfortable for your child.

ALLERGIES, FOOD INTOLERANCE AND CHEMICAL SENSITIVITY

Allergies

The word 'allergy' has been used to describe many things. However, the traditional allergists insisted that elevated antibody levels or skin reaction, whereby you scratch or prick the skin and apply a drop of the allergen on it, are the only reactions that confirm allergic responses in an individual. If there is a red weal after a scratch test, then the allergist knows that the antibodies, for example to pollen, are present. The body mounts a specific antibody response to a specific antigen (house dust, cat fur, grass, food, for example). Because antibody levels never really disappear, the allergists say that once you react, even if months or years go by between exposures, you will always react.

The one problem in this argument is that when this rule is applied to foods only about ten per cent of cases of intolerance show any elevation of antibody levels, nor can any specific levels of antibodies be detected. In 90 per cent of the cases there are no antibodies present, no change in the immune system or blood. So the allergists believe that there is no known allergy. However, if your child develops a stomach-ache each and every time she eats tomatoes then you can be fairly sure she is having an allergic response to tomatoes.

The term 'fixed' allergies was used to describe those whose reactions were not affected by the time between exposures or the amount of the substance in question. The other allergies were called 'cyclic' allergies because they tend to come and go in cycles. The word 'allergy' is slowly being replaced by the words 'hypersensitivity', 'sensitivity', 'maladaptation' and 'intolerance'. It's basically up to the practitioner as to what terminology is used.

Food intolerance

Food intolerance can come from eating nutritious foods as well as excessive consumption of salt, sugar, refined carbohydrates and fat. It is usually recognised as an inability to digest a particular food due to a digestive enzyme deficiency as in lactose intolerance, or a mental or emotional disorder. Other people have a genetic susceptibility, which involves a missing digestive enzyme or having abnormal intestinal enzymes as in gluten intolerance. There is no antigen-antibody reaction, as the antigen is not ingested.

Other factors affecting food intolerance:

- In some instances, food peptides act as antigens and induce the body to make antibodies that then form immune complexes. These can cause degeneration and inflammation in the soft tissue, bones and joints such as in rheumatoid arthritis. They can also cause hypersensitivity of the bronchial passages, as in asthma, and inflammation of the skin, as in eczema. The symptoms which a patient experiences are related to the release of substances called prostaglandins and it is their release that causes pain and discomfort.

- Foods containing salicylates, preservatives, colouring. Salicylates are found in tea, licorice, almonds, herbs, spices, peppermint, all vegetables except potato, peas, beans, cauliflower, cabbage, Brussels sprouts, celery, onion and garlic; all fruits except pears, mango, pawpaw and bananas; all dried fruit, cider wine, liquor, vinegar, sauces and pickles.

- Naturally occurring toxic substances that have been shown to bring on irritability, hyperactivity, short attention span, lack of concentration, aggressive behaviour.

- Lead, mercury cadmium and other toxic mineral contaminants in food may affect balance, co-ordination, learning and fine motor co-ordination.

Additional factors that affect allergic manifestations:

- The mental and emotional state of the infant/child and mother.
- Amount of exercise, rest and nutrient intake.
- Interaction of external environmental factors including viruses, bacteria, temperature, weather changes (wind, rain, etc.) fungus, house dust, yeasts, pollens, chemicals and moulds.

Day-to-day changes

Most food intolerances are not 'fixed', they are what is known as 'cyclic' allergies and are not consistent at all. One week your child could have a reaction to a particular food and another week there will be no reaction at all. If your child doesn't eat a food for weeks at a time and then suddenly consumes great quantities of it, she may start to react because of the increased exposure to the food. However, there may only be a reaction if she has also been exposed to an inhalant allergen (see page 90). Any food eaten on a daily basis may eventually lead to food intolerance depending upon the individual. In the United States the food intolerances point more in the direction of corn and soya products since there is a rapid increase in the use of these two foodstuffs in most processed foods.

When a child shows an intolerance to one food it is not uncommon that she may also exhibit a sensitivity to other foods that are in the same family group. For example, a child who has an intolerance to tomatoes may also be sensitive to potatoes, eggplant, and capsicum (peppers). However, it is possible that single foods may cause problems, not the whole family of foods.

If your child is showing signs of a cyclic allergy as opposed to a 'fixed' allergy which requires total elimination of the suspected foods, just rotate food types so that the same foods are not eaten every day. In this way your child's body can have a break from a particular food and allow the body to heal as well as ensure that adequate nutritional requirements are obtained in a balanced way.

This type of 'rotation' diet ensures that your child is getting a sound nutritional diet and can prevent food intolerances from developing by exposing her to a greater variety of foods.

Chemical sensitivity

For thousands of years we have been adding chemicals to our food. Preserving our food through the long winter months we learned that we could use various methods such as pickling, drying, smoking, curing, salting; adding lots of salt, sugar, spices and herbs that could act in preventing unstable foods from decaying.

We are also concerned with how food looks, and so even in ancient Egypt saffron was used to colour food yellow, and as we became more sophisticated we started to use various other methods to cure meats, make cheese and colour food. For example, copper was added to vegetables to enhance the green colour, nitrates were being used to cure meats, and saltpetre (potassium nitrate) was added to meat to prevent browning and enhance its red colour.

New foods are now processed for convenience factors: preservation, cost reduction, shipping and quality control As we all demand foods that look the same, are easy to prepare, retain their freshness and are colourful, pleasant-smelling and have a long shelf life, substitute foods such as margarine have shown up. Artificial cheeses and extended meat protein products made out of chemically crosslinked corn starch or textured vegetable proteins, combined with flavourings, food colours and textures, have also made their appearance. As a result more flavouring and colouring agents, thickeners, clarifiers, bleaching agents, stabilisers and emulsifiers have made their way into the food chain.

Although food additives do help to maintain freshness and prevent deterioration, facilitate handling or processing, maintain nutritional

---

WHAT TO DO AT HOME

If your child seems to be allergic to the family pet, don't just give it away. Try to reach a compromise by not allowing it into the child's room, and have the child wash his hands after playing with it and grooming it outdoors.

If the allergy is food related, find tasty substitutes so that she doesn't feel left out. Non-dairy ice-creams and wheat free biscuits and crackers can be accepted with great enthusiasm.

quality and enhance sensory qualities, over the last fifteen years there has been a growing concern about the possible effect of food additives and behaviour patterns in children. Symptoms such as short attention span, poor sleeping habits, poor muscle co-ordination, hyperactivity and fidgety, disruptive or excitable and aggressive behaviour have shown up amongst children.

There will always be some food chemicals that prove to be a problem for some children — they can cause, or affect already existing conditions such as asthma, migraine, hyperactivity, skin disorders, cancer, learning difficulties and other disorders. However, if we are aware of the situation and know the difference between the potentially harmful chemicals and those that are safe, we can have a greater control over food selection by avoiding specific troublesome food additives as well as naturally occurring food toxins.

Identifying a Child with Allergy, Intolerance and Sensitivity

It's usually easy to figure out the link between a food that doesn't agree with your child and a stomach-ache or indigestion. However, it's much harder to recognise that repeated exposure to certain substances, such as particular foods, medications, mould, pollen, plants, food additives and preservatives, dust, gas (usually ethylene gas, a petroleum derivative), electric appliances, pets, herbicides, drugs or pollution can cause children constant discomfort. They could be the underlying cause of anything from headache to diarrhoea, nausea, vomiting, fatigue, insomnia, bed-wetting, learning disorders, poor memory, hyperactivity, respiratory problems, arthritis or asthma.

In many instances your child may only react to a food if she is exposed to an inhalant allergen, such as a pollen, house dust, dog or cat fur, mental or emotional stress.

If you suspect that your child has an allergic foundation for the symptoms she is displaying, consider all of the potential causes that might exist in the child's environment, eliminate them one by one and see whether or not the symptoms disappear. Sometimes there may be two causes of one reaction. For example, eczema can be set off by active chemicals in foods as well as by natural food proteins that affect the immune system.

The drugs commonly used in the treatment of allergic conditions have many potentially harmful side-effects. For example, Phenergan or Teldane may cause drowsiness, nausea and dizziness.

Robert Buist, Ph.D., in his book *Food Chemical Sensitivity*, says, 'A great majority of adverse food reactions are related to small chemical molecules that are associated with foods, but are not proteins or peptides, and which can cause toxic reactions through the formation of reactive free radicals or by acting directly on the tissues in the same manner as drugs.'

There is enough evidence now for us to be sure that the most critical time in the development of any food intolerance or chemical sensitivity is the first few months of life. The immune system is immature and the intestines are very permeable, making it easy for some of the large protein molecules in food to pass into an infant's body. They then can get into the bloodstream where they become a filtering system for any future foreign proteins that pass into the system.

Babies who exhibit allergies in the first few weeks of their lives usually do so about a week after the food was consumed. The most common allergic food at this age is cow's milk which can elicit such symptoms as vomiting, diarrhoea and cramps.

Breastfed babies have a much more highly developed level of immunity than other babies to foods that may cause allergies, infectious diseases, bacteria and viruses. It is possible that your baby may inherit food sensitivity before being born. For example, if you have an intolerance to cow's milk and drink it while you are pregnant, and your baby is fed cow's milk or a formula containing cow's milk, as soon as she is born, there is a much greater chance of your baby becoming sensitive to that food for the remainder of her life. If you know that you have an intolerance to certain foods it is best to avoid them during pregnancy and breastfeeding.

If your baby is totally breastfed and has diarrhoea but is still gaining weight and thriving, chances are that she is allergic to something in your diet. Any foods eaten every single day can be suspect if the diarrhoea is chronic. In this case you need to be very astute in your detective work and may need to follow an exclusion diet that includes totally different staples to those that you are regularly eating.

If the diarrhoea clears up after two weeks of the exclusion diet, foods can be introduced one by one until the offending food or foods are discovered.

It is only when your baby reaches six or seven months of age that her digestive system will have matured enough to handle the bulk of foreign proteins. So until this age, breastfeeding should be encouraged and the introduction of other foods avoided. At the very least you should avoid introducing dairy products, eggs and wheat before seven months of age. These cause more problems than any other foods.

If your child does avoid certain foods it could well be that she is sensitive to them and so it may not be healthy to force her to finish up her food. Some children won't adhere to a rigid diet. Having a special treat each week can often help children feel more excited about their daily food as does making the food look more appetising. If chips are an important food, try deep-frying vegetables yourself. Use smaller amounts of meat as in stir-fried dishes and buy meat, chicken, vegetables and fruit that are preservative-, hormone-, additive- and pesticide-free.

In children, many cases of allergy and food intolerance seem to produce different symptoms as they grow older. A sensitivity to cow's milk may produce symptoms of colic when they are very young, bronchitis as they get a little older, asthma, sinus congestion or migraine as they mature further, as well as glue ear and constant sniffles and colds.

If your child has a chemical or food intolerance she will usually have a cluster of symptoms which disappear when the food or irritants are withdrawn for a couple of weeks and reappear when the substances are reintroduced. Some health authorities believe that as many as one in four children suffer from these conditions. Psychological and social stresses may also be involved, so these should be considered in order for a child to recover more quickly.

Physical appearance

- Pale face, dark circles under the eyes, crease across the top of the nose, vacant facial expression, red scaly appearance of skin across top eyelids, puffiness of skin, especially under eyelids and cheeks, lips are often scaly and dry with corners cracked, base of ears where they join the face may be red and cracked, eyelashes may be wet

with the ends sticking together, general listlessness.

Immediate reactions

- Violently ill after drinking milk or eating eggs for the first or second time.
- Red or swollen face with hives immediately after eating fish.

Developmental characteristics

- Slow to walk, stand or crawl, often does not go through crawling stage, poor development of co-ordination.
- History of feeding and sleeping problems.

Behavioural and learning problems

- Poor social adjustment, difficult personality, motor problems, general learning difficulties, poor handwriting, good vocabulary but poor comprehension.
- Avoids ball sports, trips a lot, awkward pencil grasp, print blurs or doubles while reading, poor attention and concentration, high activity level followed by lethargy and fatigue, irritable and aggressive, depressed, mood swings, forgetfulness.
- Bed-wetting.

Physical symptoms

- Nausea, abdominal pain, diarrhoea or constipation, colic, flatulence or bloating, cystitis, vaginal inflammation, repeated colds and chest infection, chronic cough, asthma, croup, runny nose or sinusitis, frequent bleeding nose, palpitations, aching joints and muscles, headaches, migraines, high temperature with no apparent cause, sore throat, many acute ear infections, chronic glue ear, aching joints and muscles.

NOTE: These symptoms may also be caused by other factors. The presence of any number of them does not guarantee a diagnosis of allergy, intolerance of sensitivity. The only real proof, if other factors have been ruled out, lies in the use of the elimination diet.

Main areas of the body affected

- Skin and membrane tissues — these symptoms are particularly noticeable at the base of the ears and around the mouth, and include swelling, flushing, eczema, rashes, hives and a severe swelling in the throat area — which can cause difficulty in breathing.
- Respiratory system — commonly affects the

lungs; throat and nose manifesting such symptoms as sneezing, runny nose, coughing, wheezing, bronchitis and asthma.
- Digestive system — the intestines and stomach are affected and produce such symptoms as spitting up food, pulling away from the breast, colicky behaviour, stomach-ache, diarrhoea, vomiting, blood in the stools, abdominal pain and poor appetite.
- Circulation — low blood pressure and possible collapse.
- Inflammation of the middle ear (otitis media).

The Elimination Diet

As the name suggests, this diet is one in which particular foods or groups of foods are removed in order to determine whether they are allergy-causing. The aim is to eliminate specific proteins, lactose, food colourings or preservatives or biologically active chemicals such as salicylates (see page 81). If the symptoms do not not subside on the elimination diet, you can assume that either the food or chemical producing the allergy has not been eliminated or that allergy may not be the cause and some other factor exists.

The second half of the diet, called the 'challenge' phase, is a follow-up to see if the improvement was indeed due to the elimination of the suspected food. The food is reintroduced to see whether it will induce the allergic reaction. Because children are rapidly changing and may be able to grow out of 'intolerances', re-challenge should be done at regular intervals.

This diet eliminates the most common problem foods and should be followed carefully for two weeks before any particular foods are tested. Withdrawal symptoms can occur in the first few days and should be allowed to subside so that the effects of tested foods can be determined.

Foods allowed on elimination diet

FRUITS all except oranges and apples
FISH including tinned fish
CHICKEN preferably organic/free range
LAMB OR MUTTON
LEGUMES lentils, adzuki beans, mung beans, peas, borlotti beans, lima beans, navy beans, no soy beans
NON-GLUTEN GRAINS AND FLOURS millet, buckwheat, sago, brown rice, arrowroot, besan (chickpea flour), potato, tapioca
NOODLES rice noodles, buckwheat noodles,

CAUTION

The elimination diet is not a nutritionally balanced diet. It is to be followed for a short time only. The aim of the diet is *only* to discover which of the eliminated foods on reintroduction or 'challenge' is found to cause symptoms. This treatment is best done under professional supervision.

green bean threads, mung bean noodles
VEGETABLES all allowed
NUTS all except peanuts
DRINKS — water, mineral water, fruit juice (if freshly squeezed with no preservatives), almond, cashew or coconut milk

Foods to be eliminated

SUGAR
GRAINS AND CEREALS wheat, rye, corn, barley, oats
CHOCOLATE
FERMENTED FOODS pickles, vinegar, miso, soy sauce, etc.
EGGS
MEAT beef, veal, pork, ham, bacon
ARTIFICIAL COLOURINGS, FLAVOURINGS AND PRESERVATIVES
SOY PRODUCTS
ALCOHOL
TEA
COFFEE
CIGARETTES from the child's environment

Reintroduction of foods

After the exclusion period, reintroduce one food at a time allowing two days for each new food. Introduce each new food on its own, for example wheat separate from yeast (do not use bread, instead use whole wheat berries, porridge, noodles, damper), milk separate from cheese (as there are yeasts in cheese), butter and cream separate from milk, eggs alone, not in baked goods.

To observe a reaction look for a recurrence of the old symptoms or the development of a new symptom. You can also test and compare a child's writing, ball catching, reading or general motor co-ordination (gross and fine motor skills) as all these may deteriorate quite dramatically on exposure to the offending food. Look for obvious but unexplained changes in the child's mood and behaviour.

Being successful on the diet

Spend some time developing alternative meal recipes that the whole family will enjoy. Most families need about five or six different evening meals to prevent boredom. Your child will need four or five different lunches and two or three breakfasts, and don't hesitate to explore new and different foods.

Changing the Constitution of the Child With Allergies

There is some controversy about whether allergic children can grow out of their sensitivities and intolerances. It is felt by some authorities that symptoms merely change and the intolerance or sensitivity remains as long as it continues to be an ongoing part of the diet. For example, eczema may disappear to be replaced by asthma, which can later manifest as learning difficulties. In adulthood it may become hypoglycaemia or arthritis. The exclusion of the offending substance is an important first step in helping the body overcome intolerances.

It does seem that the body is able to recover from intolerance and sensitivity as the general health and balance of other organ systems are restored. If a child suffers from a true immunological allergy it shows up as an immediate reaction to the substances, it is inherited, and tends to stay for the whole of the child's life.

To alter the constitution of a child with allergies, food intolerance or sensitivity, it may be necessary to use herbs and supplements to strengthen and balance the immune system, the digestive system, the adrenals or liver.

The liver is the organ responsible for breaking down chemicals and toxic substances in the body via certain enzyme systems and specialised cells. A number of people working in the field of allergies now believe that if the liver detoxification system is made more effective any allergy, intolerance or sensitivity may be eased.

The liver's enzyme systems are dependent on a number of nutrients including some of the B complex vitamins, trace minerals and amino acids. If these nutrients are deficient, and then given in the correct dosages, it may be enough to help some children overcome their reactive state.

Severe stress is known to eventually suppress the adrenal glands and, in animals, actual shrinkage of the adrenal glands has been shown to follow prolonged stress. Allergy and intolerance reactions create a stress response in the body. For this reason, we need to be mindful of weakened adrenals in prolonged allergy situations and to eliminate continued exposure to reactive substances as a way of protecting the adrenals from exhaustion.

Avoid processed and refined foods, including sugar, white flour and food that contains additives of any kind. All these foods and additives weaken the immune system, liver and general vitality of the child. Also, exercise and stress reduction need to be introduced. Children thrive best in an ordered, structured environment with an abundance of love and focused attention.

The Chinese viewpoint

In Chinese as well as naturopathic medicine, some form of weakness, immaturity or malfunction is believed to be one of the reasons for the development of intolerance and allergy. In Chinese medicine it is observed that one of the main causes of allergy is weak 'kidney function'. In children this is seen as a constitutional state inherited from the parents and made worse by conditions of stress.

If you chose to consult a practitioner using Chinese herbal medicine, she would prescribe a formula made up of a number of herbs that fit the constitution of your child.

Herbal Remedies

Chamomile

Chamomile has anti-allergenic and anti-inflammatory properties and is likely to reduce the severity of an allergic reaction.

Infusion: use 1 teaspoon dried flowerheads to 1 cup of boiling water. Let steep for 5 minutes, strain. Can be sweetened with honey or rice malt. Dilute with water for smaller children.

DOSE

1-2 years: 20-40 mL ($^2/_3$-1$^1/_3$ fl oz) 3-4 times daily
3-4 years: 50-80 mL (1½-2$^2/_3$ fl oz) 3-4 times daily
5-6 years: 100-125 mL (3-4 fl oz) 3-4 times daily
7 years and older: 150-200 mL (5-6$^2/_3$ fl oz) 3-4 times daily

Ginger

A stimulant of digestive function and circulation. Ginger is useful if food allergy is related to impaired digestive function. Hayfever and allergies producing sinus trouble will also benefit from this herb.

Infusion: use 3 slices (2-3 cm/1 inch in diameter and 3 mm/⅛ in thick) of fresh Ginger to 1 cup of boiling water. Let steep for 5 minutes. Sweeten with honey or rice malt. Dilute with water for small children.

DOSE
2-3 years: 20 mL (⅔ fl oz) 2-3 times daily
4-5 years: 30-50 mL (1-1½ fl oz) 2-3 times daily
6 years and older: 60-80 mL (2-2⅔ fl oz) 2-3 times daily

Licorice

Licorice has anti-inflammatory and anti-allergenic properties resembling the powerful corticosteroid drugs (such as cortisone). Licorice, however, acts by inhibiting the breakdown of our own corticosteroid hormones, thus increasing their effect. Prolonged use of Licorice may lead to oedema, and a low salt diet should be followed when Licorice is taken. Licorice is contraindicated in oedema, hypertension and diarrhoea.

Decoction: use ½ teaspoon chopped Licorice root to 1 cup of water. Simmer covered for 10 minutes.

DOSE
1-2 years: 20 mL (⅔ fl oz) 3 times daily
3-4 years: 30-50 mL (1-1½ fl oz) 3 times daily
5-6 years: 60-80 mL (2-2⅔ fl oz) 3 times daily
7 years and older: 100-120 mL (3-3⅔ fl oz) 3 times daily

Golden Seal

This herb has profound healing and anti-inflammatory effects on mucous membranes both in the digestive tract and in the upper respiratory system. It is also a digestive stimulant.

Decoction: use ½ teaspoon of chopped root and rhizome to 1 cup of water, simmer covered for 5-10 minutes, strain. Can be sweetened with honey or rice malt. Dilute with water if necessary.

DOSE
2-3 years: 15-20 mL (½-⅔ fl oz) 3 times daily
4-5 years: 30-40 mL (1-1⅓ fl oz) 3 times daily
6-7 years: 50-60 mL (1½-2 fl oz) 3 times daily
8 years and older: 80-100 mL/(2⅔-3 fl oz) 3 times daily

Marshmallow

A soothing remedy for the lining of the gut, Marshmallow is indicated in food allergy with diarrhoea and inflammation of the gut

The root is prepared as a decoction, use 1-1½ teaspoons of chopped root to 1 cup of water, simmer covered for 5-10 minutes.

The leaf is prepared as an infusion: use 2 teaspoons of dried leaf to 1 cup of boiling water, let steep for 10 minutes. Can be diluted with water.

DOSE
½-1 year: 15-30 mL (½-1 fl oz) 3 times daily
2-3 years: 40-50 mL (1⅓-1½ fl oz) 3 times daily
4-5 years: 60-80 mL (2-2⅔ fl oz) 3 times daily
6 years and older: 80-120 mL (2⅔-3⅔ fl oz) 3 times daily

Slippery Elm bark

Another soothing and slightly astringent remedy for an inflamed digestive tract. Slipper Elm bark has considerable nutritive value in itself. Indications as for Marshmallow (see above).

Use 2-3 teaspoons of powdered bark to ½ cup of hot water; this will form a paste that can be sweetened with honey or rice malt or mixed with fruit, porridge, etc.

DOSE
½-1 year: 2-4 teaspoons of the paste 3 times daily
2-3 years: 2-3 tablespoons of the paste 3 times daily
4-6 years: 4-6 tablespoons of the paste 3 times daily
7 years and older: 6-8 tablespoons of the paste 3 times daily

NOTE: Do not give the dried powder internally!

Echinacea

Echinacea is an immuno-stimulant herb, that is, it enhances the function of the immune system in a number of ways. Since most allergies are associated with a malfunctioning immune system, Echinacea is indicated in most cases. It should be given over a longer period (3-6 months) for best results.

Decoction: use 1 teaspoon of dried root and rhizome to 1 cup of water, simmer covered for 5 minutes. Dilute with water if necessary. Can be sweetened with honey or rice malt.

DOSE
1-2 years: 10-15 mL (⅓-½ fl oz) 3 times daily
3-4 years: 20-30 mL (⅔-1 fl oz) 3 times daily
5-6 years: 40-50 mL (1⅓-1½ fl oz) 3 times daily
7 years and older: 60-100 mL (2-3 fl oz) 3 times daily

Eyebright

Eyebright is an anticatarrhal, especially for rhinitis, hayfever and sinus trouble and is topically applied to the eyes for conjunctivitis and itchy eyes.

Infusion: use 1 teaspoon of dried herb to 1 cup of boiling water. Let steep for 5 minutes, strain. Can be sweetened with honey or rice malt. Dilute with water if necessary.

DOSE
1-2 years: 15-30 mL (½-1 fl oz) 3 times daily
3-4 years: 40-60 mL (1⅓-2 fl oz) 3 times daily
5-6 years: 70-90 mL (2⅓-3 fl oz) 3 times daily
7 years and older: 100-150 mL (3-5 fl oz) 3 times daily

Golden Rod

Golden Rod is used as an anticatarrhal for the upper respiratory tract, especially when a nervous element is present.

Infusion: use 1 teaspoon of dried herb to 1 cup of boiling water. Let steep for 5 minutes, strain. Can be sweetened with honey or rice malt. Dilute with water if necessary.

DOSE
1-2 years: 10-20 mL (⅓-⅔ fl oz) 3 times daily
3-4 years: 30-40 mL (1-1⅓ fl oz) 3 times daily
5-6 years: 50-60 mL (1½-2 fl oz) 3 times daily
7 years and older: 70-100 mL (2⅓-3 fl oz) 3 times daily

Catmint

Catmint is an anticatarrhal for the upper respiratory tract and a decongestant. It is relaxing, carminative (relieves flatulence) and stimulates digestion.

Infusion: use 1 teaspoon of dried herb to 1 cup of boiling water. Let steep for 5 minutes, strain. Can be sweetened with honey or rice malt. Dilute with water if necessary.

DOSE
1-2 years: 15-30 mL (½-1 fl oz) 3 times daily
3-4 years: 40-60 mL (1⅓-2 fl oz) 3 times daily
5-6 years: 70-90 mL (2⅓-3 fl oz) 3 times daily
7 years and older: 100-150 mL (3-5 fl oz) 3 times daily

Homoeopathic Remedies

Food allergies are regarded as a constitutional problem and should be referred to your homoeopath.

Chinese Remedies

'Deficiency'

Yellowish or pale complexion. Poor appetite. There may be a yellow tint in the area between the eyelids and eyebrows. The whites of the eyes may be yellowish. There may be a blue vein or dark tint between the eyebrows at the bridge of the nose. The lips are pale. The tongue is pale. The child may sleep with eyes slightly open. Stools are often loose.

QIAN BHI BAI ZHU SAN
LI ZHONG WAN (cold hands, feet or abdomen)
XIANG SHA YANG WEI TANG (bloating after eating)
XIANG SHA LIU JUN ZI TANG (mucus discharge from nose or throat)
SHEN LING BAI ZHU TANG (diarrhoea and vomiting)

2 'Food stagnation'

See 'Abdominal Pain' for symptom picture.

BAO HE WAN (normally healthy child)
REN SHEN JIAN PI WAN

ASTHMA

Approximately 20 per cent of school age children have some degree of wheezing. The incidence of asthma in America is on the increase, possibly indicating that certain factors such as diet, pollution of our homes, environment and chemical additives in our food may be contributing causes.

Children with asthma will usually have a history of frequent respiratory infections. These can often trigger an asthmatic attack.

Although asthma is usually allergic in origin, it is more confusing than other allergic diseases because its onset is inconsistent and sometimes unrelated to specific food or environmental allergens. The attacks can be provoked by colds and other infectious illnesses, emotional trauma, anxiety, disappointment and other psychological conditions. The frequency of attacks can also vary with activity, food, climate (especially cold weather) and the environmental conditions of the home.

Asthma occurs when the passageways in the lungs become blocked to the flow of air. The muscles in the airway walls then go into spasm and narrow the tubes quite considerably. The passageways can become blocked because of an over-production of mucus, as they do when there is a respiratory infection. In an infant, because the airway walls are soft, they may collapse, but in older children the muscles can easily go into spasm, especially if the child is in a tense situation that makes her nervous and upset.

The body of a child with asthma often shows a lot of tension, because she has to put extra effort into breathing. The chest wall becomes rigid and does not move easily to allow the flow of breath into the lower chest and diaphragm area. The muscles of respiration stay tense even when there is no acute breathing difficulty. This maintains an abnormal pattern in the neuro-muscular system associated with breathing. The nerves to the muscles of the chest wall have connections to the nerves that control the spasm in the lungs and asthmatics have patterns of excessive excitation in these nerves.

Chronic mucus congestion also exists in asthma and if not expelled leads to further irritation of the lungs. Even though mucus may not be obvious on a daily basis, in Chinese medicine it is believed that phlegm is always present in asthma. Some children may have a cold or other form of nasal discharge whereas others may only have a sore throat or swollen glands prior to an asthma attack.

It is important to strengthen the immune system to prevent the occurrence of respiratory infections. However, in most cases allergy or hypersensitivity often accompanies and predisposes children to bronchitis as well as asthma. Allergies weaken the immune system and create the characteristic spasm of the bronchial smooth muscles that occur in asthma, which can be dangerous and life-threatening. Psychological factors alone do not cause asthma although they can trigger asthma in a susceptible child. Natural medicine can be used to help prevent the asthmatic attacks and decrease their intensity. However, a severe attack may require orthodox drugs, in which case you should consult a practitioner of your choice immediately.

If you have selected the right treatment with the help of a qualified practitioner, then you should see results within one to two weeks of starting a treatment. Your child's energy level should increase and the time in which it takes to recover from an attack should be shorter and easier.

Allergies and Asthma

While most children do not have major genetic defects and can happily cope with their environment without having an asthma attack, there are some children who cannot because of a genetic or environmental reason handle specific chemicals ingested with food. Some of these chemicals are food additives.

A variety of sulphiting agents including sulphur dioxide and some inorganic sulphites are being used as preservatives. They act as antioxidants and prevent microbial spoilage. Sulphites are also used to sanitise containers in the fermentation industry. There are actually six different sulphite substances. They are presently sprayed on fresh fruit, chicken, shellfish, bread, vinegar, frozen pizzas, olives, French fried potatoes, to name just a few.

Due to accumulating evidence, it is now thought that when an acid solution containing bisulphite or sulphur dioxide is taken by asthmatics, an asthma attack can be promoted within minutes of ingestion in some children and adults. Robert Buist reports in his book, *Food Chemical Sensitivity*, 'A recent study at a children's hospital in Sydney, Australia, showed that asthma in up to 65 per cent of patients, both children and adults, was provoked by ingestion of foods or beverages containing metabisulphite.' Metabisulphite is found in dried tree fruits such as apples, pears and apricots, fruit bars, fruit yoghurt, cheese pastes, cordials, soft drinks, sausages, uncooked fresh prawns and shellfish and some potato crisps.

Air pollutants are another factor in asthmatic attacks. In industrial countries power plants that use oil or coal probably account for 75 per cent of sulphur dioxide emission, according to Robert Buist (*Food Chemical Sensitivity*).

In a newspaper article in the *Sydney Morning Herald* on 31 October 1985, it was reported that 40 per cent of children attending a public school that was situated between two large power stations, had some form of respiratory complaint contracted after moving into the area. (The figures from school records were presented to the NSW Commission of Inquiry into power generation at Gosford.) Three doctors estimated that the incidence of asthma in children under twelve is 30 per cent — twice the national average. Adults also reported that they suffered from recurrent bronchitis even though they didn't smoke. The fallout arising from the power stations and possibly causing asthma and other bronchial problems is thought to be sulphur dioxide gas.

You don't have to pack up the whole family and move to Arizona or Alice Springs if your child suffers from asthma. A warm, dry climate will definitely help, but finding the perfect climate isn't that easy any more, and is not the only answer. 'Asthma is a reversible disease. and in the under 40 age group, probably 90 per cent of asthma is triggered by an allergy,' says Dr Ziering, an allergist in private practice in Fresno, California. There's plenty you can do at home to reverse your child's condition.

Children can be allergic to inhaled substances such as dust, dust mites, moulds, pollen, animal dandruff, pesticides and fumes. These should be controlled diligently around the home. You should also control food allergies. There are two types of foods which commonly cause asthma:

- Those that cause an immediate reaction and are therefore easily recognised. The most common, in order of prevalence, are eggs, fish, nuts, peanuts.
- Those that have a delayed reaction. These are harder to identify until they have been eliminated and reintroduced through the elimination diet. The most common, in order of prevalence, are milk, chocolate, wheat, citrus, soy, beef.

The control of food additives in the diet is another vitally important factor in the management of childhood or adult asthma. Other well-known provokers of asthma are the sulphites used as preservatives in dried fruits and vegetables, fruit juices, wine, pickles, sausage meats, vinegar, jams, beer, desiccated coconut, raw peeled potatoes used in chips, flours and uncooked prawns. Tartrazine, a commonly used yellow food colouring, also causes asthma. It is found in some brands of butter, margarine, confectionery, cakes, noodles, soft drinks, packet desserts, canned peas, marzipan, pickles, brown sauce, canned fruit and flavoured pie filling.

Air pollutants are another factor in asthmatic attacks. Ozone, especially when mixed with sulphuric acid from car exhaust fumes, leads to asthmatic attacks. 'In humans, there's strong evidence that ozone exposures seen in many cities kill the outer layer of cells in the lung, causing redness and water buildup, and the layer of tissue is sloughed off in a way analogous to sunburn,' stated Donald Horstman, an air pollution expert at the Environmental Protection Agency's Health Effects Research Laboratory in North Carolina. Sulphur dioxide and nitrogen oxides weaken the lungs, leading to infection.

Another possible cause for the increase of deaths from asthma might be the drugs used to treat the disease. While in the short-term there is no doubt that they save lives, their long-term use may be contributing to the death rate. Several studies have implicated drugs known as beta-2-agonists, which are common ingredients in asthma treatments, according to

Graham Phillips, journalist for the *Sunday Telegraph* newspaper, 12 January 1992. The strongest evidence was a study, the results of which were published in the *Lancet*, December 1990, with two groups of asthmatics. One group was given inhalers which contained beta-2-agonists; the other group were given placebos. After six months the asthma in the group taking the beta-2-agonists had worsened.

Prevention

- Magnesium — Adequate levels of Magnesium are required in asthmatics. It helps prevent spasm in the bronchials.
- Carotenes — Those Carotenes that are found in green and yellow vegetables, help to protect the lungs of children with asthma.
- B6 Pyridoxine — This vitamin has been shown to be low in asthmatics. Supplementing with 50 mg per day over a few months can lead to dramatic reduction in wheezing frequency and severity.
- Vitamin C — Asthmatics also show low levels of this vitamin. Treatment with vitamin C at a moderately low dose, of 500 mg per day over the age of three, is very helpful for some children in reducing the severity of asthma. Smaller doses do not appear to have such protective effects.
- Quercetin — This is a bioflavinoid found in some brands of vitamin C. It has a vitamin C sparing effect but on its own is a very important treatment for asthma. The dosage must be at the level of 500 mg per day. It is an inhibitor of histamine and also prevents the release of some powerful chemicals known as leukotrienes, which are responsible for the spasm of the bronchials.
- Vitamin B 12 — Studies of this vitamin show that it is effective in younger individuals for the treatment of asthma. Weekly injections of 1000 mg are required. It is also useful in individuals who have sulphite sensitivity as it helps to inactivate this substance.
NOTE: Consult a practitioner of your choice for guidance on preventative treatments.

Remedial treatment

A combination of physical therapies, chiropractic, osteopathy and physiotherapy can achieve the following:
- relaxed muscles
- relaxation of nerves
- free movement of chest

- pattern of breathing becomes even and full with the use of the whole chest and diaphragm
- mucus loosened and expelled

Spinal manipulation and mobilisation will increase the mobility and release fixation in the chest wall. Chiropractic and osteopathy aim to normalise nerve action to the lungs by releasing nerve pressure and altering the electrical potential to the nerves.

CAUTION

Spinal manipulation should only be done by a qualified practitioner.

Massage and vibrator therapy also work to relax muscles and change the patterns in the neuromuscular system. A vibrator is often used to help loosen mucus in the lungs and to normalise the nerve impulses to the lungs. Shaking and vibration of the chest is also applied manually to loosen mucus.

BREATHING EXERCISES

A good series of breathing exercises will teach the child how to do deep, relaxed abdominal breathing, which will increase the efficiency of breathing and induce calm. Minor asthma attacks can sometimes be controlled with breathing exercises alone. Encourage some strong forceful expiratory breathing as a way of loosening mucus and increasing the effi-

---

CAUTION

Trying to treat asthma can be very wearing, especially if you are expecting the treatment to 'cure' the problem very quickly. It can take a long time to cure asthma — anywhere from six months up to one or even two years. It is not uncommon for children to need to go back to using orthodox drugs and inhalers for a period of time. A small dose of orthodox medicine early in the attack can sometimes avoid the necessity of a larger dose later on. Do not stop orthodox drugs immediately upon beginning to use natural medicines. The reduction of the dosage of orthodox medicine must be done gradually over a period of many weeks and even months and with the support of a qualified medical practitioner. Remember that asthma can be a life-threatening disease.

---

ciency of expiration as asthmatics have a hard time getting air out. Exercises that mobilise the thoracic spine and rib cage should also be included.

Some sort of body work and exercise should be done daily with the child who has asthma. These can be taught by a physiotherapist, chiropractor or osteopath and be carried out at home with the supervision of the parent.

Home Remedies After an Attack

- Give your child plenty of liquids to drink to loosen the bronchial secretions.
- Add 100 g (3½ oz) of thyme leaves to 2 cups boiling water. Mix into the bath.
- Try using a vaporizer with eucalyptus or thyme leaves.

Herbal Remedies

Licorice

Licorice has anti-inflammatory and anti-allergenic properties resembling the powerful corticosteroid drugs (such as cortisone). Licorice, however, acts by inhibiting the breakdown of our own corticosteroid hormones, thus increasing their effect. Prolonged use of Licorice may lead to oedema, and a low salt diet should be followed when Licorice is taken. Licorice is contraindicated in oedema, hypertension and diarrhoea.

Decoction: use ½ teaspoon chopped Licorice root to 1 cup of water. Simmer covered for 10 minutes.

DOSE

1-2 years: 20 mL (⅔ fl oz) 3 times daily
3-4 years: 30-50 mL (1-1⅔ fl oz) 3 times daily
5-6 years: 60-80 mL (2-2⅔ fl oz) 3 times daily
7 years and older: 100-120 mL (3-3⅔ fl oz) 3 times daily

Elecampane

Elecampane is a rejuvenating tonic for the lungs and relieves congestion. It is not a remedy for acute attacks but should be taken as a preventative over a longer period.

Decoction: use 1-1½ teaspoons of chopped root to 1 cup of water, simmer covered for 5-10 minutes.

DOSE

1-2 years: 15-30 mL (½-1 fl oz) 3 times daily
3-4 years: 40-60 mL (1⅓-2 fl oz) 3 times daily

5-6 years: 70-90 mL (2⅓-3 fl oz) 3 times daily
7 years and older: 100-150 mL (3-5 fl oz) 3 times daily

Mullein

This herb has anti-spasmodic and sedative actions and also acts as a bronchial decongestant. It can be used both as a preventative and to reduce the severity of acute attacks.

Infusion: use 2 teaspoons of the dried leaves or ½ teaspoon of the dried flowers to 1 cup of boiling water. Let steep for 5-10 minutes, strain. Can be sweetened with honey or rice malt.

DOSE

1-2 years: 15-30 mL (½-1 fl oz) 3 times daily
3-4 years: 40-60 mL (1⅓-2 fl oz) 3 times daily
5-6 years: 70-90 mL (2⅓-3 fl oz) 3 times daily
7 years and older: 100-150 mL (3-5 fl oz) 3 times daily

Thyme

Thyme exerts marked anti-spasmodic effects on the respiratory system and is also anti-bacterial. A good preventative; in acute attacks steam inhalations with Thyme can be very useful.

Infusion: use 1 teaspoon of dried herb to 1 cup of boiling water. Let steep for 5 minutes, strain. Can be sweetened with honey or rice malt. Dilute with water if necessary.

DOSE

1-2 years: 15-30 mL (½-1 fl oz) 3 times daily
3-4 years: 40-60 mL (1⅓-2 fl oz) 3 times daily
5-6 years: 70-90 mL (2⅓-3 fl oz) 3 times daily
7 years and older: 100-150 mL (3-5 fl oz) 3 times daily

Homoeopathic Remedies

In homoeopathy asthma is regarded as a constitutional problem with a number of different causes. It is usually a chronic condition and so should be referred to your homoeopathic practitioner.

Where there is an acute episode of the condition the following medicines may be considered:

Where the attack is brought on by a cold, dry wind and accompanied by fear and restlessness **Aconite** 30C may be applied.

You may note that your child is unable to lie down and must sit or bend forward during an attack. If this is associated with fear and suffocation **Arsenicum** 12C would be the best indicated medicine.

Asthma after long spasmodic cough indicates **Carb-veg** 12C. Your child may also crave the open air and the skin may be cold to touch.

Periodic occurrences of asthma associated with a cough often indicate **Ipecacuana** 12C. Like the **Arsenicum** child you will find they must sit up.

Where the asthma is characterised by swelling in the throat and air passages **Apis** 12C may be given.

Dose: One dose up to every 15 minutes in a severe situation and three times daily for up to three days where the symptoms are mild.

Chinese Remedies

BELOW THE AGE OF SIX

1 'Cold Type'

Asthma with sneezing, runny nose, clear and copious mucus, Urination is frequent, clear and copious. Fever and chills (chills predominant). Absence of sweating. Dark complexion. Red fingernails. Red vein at 'San Guan'. Tongue is pale with a white coating. Increased sensitivity to cold. Child requires warm clothing or coverings.

XIAO QING LONG TANG
XIAO CHAI HU TANG taken together with BAN XIA HOU PU TANG (loss of appetite, diarrhoea, symptoms aggravated by stress, emotional factors, cold foods and sugar)

2 'Hot Type'

Asthma with thick yellow mucus (in severe cases mucus may be green and contain pus). Fever with sweating. Red complexion. Finger-nails are purple. Eyes are red. Veins at the back of the ears are prominent. Purple vein at 'San Guan'. Mouth is dry. Tongue is red with a yellow coating. There may also be eczema and bed-wetting. Urine is dark in colour and reduced in quantity.

XIE BAI SAN
QING FEI YI HUO TANG (severe symptoms with coughing up of blood-streaked sputum, constipation)

ABOVE THE AGE OF SIX

For child six years or older the symptoms tend to occur in more complex patterns than those listed above. It is recommended that you take your child to an experienced practitioner for professional diagnosis and treatment.

Massage

Massage should be done preceding or at the very beginning of an asthma attack.

1 Have the child sit on a chair in front of you. Roll up small hand towel and place on right shoulder.
2 Place your forearm on towel and slowly but firmly press straight downward towards the floor. At the same time have your child resist and try to push upward towards the ceiling. This is a slow isometric stretch. Do this three times (pressing down and child pushes up), pause, then repeat for three times, slowly. This helps to open bronchial tubes and allows drainage of fluid.
3 Repeat on left shoulder.
4 As you do this exercise say to your child in a relaxed tone, 'There is enough room in your body to breathe. It's becoming easier and easier for you to breathe.'

and/or

5 On the bottom of both feet in the centre of the ball of the foot, press in with your thumbs, towards your child's head, following her in breath, then pull toes toward you as child exhales. Do this four or five times.

BED-WETTING

Potty training can provide endless hours of 'patience training' for parents, but when it comes to bed-wetting it's a different kettle of fish! Although most parents are aware of the importance of not punishing children for bed-wetting accidents which are not under a child's conscious control, the constant tedium of washing sheets and pyjamas daily can lead to anger and hostility. Children can all too easily become aware of such feelings, and combined with the teasing from siblings and friends can lead to feelings of embarrassment and shame.

Bed-wetting is twice as common in male children as it is in female children. For both sexes the incidence is generally much higher than people realise, as the following figures show:

three years — one in three children wet the bed

four years — one in four children wet the bed

six years — one in six children wet the bed

eight to nine years — one in fifteen wet the bed

twelve to fourteen — one in twenty-five wet the bed

Causes

There are some medical causes of bed-wetting, including inflammations of the urinary tract and malformations of the urinary system. These generally make up a very small number of cases. Immature development of the nerves that allow bladder control is another reason for bed-wetting.

Psychological factors may play a role but should not be over emphasised. Studies done on the use of psychological counselling in the treatment of bed-wetting show very poor results. If a child who has been dry at night for a prolonged period of time suddenly starts to wet the bed again causes such as stress or excess fatigue should be considered.

Childhood allergies, food intolerance and chemical sensitivities can also be the cause of bed-wetting. There are children who will inevitably wet the bed if given too many foods containing salicylates (see page 81) and sometimes children who are allergic to wheat wet the bed if they eat any wheat products. The offending substance probably leads to local irritation of the urinary tract or over excitation of the peripheral nerves.

An Overview of Current Remedies

Many home remedies exist for bed-wetting, including raising the foot of the bed, excluding draughts, withholding fluids for a period of time. Most of the time these do not really make a difference. When the child is ready to sleep through the night without wetting the bed she will do so. However, a young child may be supported by being taken to the toilet after she has been sleeping for three or four hours.

Many behavioural techniques have been developed for training the child to control their bladder function. These can be very successful but are best carried out under the guidance of a trained behavioural psychologist as some involve quite complicated procedures. The simplest technique is the use of the pad and buzzer. These tend to be more successful for the child over five years. They can be rented from some drugstores and early childhood health centres, and are simply a moisture sensitive pad which sounds an alarm when your child begins to urinate. If all goes to plan she wakes and goes to the toilet, and over a period of time learns not to do it in her sleep.

Chiropractic, osteopathy, acupuncture and massage treatment are very successful in treating some children, probably because of the effect they have on the autonomic nervous system that controls the bladder.

Chinese herbal medicine has developed some successful treatment for bed-wetting based on using traditional formulas.

Herbal Remedies

Horsetail

This herb is used to strengthen the bladder.
Decoction: use 1 1½ teaspoons of the dried herb to 1 cup of water. Simmer covered for 10-15 minutes, strain. Can be sweetened with honey or rice malt.

DOSE

1-2 years: 15-30 mL (½-1 fl oz) 3 times daily
3-4 years: 40-60 mL (1⅓-2 fl oz) 3 times daily
5-6 years: 70-90 mL (2⅓-3 fl oz) 3 times daily
7 years and older: 100-150 mL (3-5 fl oz) 3 times daily

Homoeopathic Remedies

In homoeopathy this is a constitutional problem with a number of different causes. It is usually a chronic condition and should be referred to your homoeopathic practitioner.

Chinese Remedies

(See pp. 39–43)

1 'Deficiency' — 'Cold'

Easily fatigued. Lack of energy. Pale complexion. Frequent urination. Poor appetite. Tongue is pale with a thin white coating. Cold hands and feet. Dry mouth and throat.

XIAO JIAN ZHONG TANG

2 'Heat'

Thirst. Sweating. Red complexion. Red tongue. Purple vein at 'San Guan'. Rapid pulse. Child feels hot and may also have a mild fever. Prefers light clothing or coverings.

ZHU YE SHI GAO TANG

3 'Deficiency'

Nervousness. Frequently catches colds. Poor appetite. Frequent stomach upsets, indigestion and diarrhoea. Complexion tends to be pale. Low energy.

XIAO CHAI HU TANG together with GUI ZHI TANG

4 'Deficiency' of Kidneys

Obesity. Pale complexion. Thirst. Loss of appetite. easily tired. Low energy. Frequent constipation. Frequent passing of clear, pale urine in large quantity. Sleeps more than normal. Dark complexion. The lower abdomen below the navel may feel cold and/or lacking in tone or firmness.

JIN GUI SHEN QI WAN

5 'Deficiency' of Lungs and Digestive System

Stiff muscles of neck, shoulders and upper back. Frequent loss of appetite. Occasional diarrhoea or loose stools. Frequently catches colds.

GE GEN TANG

Massage

A foot massage before bedtime can be very relaxing for a child who may be anxious about wetting the bed.

1 Press just above the heel on the instep of both feet. Press softly, first on one foot then the other working in gradually until you can go in no further or until your child says 'ouch'. Hold for thirty seconds maintaining even, gentle pressure just below her pain threshold.

2 Press in with your thumb, making thumb prints, along instep on side of each foot from heel to big toe. These are bladder and kidney reflex points. While you are doing this have your child breathe in slowly, then exhale, telling him he is safe and loved.

and/or

3 Hold one hand at base of spine and the other hand on lower abdomen over bladder, direct warm loving energy through your hands.

DRY OR WET

It's not unusual for five year olds to wet their bed two nights per month, says child urologist Dr H. Gil Rushton (Washington). He says that 15 to 20 per cent of all children in this age bracket are afflicted by this condition. As the child gets older, the number of times that this occurs naturally decreases.

BITES AND STINGS

Sooner or later your child is bound to get bitten or stung by some creeping, flying, walking, crawling, running, swimming or slithering insect or animal. Most of the time there is no reason to worry, but sometimes all caution must be taken and the sooner the response to the bite, the better.

The treatment varies depending on what has actually done the biting. However, for most dangerous bites a pressure bandage is the most important initial response.

Pressure and immobilisation techniques are used in situations where it is essential to prevent the spread of poison from a bitten area to the rest of the body. Recent research has shown that if firm pressure is applied immediately to the bitten area, very little venom reaches the blood stream. The patient is then immobilised to further prevent the poison from circulating in the blood stream.

Emergency Treatment

1 Keep the bitten area still.
2 Apply a broad bandage, wrapping it as tightly around the bitten limb as you would apply to a sprain. If no bandage is available, tear up clothing or any other material into strips. Wrap the bandage from the wound towards the body, to further decrease the circulation.
3 Immobilise the limb by binding it to the body in the case of the arm, or to the other leg in the case of a leg. Bind the limb to a splint if possible — use anything that is rigid, for example, a piece of wood. Immobilise the child's body by wrapping her tightly in a blanket or similar large cloth.

If the bite is to the body or face there is nothing that can be done, other than immobilising the child to prevent the rapid spread of the poison, and summoning immediate medical help. You can apply pressure to the bitten area by pressing with your hand but it is not nearly as effective as a pressure bandage. A pressure bandage can be used on the body and, if it will

---

> **CAUTION**
>
> **Do not wash or cut the bitten area, and do not apply a tourniquet if bitten by a snake or spider.**

not obstruct the airways, on the head as well.
4 Bring help to the injured child wherever possible, but if necessary, carry the child to where she can be tended until medical help arrives.
5 Seek urgent medical help and do not remove the pressure bandage until that help arrives. Continue to keep the child immobilised.

Snakes

There are more non-venomous snakes than venomous snakes in America. However, if you are not absolutely sure it is not venomous, treat it as if it is and seek medical attention urgently. It is helpful to be able to identify the snake but if not, a general antivenene can be administered.

Treatment
Choose one:
1 Localise the venom with a pressure bandage.
2 Immobilise the child until medical help arrives.

Spiders

Most spiders are shy and non-aggressive and do not bite even when handled roughly. There are no spiders native to America whose bites are known to be consistently fatal. However, if your child gets bitten by a black widow or a brown recluse spider, it is best to seek medical attention. It is also helpful if you can capture and deliver the spider to the doctor.

Black Widow

Only the female, marked with a red dot on her shiny black abdomen, is venomous to humans. Most symptoms begin within 30–60 minutes.

1 Keep the child quiet
2 Seek medical attention as soon as possible

Brown Recluse

The bite of this spider either may go unnoticed with no after-effects or may be followed by a severe localized reaction. If you suspect a brown recluse bite:

1 Keep the child quiet
2 Apply ice compresses
3 Seek medical attention

Sea Creatures

Portuguese man-of-war

These swimming creatures can be found on most Australian beaches at some time of the year and contact with the tentacles can be very painful.

1 Apply vinegar, which helps neutralise the venom, but do not wash, as this spreads the venom.
2 Carefully remove the tentacles from the skin, flicking them off with something like a towel to avoid being stung yourself.
3 Apply ice wrapped in a cloth to the stung area;. use an ice compress if possible.
4 Seek medical attention.

Jellyfish

1 Apply vinegar, which helps neutralise the venom, but do not wash, as this spreads the venom.
2 Carefully remove the tentacles from the skin, flicking them off with something like a towel to avoid being stung yourself.
3 Seek medical attention.

Other stinging fish

1 Apply ice wrapped in a cloth to the stung area, making an ice compress and binding it to the wound if possible.
2 Seek medical attention immediately.

Sea snake

These creatures, like the sea wasp, can kill in minutes.

1 Apply a pressure bandage.
2 Seek *urgent* medical attention.

Insects

With insect bites, there are so many different kinds, from big, puffy swellings down to a small little spot without any noticeable swelling. Most bites will have a tiny hole or bump in the centre where the stinger has penetrated the skin.

Medical attention should be sought if pain is severe or there is any sign of allergic reaction or illness. However, most bites and stings can be treated relatively simply.

Treatment

- Apply ice to the area.
- Apply a paste made with a few drops of water mixed into one teaspoon of bicarbonate of soda. Tea-tree oil or any soothing ointment is also useful.
- Pain may also be relieved by washing the area with one of the following: vinegar, lemon juice, onion or shallot juice, a clove of garlic or a clay compress (see Appendix 7).

Bee stings

Bee stings should be removed with tweezers or fingernails. It is important to remove the sting as quickly as possible to prevent more poison being injected into the tissue. A bee sting has its own 'pump' and will continue to inject poison long after the initial piercing of the skin. If your child has been stung near or on the neck, nose and mouth or genitals seek *urgent* medical attention. Do not squeeze the stung area as it spreads the poison. Bee stings can be bathed with a paste of baking soda and water. If the area still becomes inflamed or sore, strips of fresh papaya are full of healing enzymes and anti-inflammatory agents.

Ticks

There are many kinds of ticks and all should be treated with care, as some can be quite dangerous.

- Remove the tick with tweezers, or fingers, trying to get hold of it as close to the head as possible.
- If the head is left in, it will simply fester and come out like any other foreign body.
- Ticks can be killed first by applying a few drops of one of the following fluids to the insect: methylated spirits, turpentine, kerosene or sal volatile. Use these fluids carefully as they can burn young skin, causing more pain than the tick bite.

• If there are any symptoms such as paralysis of limbs or blurring of vision, seek medical attention immediately.

Animal and Human Bites

1 Wash the bite under cold running water.
2 Dry it and apply an ointment such as calendula cream or tea-tree oil.
3 Wrap in a clean dry bandage.
4 Inspect the bite over the next few days for redness, which could indicate infection.
5 If the bite is deep or signs of infection develop, consult a medical practitioner immediately. In the case of animal bites the possibility of contracting rabies should not be discounted.

Home Remedies

Leeches and ticks

• Apply pure tea-tree oil to kill the animal then dab on the bite.
• Apply salt to remove the leech.

Fleas

• Eating raw garlic daily keeps fleas at bay.
• Pennyroyal, citronella, bay, and eucalyptus oils sprinkled around sleeping areas, and on bodies may help stop fleas from biting.
• If bitten, rub lemon juice, vinegar, vitamin E oil or aloe vera juice on affected area.

Bites

• Mosquito and sandfly bites can be treated by rubbing green leaves on them, especially crushed plaintain leaves or common dock leaves. Relief is also available from the gel of the aloe vera leaf.
• Wasp stings should be treated with an acidic substance such as lemon juice or vinegar. Later, papaya can be applied.

Herbal Remedies

Insect stings

Compress with Chickweed (especially if itchy) or Parsley (see below).

Fresh juice of Aloe Vera (gel), Ribwort or Plantain can be used. Aloe grows readily indoors as well as in the garden in frost-free areas (avoid direct sun). Both Ribwort and its close relative Plantain are very common weeds in urban as well as rural areas.

CHICKWEED COMPRESS

First make up an infusion using 2 teaspoons of dried herb or 6-8 teaspoons of fresh, chopped herb to 1 cup of boiling water. Let steep for 5-10 minutes, strain. Dip a piece of cotton (such as a handkerchief) in the infusion, fold it a couple of times and apply to affected area. Reapply a number of times, then cover with a dry tea-towel or handkerchief and secure with a bandage.

PARSLEY COMPRESS

First make up an infusion using 2 teaspoons of dried herb or 4-5 teaspoons of fresh, chopped herb to 1 cup of boiling water. Let steep for 5-10 minutes, strain. Dip a piece of cotton (such as a handkerchief) in the infusion, fold it a couple of times and apply to affected area. Reapply a number of times, then cover with a dry tea-towel or handkerchief and secure with a bandage.

Bites of poisonous spiders and snakes

Seek immediate medical help. Keep calm, reassure the child and keep her as still as possible. Do not delay the departure for hospital or the doctor, but if, for some reason, there is waiting time, give a cup of Echinacea and/or Scullcap tea and apply Echinacea topically to the bite (see below).

Don't forget to take a good look at the aggressor; this may enable you to identify the species and therefore the antidote.

ECHINACEA

This herb was used by North American Indians to treat snake bite. It is anti-infective and supports immune function. Apply topically as well as taking it internally.

Decoction: use 1 teaspoon of dried root and rhizome to 1 cup of water, simmer covered for 5 minutes. Dilute with water if necessary. Can be sweetened with honey or rice malt.

DOSE

1-2 years: 10-15 mL (¼-½ fl oz) 3 times daily
3-4 years: 20-30 mL (⅔-1 fl oz) 3 times daily
5-6 years: 40-50 mL (1⅓-1½ fl oz) 3 times daily
7 years and older: 60-100 mL (2-3 fl oz) 3 times daily

SCULLCAP

A calming herb, Scullcap may reduce the fear and panic which may accompany a bite.

Infusion: use ½-1 teaspoon of the dried herb to 1 cup of boiling water. Let steep for 5-10 minutes, strain. Sweeten with honey or rice malt. This herb has an unpleasant bitter taste and should be mixed with a suitable pleasant-tasting herb such as ½–1 teaspoon Fennel Seed, Aniseed or Licorice Root.

DOSE

1-2 years: 15-30 mL (½-1 fl oz) 3 times daily
3-4 years: 40-60 mL (1⅓-2 fl oz) 3 times daily
5-6 years: 70-90 mL (2⅓-3 fl oz) 3 times daily
7 years and older: 100-150 mL (3-5 fl oz) 3 times daily

Homoeopathic Remedies

Bites and stings of bees, bluebottles, insects

Apis mellifica 12C is specially indicated where there is marked swelling associated with the sting and the part is hot to touch.

Ledum 12C is used where there is pain that shoots away from the site with the part feeling cold or numb. The site is better for cold applications.

Dose: One dose three times daily. Half-hourly at first if the sting is severe.

Puncture wounds

Hypericum 30C is very useful for the effects of puncture wounds and specially where there are shooting pains in or extending from the wound.

Ledum 12C is also indicated and should be used when the wound is puffy and/or feels cold and is relieved by cold applications.

Dose: Three times daily for up to three days.

BLEEDING

'But Mommy, it's bleeding' is a common cry of children everywhere. Blood seems to prove, in children's eyes, the seriousness of an injury. Many people hate the sight of blood, especially their own, so it's best to always be calm and reassuring. Assess the severity of the wound and treat appropriately.

Emergency Treatment

Minor cuts and scrapes

(See Cuts and Grazes)

1 Wrap ice in a cloth and press to the affected area, or wash with cold water and apply pressure to stop the flow, or wash the wound with Tea-Tree oil, to clean it, then if possible, leave it open to the air to help it heal.

2 Apply ointments such as Calendula cream, Chickweed ointment and diluted Tea-Tree ointment (available from health food stores) or apply tincture of Calendula, Echinacea or Hypericum diluted 5:1 with water.

Larger cuts

1 Apply pressure to the wound by pressing on it firmly with a clean cloth or dressing until it stops bleeding.

2 Bind it with a gauze dressing.

3 If blood is still oozing, apply further dressings on top of the first one and bandage firmly. Do not use cotton wool, which will adhere to the wound.

4 Take your child to a doctor in case stitches are required, or if there are any foreign bodies left in the wound.

5 Continue to apply pressure and if the wound is on a limb then elevate it to help staunch the blood flow on the way to the hospital or medical centre.

6 Chickweed is particularly helpful if the wound is itchy.

Arterial bleeding

If blood spurts from a would, an artery may be severed. *This is an emergency.*

1 Hard pressure should be applied immediately on the wound and just next to it towards the heart.

2 If possible, raise the injured part above heart level to help reduce the flow of blood.

3 Do not relax the pressure on the wound at any time. If you cannot get help without releasing the pressure, replace your hand with something like a spoon or bowl, pressed on the wound with the smooth side, or, if you are outside, use a smooth stone. Then bandage tightly with whatever can be found.

4 It is imperative that the bleeding be controlled and medical attention sought immediately.

Mouth injuries

Many toddlers seem to be continually falling and splitting open their lips or mouths. Such cuts are not usually serious but can produce a lot of blood for the size of the wound. Press ice on the wound or get your child to suck ice, which helps to control the bleeding quickly, and can provide an interesting diversion from the injury.

Nosebleeds

1 Pinch on the bridge (bony part) of the nose for about ten minutes or until the bleeding stops.

2 If the bleeding persists, consult a doctor or your local hospital.

3 Don't let your child pick or fiddle with their nose for at least an hour after the nosebleed stops in case it starts again. (See Nosebleeds).

Herbal Remedies

Yarrow or Calendula

Compresses: use 2-3 teaspoons of dried herb to 1 cup of boiling water, let steep 5-10 minutes, strain. Dip a piece of cotton (such as a tea-towel) in the cold decoction, fold it a couple of times and apply to affected area.

Other herbs to stop bleeding:

Prepare American Cranesbill, Sage, Yarrow, Shepherd's Purse, and Witch Hazel leaf as infusions (see page 15). Prepare Tormentil and Witch Hazel bark as decoctions (see page 15). Use 2 teaspoons of dried herb or 5 teaspoons of fresh, chopped herb to 1 cup of water. Apply to the wound with a clean handkerchief or tissue, apply pressure for a couple of minutes or more if necessary.

Homoeopathic Remedies

Bleeding from cut or injury

Arnica 30C is a remedy that is often used in injury and which will assist in stopping bleeding.

Where bleeding associated with an injury is not easily controlled then **Phosphorus** 12C will probably be useful. **Phosphorus** is also indicated for bleeding after dental work.

Ipecacuana 12C may be given for bleeding from orifices such as the nose or where there is bright red blood associated with vomiting.

Dose: Every 10 to 15 minutes where there is profuse flow of blood or hourly if bleeding is slow.

Nosebleeds

A few doses of **Phosphorus** 12C given every 5 minutes or so will usually stop a nosebleed. It is specially indicated when the bleed comes after blowing the nose and if the blood is bright red. Where this is a chronic condition it should be referred to your homoeopathic practitioner.

Massage

Nosebleeds

Hold a cold wash-cloth at base of nose and press with your finger into the centre of the upper lip just below the nose.

Chinese Remedies — Nosebleeds without provocation.

1 'Heat'

Red complexion. Red nose and lips. Red tongue with a yellow coating. Fingernails are purple. Child may grind teeth when sleeping. Prominent veins at back of ears. May be prone to mouth ulcers. Dry mouth. Thirst with desire for cold drinks. Dark urine in reduced quantity. Rapid pulse.

HUANG LIAN JIE DU TANG

2 'Deficiency'

Weak constitution. Poor sleep. Irritability. Dry mouth and throat. Tendency toward constipation. Pale complexion. Poor appetite. Usually underweight. Tongue is red without a coating.

ZHI GAN CAO TANG

BOILS

Boils are highly contagious, very painful and unfortunately quite common in childhood. Although a boil initially is only a raised patch of skin, it will turn a deep reddish or purple colour, become more painful and swollen and then a head will appear where there is a collection of pus.

Boils are usually the result of an infection caused by staphylococcal bacteria under the skin or in the hair follicle. The bacteria usually exist initially in the nose or throat and can also be present in children who do not suffer from boils. Your child's immune system will react by fighting the bacteria with white blood cells, which die in the process and form the pus in the boil. It seems that once a boil is broken, the pus can easily spread the infection.

CAUTION

Boils can actually cause blood poisoning. If the bacteria from the boil enter the blood stream causing symptoms such as fever, swelling of the lymph nodes or red radiating lines, seek medical advice immediately. It is also important to get your doctor to treat any facial boils as complications can allow the infection to spread to the brain.

The imbalance in your child's system that has allowed this boil to occur in the first place can be caused by poor fat metabolism. Your child's metabolism will be affected if too much rich, fatty food is eaten in relationship to the amount of exercise that is being done. The weather also affects the ability to metabolise fat. The warmer it is the more exercise is required to metabolise fats and proteins as they do not get utilised as quickly as when the weather is cold.

It is best to avoid eggs, chicken, dark meats, fried and fatty foods, and peanuts. Eat more fresh fruits and vegetables if this condition occurs.

Lancing a Boil

When there is a head on the boil with associated pressure it means that the boil is 'ripe' and should be lanced.

1 Sterilise a very fine, sharp needle in a flame, allow the needle to cool and then gently pierce the skin.

2 Wipe up the pus and cover with a clean pad. Be careful not to spread any seepage from the boil when cleansing and change the dressing frequently. If the boil looks as if it is not healing and is becoming infected, consult a practitioner of your choice as soon as possible.

Home Remedies

Apply any one of the suggested poultices below to the boil to calm the pain and bring the boil to a head more quickly. Change the poultice three to four times a day, more frequently if there is a discharge. Keep applying the poultice until the pain eases and the boil has gone down.

If any sign of infection occurs, seek medical advice immediately.

- Potato poultice (see Appendix 7: Compresses, Poultices and Baths).
- Fenugreek poultice (see Appendix 7: Compresses, Poultices and Baths).
- Grated potato mashed with cabbage or parsley can be applied directly on the boil (2:1).
- Apply miso directly to the boil and cover with a bandage. Change every hour or two. When the boil breaks, clean it and re-bandage without miso. Change this bandage daily, exposing the boil to the air as frequently as possible.
- White cabbage leaves can be used to draw pus. The outer leaves of the cabbage can be dipped in water and applied to any sores. Replace the leaf as it becomes warm.
- To encourage drainage of the boil, use warm Epsom Salts solution (about a 1 in 8 dilution) or a Linseed poultice (mix together 4 teaspoons of Linseed meal and enough warm water to make a paste. Apply to boil and change every 30 minutes).

Keep applying one of these until the boil drains, ensuring that the pus is caught up in a sterile bandage.

If the child is over three years of age, cleanse both the surrounding skin and boil area with undiluted tea-tree oil. If they are younger, dilute it.

Herbal Remedies

For skin infections generally where pus is present, apply a tincture consisting of 1 cup of water mixed with 1 teaspoon of one of the following substances: Hypericum, Golden Seal, Calendula, or use strong, cooled tea or a Fenugreek poultice (see Appendix 7).

Homoeopathic Remedies

In the early stages of an infection where there is inflammation, heat, burning and throbbing **Belladonna** 30C may be used.

If the site of infection is characterised by great sensitivity to touch or cold and there are offensive discharges **Hepar sulph** 12C will be the medicine of choice.

Mercurius 12C is indicated where the infection is accompanied by unusual salivation and sweating. Discharges are offensive like in **Hepar sulph**. Pains are often worse at night.

Dose: every hour when the symptoms are intense and twice daily when the symptoms are mild.

Chinese Remedies

1 'Deficiency'

Weak constitution or weakness after a prolonged febrile illness. Low energy. Pale complexion. Pale lips. Dull eyes. Pale tongue. Poor appetite. Speaks little. Quiet voice.

TUO LI XIAO DU YIN (early stage — before eruption)
QIAN JIN NEI TUO SAN (erupted with 'head')

2 'Excess'

Robust constitution. Fever and chills.

JIN FANG BAI DU SAN (chills more than fever, no sweating, general body aches and pain, muscular stiffness, tongue normal colour with a thin white coating)
WU WEI XIAO DU YIN (fever more than chills, red tongue with a yellow coating, pulse is rapid)

BUMPS AND BRUISES

Unless you wrap your children up in cotton wool, bruises are part and parcel of every childhood. They occur when the blood vessels under the skin are crushed and blood escapes into the tissue and can range in severity depending upon the cause.

General Treatment

1 Raise the affected limb if possible.
2 An ice compress or pack should be applied as quickly as possible and then at fifteen minute intervals for the next twenty-four hours. This will constrict the blood vessels, minimise swelling and also help to numb the area.

After twenty-four hours, warm applications (warm towel or heat pack) will hasten the reabsorption of the bruise by dilating the blood vessels and improving circulation.
3 Apply Arnica ointment (available from most health food stores) to the bruise if the skin is not broken. This can be done immediately and continued until the bruise is healed (three times daily). It will stop the bump from growing and the bruise from spreading.
4 If the child bruises very easily consider giving extra vitamin C with bioflavinoids. Give one tablet per day until the condition improves with 50-100 mg of Vitamin C that has bioflavinoids included in the formula. This will help build strong collagen tissue in blood vessels in the skin.

Bruising is rarely serious but if the bruise is very large you can reassure yourself with medical attention.

Herbal Remedies
Topical applications

Arnica ointment or tincture (do not give Arnica tincture internally), Calendula ointment, compress or poultice.

Calendula (Marigold)

Compress (infusion for topical use): use 2-3 teaspoons of dried flowers to 1 cup of water.

Let steep for 10 minutes, strain and let cool. Dip a piece of cotton (such as a tea-towel) in the cold decoction, fold it a couple of times and apply to affected area. Cover with a tea-towel or handkerchief and secure it with a bandage.

Homoeopathic Remedies
Bruises

An excellent remedy for bruises and any injury to soft tissue is **Arnica** 30C. It should be administered three times daily for up to five days, stopping on marked improvement.

Bumps

Where there has been a hard bump to soft tissue which results in soreness then **Arnica** 30C is the right medicine. It also serves as first aid in injuries to the head. Give one dose three times daily for up to five days.

Sprains

The first remedy to by applied in sprains is **Arnica** 30C. This may considerably relieve the pain and weakness. Should there be little progress after the first day then **Rhus-tox** 12C should be administered three times daily for up to three days.

Injuries to shins or joints

The outstanding medicine in this instance is **Ruta grav** 12C which can be given twice daily for up to three days.

Eye injuries

Symphytum 6C is an excellent remedy for a black eye and may be given three times daily until there is marked improvement.

If there has been injury to the eyeball professional advice should be sought immediately. **Aconite** 30C may be useful as there is usually great fear associated with such an injury.

Fall on the coccyx (tail bone)

When a fall on the coccyx causes pain or discomfort then **Hypericum** 30C may be used to heal the damage to nerves and shock to the spine. Give a dose twice daily for up to three days.

Crushed fingers or toes

These unfortunate accidents often call for **Arnica** 30C if there is shock involved but this should be quickly followed by doses of **Hypericum** 30C which is excellent for the pain and may be administered as often as required (even as often as every 5 minutes) to alleviate the pain. No more than five to six doses should be required before there is a marked decrease of pain. However, when pain returns or increases a further dose can be administered.

Massage

A very simple effective technique for treating bumps and bruises is a V-spread. For a bump, place one hand on the bump forming a 'V' with your fingers around the area, then find a spot behind the bump (for a skinned knee the V is over the bruise and the other hand is behind the knee). Hold for one to four minutes. You may feel a warm and tingling sensation on the injury; if so, hold until this lessens or stops.

BURNS AND SCALDS

Knowing the extent and degree of burns is important for proper treatment. Burns that cover a large part of the body may endanger the child and you should seek immediate medical attention.

- First degree burns redden and blister after a period of time.
- Second degree burns redden and blister immediately. These should be treated professionally if they cover more than ten per cent of the body. (This is an area more than twice the size of the child's palm.)
- Third degree burns should receive immediate professional attention. The skin is burnt to its full depth and may appear blackened, blistered or white in appearance.

Emergency Treatment

Minor burns (first degree)

1 Cool the burnt area immediately in cold water for at least ten minutes or until the pain has subsided. If the burns or scalds are extensive, place the child in a cold bath or pour on jugs of cold water. The cold water restricts the blood flow to the area and helps reduce the pain, as well as cleansing the skin. An ice pack can also be applied.

2 If the skin isn't broken, apply Aloe Vera gel, honey or Tea-Tree oil and cover with a sterile adhesive dressing to prevent rubbing. If the skin is broken, use Calendula, from a tube rather than a jar to avoid cross infection.

3 Do not get the burnt area wet for a few days as it needs to be dry to heal.

Major burns (second and third degree)

Many burns and scalds are more serious than they seem as there can be extensive damage to the tissues under the skin that may not be visible to the naked eye. All such burns should be assessed by a medical practitioner — see your doctor or local hospital.

- Immerse the burnt area in cold water for at least ten minutes. You can add ice to the water if practical, to speed up the cooling. This is to prevent further damage to the tissue. You can also grab something like a packet of frozen vegetables from the freezer and press it to the burnt area with an appropriate barrier such as a dishtowel.
- Wrap the child in a clean sheet or blanket and seek immediate medical attention.
- Do not use cotton wool or any fluffy material on the wound as it will stick to the burn and make treatment harder. Also, do not attempt to remove any clothing as it may have adhered to the skin and will create more damage if removed.
- Treat for shock with Bach's Rescue Remedy, which is helpful. A few drops are taken internally. However, it is optional, unlike the need to immerse the burn in cold water.

Fire

1 If your child's clothing catches fire, lie her down and extinguish the fire immediately by smothering it with a blanket or a rug, or with water or any other available liquid such as milk. If necessary, use your own body to smother the flames.

2 Do *not* remove charred clothing. Immerse the affected area in cold water immediately, for at least ten minutes.

3 Wrap the child in a clean sheet or blanket.

4 Seek urgent medical attention.

Electrical burns

- Do not touch the child until she has been removed from the electric current. Either turn off the switch, or else push the child free with something like a wooden broom handle.
- Seek medical attention immediately.
- Electrical burns can be deceptively serious as often there is only a small mark on the skin and substantial tissue damage beneath the skin. The burnt area is treated by immersing it in cold water for ten minutes.

Emergency resuscitation may be required; both artificial respiration and cardiac massage, should the child have stoped breathing, or should her heart have stopped, due to the electrical shock. If the child is unconscious, but breathing, lay her in the recovery position (see page 156) while seeking urgent medical attention. Obviously treatment for a burnt area takes second place to saving a child's life, if her heart or breathing is being affected by the electrical shock.

Chemicals and liquids

In the event of a chemical burn, first run cold water over the affected part for at least five minutes, allowing someone else to call an ambulance. If you are alone apply water first and then call for help.

If your child's clothing is saturated with a burning liquid or chemical, tear it off as you turn on the cold water tap, otherwise the burning will continue. Immerse your child in cold water for ten minutes. If an eye is affected, hold open the eyelid with your fingers and pour water from the side of the eye closest to the nose to the outside and downwards to avoid washing the chemical into the other eye. Continue for at least ten minutes and seek medical attention immediately.

Home Remedies for Minor Burns

- Adding salt to the water in which you are to immerse the burn can help prevent blisters forming. If the skin is broken from the burn, immersion in water or salt water will sting. The important thing is to rapidly cool the burnt area to prevent further damage to the surrounding tissue.
- Exclude air from the wound with substances such as honey and egg white. This will help minimise infection by excluding airborne bacteria. It also helps relieve the stinging and has a placebo effect, especially for a child with a *minor* burn. Anything more serious should be treated by a medical practitioner.
- Fresh pulp from the inside of the Aloe Vera leaf can be applied as well as Calendula ointment, Pawpaw ointment or Plantain cream.
- Tofu plaster will take the heat out of a burn

and promote healing. Crush the tofu and bind together with a little white flour. Apply to the burn. The plaster will be cool and damp, then as it draws the heat out of the burn it will become hot and dry. This will take about half an hour and once it gets to this stage the plaster will need to be replaced with a new batch. Continue this process until all the heat has been removed from the burn.
- Except for Vitamin E oil squeezed directly onto the burn from the capsule, do not apply any oil or grease to the burn. Vitamin E reduces pain, scarring and damage and accelerates the healing of many kinds of burns.
- Combine 2 teaspoons slippery elm bark and 1 teaspoon vitamin E oil in a jar and stir till they form a paste that clings to your fingertip without sliding off (best to mix with your fingers), spread onto burns, cover with a bandage to prevent it from getting wet. Leave for 7-10 days at which time the scab will fall off leaving a healthy skin underneath.

Home Remedies for Electric Shock

- Honey is an antiseptic and healing substance. Immerse the burn in water until the pain has stopped, coat with Honey and cover with gauze. Reapply after a few hours.
- Squeeze the gel of one Aloe Vera leaf over the burn. This will lessen the pain and reduce the chances of infection or scarring.

Homoeopathic Remedies

Minor burns

Cantharis 30C will alleviate the pain of burns and the dose can be repeated whenever the pain returns. It is useful for the rapid healing of first and second degree burns and will often prevent blistering if administered immediately.

Calendula cream is an excellent external aid to the healing of wounds.

Electric shock

Where electric shock has been suffered **Phosphorus** 12C will often relieve the symptoms.

Dose: Three times daily for one to three days (stop on marked improvement).

CHICKENPOX

Chickenpox is very common in children. The first signs are irritability, loss of appetite, headache, runny nose, sneezing, slight fever and possible lower backache. After one or two days small red spots begin to appear, usually on the chest, and within a few hours change to very itchy, watery blisters. More spots will appear over the next few days and in severe cases the whole body will be affected. A cough is very likely to occur at this stage.

Encourage your child not to scratch the sores. Infection can also occur and result in scarring. They will leak out watery fluid and will still continue to itch after scratching.

Gradually the symptoms will subside and complete recovery takes about two weeks. There is no orthodox medical treatment for chickenpox, so it is not usually necessary to seek out medical attention. Complications are uncommon, although occasionally the blisters can become infected.

Keep your child quiet when there is a fever and let her drink lots of fluid to prevent dehydration from the fever. The fever that is often associated with viral infections such as chickenpox is actually helpful. It is a sign that a strong immune system is at war with the virus. Viruses are unable to live in high temperatures, so do not panic if you see a fever. (For more information see the section on Fever.)

The incubation period of this viral infection lasts anywhere from two to three weeks. It is usually caught by contact with infected children or people. Your child will be contagious for about two weeks, beginning twenty-four hours before the rash appears, until all the blisters have cleared.

Even a healthy child will get chickenpox. If your child is strong and healthy, her immune system will react vigorously to the virus and the disease will pass through without complications.

Prevention

Even though you cannot really prevent chickenpox you can do some things to reduce the severity. The most obvious is to minimise the exposure of your child to anyone who has chickenpox. The more they are exposed to the virus, the more severe the attack will be. Try to keep your child's immune system healthy by reducing her intake of sugar, processed food, chemical additives and fatty food. If your child has allergies, do try to minimise her exposure to the substances that cause them.

General Care and Cautions

A child with chickenpox, despite her dramatic red and spotty appearance, usually is not all that sick. She may not want to go to bed and there is no need to force her. The main discomfort is usually the itchiness of the rash. It is a good idea to cut her fingernails to minimise the damage that could be done by scratching.

You can help relieve the itch by bathing her in tepid water with cornstarch or arrowroot. Be careful when drying the child not to break the blisters or disturb the scabs.

Herbal Remedies

Golden Seal and Yellow Dock relieve itching and reduce infection and inflammation. The Calendula will help with infection as will Tea-Tree

---

CAUTION

Complications may occur if the child suddenly shows a very high fever with headache, vomiting or convulsions. If the lymph glands under the arms, groin or neck become red or tender you should seek medical attention. Also watch for any broken blood vessels or spontaneous bruising under the skin, as these are also a sign of possible complications.

oil dabbed on the sores. You can also use cold Witch Hazel tincture directly on the itchy spots; pat them dry and then apply some cornstarch or arrowroot directly to the area.

Echinacea

Echinacea stimulates the immune system and is indicated in all infections so that they may be dealt with quickly and effectively by the body's own defence mechanisms.

Decoction: use 1 teaspoon of dried root and rhizome to 1 cup of water, simmer covered for 5 minutes. Dilute with water. Can be sweetened with honey or rice malt.

DOSE
1-2 years: 10-15 mL (⅓-½ fl oz) 3 times daily
3-4 years: 20-30 mL (⅔-1 fl oz) 3 times daily
5-6 years: 40-50 mL (1⅓-1½ fl oz) 3 times daily
7 years and older: 60-100 mL (2-3 fl oz) 3 times daily

Golden Seal

Decoction for topical application: use 2 teaspoons of chopped root and rhizome to a cup of water, simmer covered for 5-10 minutes, strain.

Yellow Dock

Decoction for topical application: use 2 teaspoons of chopped root to a cup of water, simmer covered for 5-10 minutes, strain.

Calendula (Marigold)

Infusion for topical use: use 2-3 teaspoons of dried flowers to 1 cup of water. Let steep for 10 minutes, strain.

Homoeopathic Remedies

If the eruptions are large or pusy and the child is drowsy with a thick tongue then **Antimonium tart** 12C will be indicated. It is specially indicated if associated with bronchitis.

If the child is weepy and thirstless despite the fever then **Pulsatilla** 12C should be your choice.

Rhus-tox 12C is needed when there are itching and burning eruptions on the skin. Extreme mental and physical restlessness will confirm this choice of remedy.

If your remedy choice is not clear you should make a further study of the remedies mentioned in the Materia Medica. Other indicated medicines are Aconite, Apis, Belladonna, Ferrum-phos, Gelsemium, Mercurius and Sulphur.

Dose: One dose twice daily.

Chinese Remedies

Symptoms are due to 'Dampness', 'Heat' and 'Toxins' which need to be eliminated from the system.

WU LING SAN
GE GEN TANG (mild symptoms, delicate constitution)

CHOKING

Choking can be very frightening especially for your young child, so it is imperative that you keep your cool. Choking happens when a foreign body such as a button, small toy, or food such as peanuts enters into the passage to the lungs instead of the stomach. In most cases your child will still be able to breathe. Coughing or gagging is the body's first natural reaction. Most of the time this will regurgitate the offending object so that no further treatment is needed.

Emergency Treatment

- If the child can speak or cry, but is coughing or wheezing, the air passage is partially blocked. In this case take your child to a doctor or hospital or call an ambulance. Do *not* take the following measures of slapping on the back, as it might dislodge the object and completely constrict the airway.

- If the object can be easily seen and your child starts gasping and going blue or grey, try to hook out whatever is blocking the throat with your fingers. This should be done while holding the infant upside down.

- If the airway cannot be cleared, place the child, head down, across your forearm or knee and give three to four sharp blows with the heel of one hand between the infant's shoulder blades.

- If your child is still not breathing try the abdominal thrust described below, but only as a last resort, as it can damage internal organs.

For a baby

Lay the baby on a flat surface on her back with the head tilted back to open the airway. Place your first two fingers between breast bone and navel and press up and inwards in a quick movement, hard enough to dislodge the obstruction. Repeat until the obstruction is removed.

For a child

Sit the child on your lap, clench your hand and place it under her breast-bone and above her navel. Press suddenly inwards and upwards. Repeat up to four times to dislodge the blockage. Turn the child head down and hit between shoulder blades until she breathes again or help arrives.

If abdominal thrust does not seem to be working, commence mouth-to-mouth or mouth-to-nose resuscitation and ensure medical help is on the way.

If the passage is blocked, mouth-to-mouth won't really help unless it is combined with attempts to dislodge the obstruction.

Home Remedy

For an object stuck in the throat

- If a child swallows a fishbone or similar object and it becomes stuck, quickly get a piece of bread (soft white bread works best) pull out the middle and get the child to eat it. The mass of sticky dough can help move the object without pain.

- Try to get the child to sneeze — you can put pepper under the nose. A sneeze can sometimes dislodge an object stuck in the throat.

COLDS AND FLU

Colds are the most common of ailments affecting children and adults alike, and the only difference seems to be that children have more of them: six per year is considered fairly average to the age of six or seven, when the immune system matures. The symptoms of the common cold will vary from one child to another and can include runny nose, coughing, sneezing, fever, watery eyes, diarrhoea, fatigue and listlessness. Flu is a common term applied to a wide variety of viral illnesses, with similar symptoms to colds and more, for example, diarrhoea, nausea, vomiting, body aches and pains, and a higher fever in most cases.

Many of the infectious illnesses of childhood seem to manifest in the early stages as flu-like illnesses so it is important to keep a special eye on your child if she seems to have a cold. If there are nasal secretions and they are mostly clear, white or grey, there is bound to be a viral infection involved. If they turn green or yellow it is likely that there is bacterial infection as well.

While babies have a hard time breathing and eating at the same time and often exhibit poor sleep patterns while they have a cold, older children often seem quite unchanged in eating, sleeping and play behaviours.

There is a real possibility that if you take your child to the doctor, she will be prescribed an antibiotic. Antibiotics are of no real value in treating viral infections (See page 11 for more information about antibiotics.) The flu and the common cold do not require any medical treatment. The medications often suggested merely relieve the symptoms and can often interfere with the body's own efforts to heal itself. They can have undesirable or dangerous side-effects and can also be a waste of money.

We can do some things to get our children through a cold more comfortably or perhaps a little more quickly, but mild colds are hardly worth treating; the symptoms usually cause little discomfort. If the cold is quite severe, however, you should treat it, especially if there is a history of lung problems, to stop it from becoming a cough as well.

The viruses which cause colds and flu are able to take hold more easily if the immune system is weakened in any way. Thus fatigue, stress, nutritional deficiencies including vitamin A, many of the B vitamins, vitamin D, zinc and protein and a diet high in refined sugar and fat will increase your child's susceptibility to colds. You can strengthen your child's immune system and ward off at least some colds by:

- Not allowing your child to become overtired.
- Dressing her appropriately for the weather to avoid unnecessary stress on the body.
- Avoid a diet with refined sugar, too much fat and refined and processed foods.
- Provide lots of love, cuddles and reassurance daily.
- If necessary, give vitamin and mineral supplements that support the immune system, for example, zinc, vitamin C, B complex and vitamin A. A preparation which contains all of these is probably the best way to go, or you can supplement as follows:
- Vitamin C — over the age of three, up to 5000 mg of powder can be taken daily if there is no diarrhoea. If there is diarrhoea, cut back on the dose. Do not stop vitamin C too quickly as the cold can worsen due to rebound vitamin C depletion. Under the age of three, one should not exceed a dosage of 2000 mg.
- Zinc — 25 mg per day over three years. Under three take no more than 10 mg.
- Vitamin A — 10 000 units per day over three years of age. Under three years, 5000 units per day.
- Cod liver oil used to be a very popular supplement for children who always had colds. This is a good source of vitamin A and has the added benefit of containing the omega 3 fatty acids which help the activity of the immune system.

Some children seem to always have a runny or stuffed nose or sniffles. Many of these children may have allergies to either food or inhalants such as dust, moulds or pollens. Children with allergies are much more susceptible to colds and so dealing with the allergy becomes the means by which you can help them strengthen their immune system and resist colds. (See Allergies).

Diet

Is the saying 'feed a cold and starve a fever' or is it the other way around? No one ever seems to remember. The basic rule should be to let the appetite dictate. Studies done with fasting have shown that during the first thirty-six hours of fasting the immune system is stimulated in its function. After this time the opposite seems to occur and the immune system slows down a little. So if your child goes off her food, realise that this might be helpful; however, it is best not to force a fast on a child who wants to eat.

If there are signs of heat, such as fever, dryness of the mouth, thirst, very sore throat and so on, the diet should include more watery food such as cooked fruits and vegetables.

If there are more signs of cold and chill, including mild fever, runny nose with clear liquid, etc. then the child should be eating lots of warm chicken soup with garlic or ginger, stews and teas. Avoid foods containing excessive amounts of fat, sugar, spices and shellfish.

Home Remedies

- For a cold with low fever, try ginger, garlic and honey tea if your child is over three years of age: mix together a teaspoon of freshly grated ginger, 1 crushed clove of garlic, juice of ½ lemon and 2 teaspoons honey. Pour 1 cup boiling water over this, leave it for a few minutes, then strain. Drink every few hours until the body begins to feel warm.
- For small, breastfeeding babies, a humidifier is a useful thing. You can put a little eucalyptus oil in the water so the steam is antiseptic and soothing.
- Keep your child warm and dry and not over-excited.
- If your child has a stuffy nose and cannot breathe properly, try a few drops of saline solution in each nostril, wait a moment and then suck out the congestion with an infant aspirator.
- Use water-soluble Tea-Tree oil in a steam bath or vaporiser.
- Give plenty of boiled water, herbal teas, warm broths and vegetable juices to drink.
- To reduce the fever and relieve minor aches and pains try a Mint and Rosemary bath:
  125 g (4 oz) fresh or dried Peppermint
  125 g (4 oz) fresh or dried Rosemary
  8 cups cold water
  Combine the herbs and water, cover and simmer for 15 minutes. Strain and discard herbs. Pour the tea into the bathtub and fill the bath with lukewarm water. Have your child bathe at least 15 minutes. Repeat daily till symptoms disappear. (If symptoms or fever gets worse after bathing consult a practitioner.)

Naturopathic Remedies

Some tried and true Western herbs for colds include Elderflowers (for fever or hot conditions), Echinacea (especially good for chronic conditions), Peppermint and Yarrow. These can be found mixed together in cold and flu mixtures or can be in the form of tinctures or teas. Licorice and Ginger (for colds and chills) may be included to help the effects of the other herbs. Horseradish is also good for cold and chills and Fenugreek will help clear mucus.

Chronic colds

If your child is one of the many who seems to never really get rid of a cold, or seems to keep catching them just after she has become well again, she should be treated by a natural practitioner as there could be an underlying weakness that needs to be looked after and strengthened.

Herbal Remedies

Echinacea

Echinacea stimulates the immune system and is indicated in all infections so that they may be dealt with quickly and effectively by the body's own defence mechanisms.
Decoction: use 1 teaspoon of dried root and rhizome to 1 cup of water, simmer covered for 5 minutes. Dilute with water if necessary. Can be sweetened with honey or rice malt.
DOSE
1-2 years: 10-15 mL (⅓-½ fl oz) 3 times daily
3-4 years: 20-30 mL (⅔-1 fl oz) 3 times daily

5-6 years: 40-50 mL (1⅓-1½ fl oz) 3 times daily
7 years and older: 60-100 mL (2-3 fl oz) 3 times daily

Elderflowers

For fever or hot conditions.
Infusion: use 2 teaspoons of the dried flowers to 1 cup of boiling water. Let steep for 5 minutes, strain. Can be sweetened with honey or rice malt.
DOSE
1-2 years: 15-30 mL (½-1 fl oz) 3 times daily
3-4 years: 40-60 mL (1⅓-2 fl oz) 3 times daily
5-6 years: 70-90 mL (2⅓-3 fl oz) 3 times daily
7 years and older: 100-150 mL (3-5 fl oz) 3 times daily

Peppermint

Use as a decongestant and for fever or hot conditions.
Infusion: use ½-1 teaspoon of dried herb to 1 cup of boiling water. Let steep for 5 minutes, strain. Can be sweetened with honey or rice malt. Dilute with water if necessary.
DOSE
1-2 years: 15-30 mL (½-1 fl oz) 3 times daily
3-4 years: 40-60 mL (1⅓-2 fl oz) 3 times daily
5-6 years: 70-90 mL (2⅓-3 fl oz) 3 times daily
7 years and older: 100-150 mL (3-5 fl oz) 3 times daily

Yarrow

Yarrow is good for fever or hot conditions.
Infusion: use 1 teaspoon of dried herb to 1 cup of boiling water. Let steep for 5 minutes, strain. Can be sweetened with honey or rice malt. Dilute with water if necessary.
DOSE
1-2 years: 15-30 mL (½-1 fl oz) 3 times daily
3-4 years: 40-60 mL (1⅓-2 fl oz) 3 times daily
5-6 years: 70-90 mL (2⅓-3 fl oz) 3 times daily
7 years and older: 100-150 mL (3-5 fl oz) 3 times daily

Ginger

The warming qualities of Ginger are very beneficial in cases of colds and flu. The herb increases digestion and circulation and helps the patient 'sweat it out'.
Infusion: use 3 slices (2-3 cm/1 inch in diameter and 3 mm/⅛ inch thick) of fresh Ginger to 1 cup of boiling water. Let steep for 5 minutes. Sweeten with honey or rice malt. Dilute with water for small children.
DOSE
2-3 years: 20 mL (⅔ fl oz) 2 to 3 times daily

4-5 years: 30-50 mL (1-1½ fl oz) 2 to 3 times daily
6 years and older: 60-80 mL (2-2⅔ fl oz) 2 to 3 times daily

Licorice

Suitable if there is constipation or cough.
Decoction: use ½ teaspoon chopped Licorice root to 1 cup of water. Simmer covered for 10 minutes.
DOSE
1-2 years: 20 mL (⅔ fl oz) 3 times daily
3-4 years: 30-50 mL (1-1½ fl oz) 3 times daily
5-6 years: 60-80 mL (2-2⅔ fl oz) 3 times daily
7 years and older: 100-120 mL (3-3⅔ fl oz) 3 times daily

Horseradish

Horseradish is suitable for cold and chills.
　　Best given freshly grated. Grated Horseradish is available from delicatessens and supermarkets. Due to its very pungent taste it is not suitable for smaller children. Never force a child to eat it. The best way to give it is to spread a little on a piece of bread.

Fenugreek

Fenugreek will help clear mucus.
Decoction: use 1 teaspoon of the crushed seeds to 1 cup of water. Simmer for 5 minutes, strain. Can be sweetened with honey or rice malt. Dilute with water if necessary.
DOSE
1-2 years: 15-30 mL (½-1 fl oz) 3 times daily
3-4 years: 40-60 mL (1⅓-2 fl oz) 3 times daily
5-6 years: 70-90 mL (2⅓-3 fl oz) 3 times daily
7 years and older: 100-150 mL (3-5 fl oz) 3 times daily

Eucalyptus oil

This is a decongestant.
　　A few drops of the essential oil can be put in an oil-burner or in a saucepan with hot water and placed in the room. Another good way of administering Eucalyptus oil is to put a few (2-4) drops in the child's bath.

CAUTION
Never give Eucalyptus oil internally to a child and do not apply it directly to the skin.

Homoeopathic Remedies

Colds

Aconite 30C is effective if given early and especially after exposure to cold and dry winds. A hot and dry fever is often present but a chilly phase may also occur.

Arsenicum 12C for children who catch colds easily from change of weather with sneezing and watery, burning discharge. When fever develops it is accompanied by great exhaustion. You may observe a thirst for small amounts of water. Colds may move to the chest.

The **Nux vomica** 30C child has sniffles. The nose is alternately blocked or running, stuffed up at night but flowing in a warm room and better if outside. The feeling of chilliness is predominant and specially if the child is uncovered. The symptoms are often accompanied by irritability.

Belladonna, Bryonia, Ferrum phos, Gelsemium, Hepar sulph, Natrum-mur, Pulsatilla and Rhus-tox may be of benefit when their own characteristic physical and mental symptoms are indicated.

Dose: One dose three times daily for up to two days.

Flu

When you are presented with streaming watery mucus from the nose, chilliness and great weakness, then **Arsenicum** 12C should be given. You may also note burning pains, thirst for sips of water, restlessness and anxiety.

Should your child be very drowsy with heaviness of the body together with drooping or closing eyes, think of **Gelsemium** 30C. There may be associated chills, aches and pains all over the body and an absence of thirst.

Nux vomica 30C is very chilly, worse from exposure to the cold and the open air. Any movement seems to aggravate the chilliness. The limbs and back ache and the nose are stuffed up. The child is often very chilly.

Dose: Once dose three times daily for up to three days is recommended.

Other remedies such as Arnica, Bryonia, Rhus-tox and Phosphorus may be considered when the above remedies do not seem appropriate.

Chinese Remedies

Most children show a predominance of heat symptoms in the early stages of colds and flu.

However it is not unusual for a child to have a predominance of cold symptoms and then change from cold to hot fairly rapidly.

The following changes may occur when your child's condition changes from cold to hot:
- Facial colour — from white to red.
- Colour of mucus — from white to yellow.
- Temperature of hands and feet — from cold to hot.
- If vein at 'San Guan' is red, it may change to purple.

1 'Cold'

Chills and fever. Irritability. Requires warm clothing and coverings. Aversion to cold draughts. Tiredness. Loss of appetite. Runny nose with clear watery mucus. Sneezing. There may be a cough with pale, watery mucus. Tongue is normal colour with a thin white coat. Red vein at 'San Guan'.

GE GEN TANG (high fever)
JIN FANG BAI DU SAN (pain and stiffness of neck, headache, general body aches and pains)
XIAO QING LONG TANG (copious mucus and chills)
XIAO CHAI HU TANG (delicate constitution — see moon pattern page 39-40)
REN SHEN BAI DU SAN (delicate constitution with neck stiffness, general body aches and pains, headache)

2 'Heat'

Fever and chills. Aversion to warmth (both clothing and room temperature). Irritability. Tiredness. Loss of appetite. Red complexion. Head is hot. Runny nose and sneezing with thick yellow or green-grey mucus. Sore throat or cough with thick yellow or grey-green mucus. Tongue is red and may have a yellow coating (initially it may be white and then change to yellow after two to three days). Eyes are red. Urine is dark and smaller amount. Purple vein at 'San Guan'. The veins at the back of the ears may become prominent.

SANG JU YIN (early stage mild symptoms)
YIN QIAO SAN (severe)

3 'Heat' and 'Dampness'

Summer time head-cold. Abdominal pain. Vomiting. Diarrhoea. Thick 'greasy' coating on the tongue. There may be a combination of 'cold' and 'hot' symptoms and signs.

XIANG RU SAN

Massage

Colds and sinus colds

- Press into the pad of each toe with your thumb. Hold for five to thirty seconds. Do this on each foot until tenderness decreases. It's easy to hold and carry your baby while you do this. Babies seem to prefer having their feet worked on. You can repeat this technique every half hour on infants. This helps relieve the sinuses.
- Rotate the big toe on each foot and press in with your thumb all around each big toe, from base of toe to tip.

Suggestions for older children

- Place thumbs on either side of your child's nose and press down and slightly up while following the contours of the cheekbone. Press down into tender spots just below child's pain threshold and hold for five to thirty seconds.
- Place middle fingers on either side of the midline at the base of skull, pressing into any tender spots and hold for five to thirty seconds.
- Place fingers (or thumbs) on the centre of the forehead and smoothly draw them across. Use moderate pressure, just enough to stretch the skin as you draw across. When you reach the temples use your middle finger tips to make small circles using a light touch.

Flu

Symptoms of fever, aching limbs, stomach pain and/or listlessness are most common. To relieve and assist your child through these symptoms, first bathe her feet in tepid water. Then work on each foot.

- Rotate each toe, then press into the centre of each toe and hold for a few seconds.
- On the bottom of the foot, press directly under the big toe, and hold. If there is any tenderness, continue to press until it eases.
- Press across the ball of each foot with your index finger or thumb, working under each toe as well. Under the little toe on the left foot, press in deeply from middle of foot up to base of little toe.
- Also on the left foot make thumb prints across the bottom of foot from the midline of foot into the ball of the foot.
- Make small circles around the ankle bones (of each foot). Press into any tender points. These will help the flow of lymph fluid, which is beneficial for the immune system.

COLIC

Colic occurs mainly in infants and young children, and is caused by a spasm of the muscles in the intestines. It appears as an abdominal cramp or indigestion.

Colic begins between the ages of one and four weeks and often ends as quickly as it began when your baby is three or four months old. Your infant will usually cry at least one to two hours or longer at the same time every day. She may move her arms vigorously with her fists clenched and her knees flexed towards the abdomen. She may arch her head and body backwards and her cry may be persistent and very loud. Her face may be pale, and a bluish-grey colour will often appear between the lips and the nose. She may exhibit flatulence and or burping and a rumbling noise in the abdomen, and her abdomen may be tense or distended.

Causes

Over the years an astonishing number of causes have been proposed. Research has dispelled the majority of these and to put your mind at ease, rest assured that the majority of children with symptoms of colic do not have anything drastically wrong with them physically or emotionally.

The most common causes are:
- Not burping the baby after feeding
- Overfeeding
- Breastfeeding on demand
- Excessive excitability of the nerves to the intestine and lack of proper inhibitory control by those nerves
- Exposure to cold, especially around the abdomen
- If breastfeeding, the mother eating foods which may cause an allergic reaction, such as dairy food (especially milk), wheat, gluten, eggs, and peanuts, yeast and oranges.
- Swallowing air when feeding
- Introducing too many kinds of food (after introducing solids) too quickly

- Too many foods with roughage such as wholemeal breads and raw vegetables
- Too much rich food
- Cold, refrigerated foods
- Raw bananas, cucumber, lettuce, yoghurt, celery and apple (eaten by the breastfeeding mother or the child)

Care of the Colicky Baby

- Ensure that your baby is not suffering from any other illness. check for fever, watch for changes in her bowel movement and make sure that your baby is getting enough food.
- Feed your baby slowly and prevent her swallowing air during feeding if breast or bottle feeding. Keep the baby in a semi-upright position unless your milk supply is flowing too rapidly. In that case lie down with your baby or place her on your chest, her tummy touching yours so that she has to work harder at sucking.
- Avoid the foods listed above.
- Avoid food that gives you wind if you are breastfeeding.
- If you are giving cow's milk, try goat's milk instead.
- Relax and don't try to do too much yourself.

Home Remedies

- Rhythmic movement and vibration help a child with colic. The use of a vibrating pillow under the abdomen can be very helpful.
- If you think there might be a possible deficiency in your milk which is contributing to the problem, try supplementing your diet with zinc, magnesium and calcium. The baby can also be given these minerals at about ¼ of the adult dose.
- Onion tea relaxes and soothes the spasms:
  5 thin slices of yellow onion
  2 cups water
  Combine the onion and water in a saucepan, cover and simmer 15 minutes. Strain and

discard the onion slices. When cool give 4 tablespoons of the onion tea two times daily either in a spoon, eye dropper or bottle. Discard the tea after two days if not used. If your child seems to get worse after two doses or does not respond at all, consult a practitioner of your choice.

• Gripe water can be prepared from a tea or syrup consisting of Dill or Fennel seeds by infusion (see below), with a little Ginger and Cloves (also useful for reducing flatulence).

CURE FOR COLIC

New research from St. James Hospital in Leeds shows that many babies with colic are allergic either to cow's milk or if breast fed to cow's milk products eaten by their mothers.

Some colicky babies may respond to a switch from breast or bottle milk to a lactose-fructose-and gluten-free formula.

Herbal Remedies

Any of the following herbal remedies may be given to relieve colic and wind:

Dill

Infusion: use ½-1 teaspoon of the dried seeds (best lightly crushed in a mortar) to 1 cup of boiling water. Let steep for 5 minutes, strain. Dilute with water if necessary.
DOSE
1-2 years: 15-30 mL (½-1 fl oz) 3 times daily
3-4 years: 40-60 mL (1⅓-2 fl oz) 3 times daily
5-6 years: 70-90 mL (2⅓-3 fl oz) 3 times daily
7 years and older: 100-150 mL (3-5 fl oz) 3 times daily

Fennel

Infusion: use ½-1 teaspoon of the dried seeds (best lightly crushed in a mortar) to 1 cup of boiling water. Let steep for 5 minutes, strain. Dilute with water if necessary.
DOSE
1-2 years: 15-30 mL (½-1 fl oz) 3 times daily
3-4 years: 40-60 mL (1⅓-2 fl oz) 3 times daily
5-6 years: 70-90 mL (2⅓-3 fl oz) 3 times daily
7 years and older: 100-150 mL (3-5 fl oz) 3 times daily

Caraway

Infusion: use ½-1 teaspoon of the dried seeds (best lightly crushed in a mortar) to 1 cup of boiling water. Let steep for 5 minutes, strain. Can be sweetened with honey or rice malt. Dilute with water if necessary.
DOSE
1-2 years: 15-30 mL (½-1 fl oz) 3 times daily
3-4 years: 40-60 mL (1⅓-2 fl oz) 3 times daily
5-6 years: 70-90 mL (2⅓-3 fl oz) 3 times daily
7 years and older: 100-150 mL (3-5 fl oz) 3 times daily

Cumin

Infusion: use ½ teaspoon of the dried seeds (best lightly crushed in a mortar) to 1 cup of boiling water. Let steep for 5 minutes, strain. Can be sweetened with honey or rice malt. Dilute with water if necessary.
DOSE
1-2 years: 15-30 mL (½-1 fl oz) 3 times daily
3-4 years: 40-60 mL (1⅓-2 fl oz) 3 times daily
5-6 years: 70-90 mL (2⅓-3 fl oz) 3 times daily
7 years and older: 100-150 mL (3-5 fl oz) 3 times daily

Cinnamon

Infusion: use ½ teaspoon of the crushed, dried bark quills to 1 cup of boiling water. Let steep for 5 minutes, strain. Can be sweetened with honey or rice malt. Dilute with water if necessary.
DOSE
1-2 years: 15-30 mL (½-1 fl oz) 3 times daily
3-4 years: 40-60 mL (1⅓-2 fl oz) 3 times daily
5-6 years: 70-90 mL (2⅓-3 fl oz) 3 times daily
7 years and older: 100-150 mL (3-5 fl oz) 3 times daily

Chamomile

Infusion: use 1 teaspoon dried flowerheads to 1 cup of boiling water. Let steep for 5 minutes, strain. Dilute with water for smaller children.
DOSE
1-2 years: 20-40 mL (⅔-1⅓ fl oz) 3 to 4 times daily
3-4 years: 50-80 mL (1⅔-2⅔ fl oz) 3 to 4 times daily
5-6 years: 100-125 mL (3-4 fl oz) 3 to 4 times daily
7 years and older: 150-200 mL (5-6⅔ fl oz) 3 to 4 times daily

Homoeopathic Remedies

When your child is arching the back in response to the pain, use **Dioscorea** 12C.

If, on the other hand, the child bends double in response to the pain, then **Colocynthis** 12C will be of great benefit.

Where the colic is associated with teething, the child is irritable, restless and wants to be carried, use **Chamomilla** 30C.

If the child is alleviated by being held with the abdomen pressed into the shoulder, then **Stannum metallicum** 12C is the indicated medicine.

If there is bloating of the abdomen and a large amount of belching and gas associated with the pain, then **Carb-veg** 12C may be given.

Other remedies including Bryonia, Ipecac, Mag-phos, Pulsatilla and Staphisagria may be used where the character of the symptoms and the temperament of the child are indicated.

Dose: One dose every 20 minutes if the colic is severe and one dose twice daily if it is mild.

Chinese Remedies
1 'Heat'

Red complexion. Red lips. Crying is loud and prolonged with tears. Restlessness. Constipation.

GAN MAI DA ZAO TANG
QING XIN CHA taken together with GUI ZHI TANG more pronounced symptoms of heat: fever, purple vein at 'San Guan', rapid pulse, crying sounds frightened

2 'Cold'

Pale complexion. Pale lips. Cold hands and feet. Subdued or quiet crying. Loose stools or diarrhoea.

BAI SHAO GAN CAO TANG to be taken at the time of symptoms

XIAO JIAN ZHONG TANG to be taken during the day as a general tonic

Massage

Colic can be very stressful for both babies and parents. These massage strokes can help everyone to relax. It's important to do this routine at least twice a day for two weeks to help relieve the symptoms. Don't be discouraged the first few times, if there is little relief; keep on with the routine as it takes a while for your baby's system to change.

1 With your baby lying down in front of you, on a cushion, changing table or the bed, use a small amount of oil (size of a five cent piece) and rub your hands together briskly to warm oil. Massage the tummy with hands open, one hand following the other from base of ribcage to bottom of tummy. Do this at least six times.
2 Hold your baby's knees and push them together up into the tummy. Hold for about thirty seconds.
3 Release the knees and gently pat legs, rocking them from side to side with your hands, notice when your child begins to relax (the muscles become softer), smile and praise her.
4 Massage the tummy in a clockwise direction with hands open and conforming to your child's abdomen, making a full circle with your right hand and followed by a half circle with your left hand. Do this at least six times.
5 Holding your baby's knees together, push them up and into tummy. Hold gently there for thirty seconds; child may expel wind.
6 Let legs relax, and gently rock and shake legs to loosen any tension.

Repeat this sequence three times. Some babies will respond better than others to this routine. A warm bath or warm water bottle will also help baby's tummy to relax. Try the massage after bath as well.

CONJUNCTIVITIS

Conjunctiva are the delicate layers of tissue covering the eye, including the mucous membrane on the inside of the eyelid. Conjunctivitis is a viral infection that can cause this tissue to become red, itchy and sore. When a secondary bacterial infection sets in, mucus is produced, collects in the corners of the eyes and spills over onto the cheeks. It may dry on the lashes at night, causing them to stick together. Often nasal irritation and discharge are also present.

Conjunctivitis is highly contagious, so it is often passed between family members or amongst students at school or playgroup. It can also be 'caught' at your local swimming pool, so encouraging your child to wear goggles when she puts her head under water is a great idea. It can also be caused by a sudden increase in dust, pollens or moulds in the air (an allergic reaction), or by close contact with an animal, especially cats and dogs.

General Treatment

It is important to treat conjunctivitis immediately, even though the body will normally clear the infection by itself.

- Wash the eyes with a solution made by dissolving ½ teaspoon of salt in 1 cup of warm water. Repeat regularly.
- Remove any specks of dust or other foreign bodies that may be irritating the eye.
- If one member of your family has the infection, try not to spread it. Encourage the infectious child to use only one towel, pillowcase, etc. and wash these regularly as the infection starts to heal.

Home Remedies

- Place a cool, moist teabag on each closed eye for about 5-10 minutes or as long as the child will lie still. (Try reading a story to her while she is lying down.)
- If your child will not stay still, just wash the affected area with cotton wool that has been dipped in cool tea, squeezing out several drops of tea in each eye if possible.
- A good remedy for babies with conjunctivitis is to squirt breast milk in their eyes.
- Bathe the eye in one drop of freshly squeezed lemon juice and 1-2 tablespoons boiled tepid water. This should be further diluted for infants. Test it on your own eye to make sure it doesn't burn.

Herbal Remedies

There are four herbal remedies good for treating conjunctivitis: Eyebright, used topically as an eyewash as well as internally; Calendula as an astringent and anti-inflammatory eyewash; Fennel as an anti-inflammatory and antiseptic; and Golden Seal as an astringent and anti-inflammatory eyewash.

Eyebright

Infusion: use 1 teaspoon of dried herb to 1 cup of boiling water. Let steep for 5 minutes, strain. Can be sweetened with honey or rice malt. Dilute with water if necessary. As an eyewash, use unsweetened and undiluted.

DOSE
1-2 years: 15-30 mL (½-1 fl oz) 3 times daily
3-4 years: 40-60 mL (1⅓-2 fl oz) 3 times daily
5-6 years: 70-90 mL (2⅓-3 fl oz) 3 times daily
7 years and older: 100-150 mL (3-5 fl oz) 3 times daily

Calendula (Marigold)

Infusion for topical application as eyewash: use 3 teaspoons of the dried flowerheads to 1 cup of boiling water. Let steep for 5 minutes, strain and let cool down before applying.

Fennel

Infusion for topical application as eyewash: use 2 teaspoons of the dried fruits to 1 cup of water, let steep for 5-10 minutes, strain and let cool down before applying.

Golden seal

Decoction for topical application as eyewash: use
½ teaspoon of chopped root and rhizome to 1
cup of water, simmer covered for 5-10 minutes,
strain and let cool down before applying.

Homoeopathic Remedies

When the eyes and lids are inflamed and red
with a watery burning and acidic discharge
Euphrasia 12C is called for. The discharge may
become thick and yellow.

When the discharge is profuse and yellow
and does not irritate the skin **Pulsatilla** 12C
is often indicated. This is especially indicated
if the condition is worse in a warm room.

Sometimes Arsenicum, Chamomilla and
Mercury are indicated in this condition.
Dose: One dose taken three times daily.

Chinese Remedies

1 'Heat'

Fever and chills. Aversion to warmth. Irritability. Loss of appetite. Tiredness. Red complexion.
Runny nose with thick yellow or green-grey
mucus. Sore throat or cough with similar
mucus. Eyes are red. Urine is dark and reduced
amount. Tongue is red and the coating is
initially white and changes to yellow after two
to three days. Veins at back of ears may be
prominent
SANG JU YIN
WU WEI XIAO DU YIN (high fever, deep red
tongue with a yellow coating, rapid and forceful
pulse, pussy discharge from the eye)

1 'Fire'

In contrast to the above situation there is an
abrupt onset of symptoms without the preceding and accompanying symptoms of an acute
head cold of the 'hot' type. There is usually
constipation and irritability and the child may
complain of a bitter taste in the mouth. The
tongue is red with a yellow coating. The pulse
is rapid and forceful. The complexion is red and
the left cheek may have a darker hue. The urine
is darker than normal and there may be
difficulty in passing it.
LONG DAN XIE GAN TANG

Massage

Press with thumb on the bottom of foot at the
base of second, third and fourth toes. These
points may be tender, but press in as deep as
the child can tolerate and hold for thirty
seconds. Do this on both feet.

CONSTIPATION

Because children have their own unique body rhythms, it can be difficult to decide what is the normal pattern of bowel movements for a particular child. For breastfed babies a bowel motion may happen every few days or a few times a day; both patterns are normal. Older children who are fully weaned on to a diet which contains plenty of whole grains, fruits and vegetables will usually go to the toilet daily, but for some on the same type of diet it is normal every second day. The most important thing to check is that there is no pain or discomfort and the stool is of a good consistency and buoyant.

If your baby is having anything other than breast milk and the stool is difficult to pass, hard and dry, she is most probably constipated. Breastfed babies do not often get constipated, but dehydration may result in a dry stool. Some children will have infrequent bowel movements, but because their stools are soft, they are not constipated. The child has constipation if some of the stools are hard and dry. Even if occasional small, runny stools occur, a child is constipated if the majority of their bowel motions are hard and dry or difficult to pass. If a bowel movement comes after several days and is loose and runny, this is referred to as both constipation and diarrhoea.

As a child gets older, she will have fewer bowel movements per day. However, the higher the fibre content of the diet, the more frequent the bowel movements.

It is not uncommon to find undigested food in the stools of infants and toddlers. It is perfectly normal and won't harm them in any way. Variety is very important at this stage of development, so don't restrict your child's diet in any way if you notice this happening.

Common Causes of Constipation

- Weak energy pattern — If your child sleeps a lot during the day, has a pale face, or a weak sounding cry, you can suspect that she falls into this category. Some children are born with weak energy and are thus more prone to constipation.
- The normal flow of digested material through the digestive system is impaired and food accumulates in the intestines and interferes with a normal digestive pattern. These children are quite the opposite of the 'weak' type and have red cheeks, with strong, muscular bodies and sometimes are green or grey between the nose and the lip area. Their cry is very strong, loud and almost piercing.
- In breastfed babies, stools are normally infrequent, loose and pale in colour. If the stools become hard and dry the only non-medical cause that has been discovered is an excess of protein or fat in the mother's diet. If you find that your baby does not respond to a change in your diet, it's best to consult a medical practitioner.
- In bottle fed babies, insufficient fluid or sugar in the formula or cow's milk.
- Excessive sweating in a baby.
- Babies who spit up or regurgitate a lot of milk (posseting) or who have episodes of vomiting may become constipated.
- Emotional upsets are common causes of constipation. A new school, or unhappy play times with friends, the arrival of a new sibling, moving house or a traumatic fright or incident can all cause constipation.

Dietary Recommendations for Children Under Three

- Eat small, regular meals daily with at least two hours in between.
- Avoid foods that are difficult to digest, such as greasy food or an excess of red meat. Wheat bran in excess or raw muesli can cause constipation in children under the age of three.
- It is best to use saucepans made from stainless steel, enamel, glass or cast iron.
- Check to make sure that your child is getting

enough to drink. If there is a wet nappy (diaper) every couple of hours and sufficient weight gain, then fluid intake is sufficient.

- Make sure that your baby gets plenty of exercise.
- Cook baby's food in prune juice, or give prune juice (diluted) in her bottle.

Constipation in the Older Child

As your child gets older she can create problems for herself by ignoring the urge to go to the toilet. This may begin at three or four years of age, but most commonly at school age. As the over-full colon starts to stretch and distend, it may lose its ability to transmit impulses to the child's nervous system signalling that it is 'time to go'. The stool becomes drier and more painful to pass and this further discourages the child from going to the toilet.

There are many reasons why a child might choose to begin ignoring the urge to defecate. The child might rebel against over-zealous toilet training where she was forced to sit on the potty. Children can often become constipated on starting school because they are reluctant to use school toilets. Some may have a rash or tear in the rectum from pushing out faeces, making them hold in bowel movements to prevent pain.

It may be very difficult at times to diagnose the cause of the constipation, and although we recommend several forms of treatment it may be necessary to consult a natural practitioner or a medical practitioner of your choice. If your child has been badly constipated you may need to use a laxative for a few days to clean out the colon so that the child can become sensitive again to the normal sensations of having to go to the toilet. This also allows you to teach her new behaviours related to sitting on the toilet. When she is taking laxatives, encourage her to sit on the toilet a few times a day, possibly in the morning after breakfast, after school and after dinner. Reward her with a star chart for just sitting on the toilet. When she has stopped taking the laxative, encourage her to continue at least one of these sitting times until new bowel habits have been established. Keep up a star chart until she is regular again.

All children start using the toilet at different stages in their development. What is most important is that you remain patient with your child and do not compare her to any other child.

Diet recommendations for children three years and over

- A diet that is too low in fibre, particularly soluble fibre, will definitely contribute to constipation. A bulky watery stool such as is formed when a child has a high fibre diet will create a strong urge to defecate, and a child will be less likely to ignore it.
- In some cases of resistant constipation, when your child has constipation that does not improve with a diet high in fruits, vegetables, whole grains and legumes, food intolerance can be the cause. Some common problem foods are milk, wheat, peanuts, yeast and eggs.

Preventing Constipation

- Begin by breastfeeding your baby if you can. The digestive system of a breastfed baby is always in better health than that of a baby which is bottle fed.
- If you do bottle feed be careful to use proper concentrations of milk for the baby's age.
- When weaning the baby take care not to introduce solid foods too early, preferably not before six months. Begin with very small quantities of solid foods or your baby may become constipated. Do not give the baby too much of any one food; try to vary its diet.
- Ensure adequate fluids.
- After the age of three, encourage a diet that includes a lot of fibre:
- Whole grain cereals — rice, barley, oats, oat bran, rye, corn, buckwheat, polenta, brown rice, millet (make up a mixture of these for a breakfast cereal). Soak several grains together overnight (3 cups water to 1 cup grain). Bring to the boil in the morning, cover and simmer 20 minutes. You may have to add more water, as each grain absorbs different amounts of water.
- Puffed whole grain breakfast cereals
- Wholemeal breads, muffins or pancakes
- Whole wheat cakes, biscuits, scones, etc.
- Fresh fruits and vegetables
- Foods that contain soluble fibre, such as legumes and special foods like linseed meal.
- Nut butters, such as peanut, tahini (sesame seed butter), almond, cashew to be used as a spread on bread or in cooking. Also whole nuts, but not for under five years of age.
- Foods with added bran
- Dried fruits, such as apricots, apples, etc.

> **CAUTION**
>
> **If you suspect that there may be a physical blockage that is causing the problem, take your baby or child to a medical practitioner immediately.**

Home Remedies

Mix a tablespoon each of lemon juice and olive oil together and ask your child to have as much as she can tolerate each time. When it's finished mix together 1 cup of warm water and 1-2 teaspoons lemon juice and have her sip it throughout the day.

You can also try prune juice if lemon is not appreciated.

Herbal Laxatives

Generally speaking, herbal laxatives fall into two categories: those that help to moisten and soften the stools; and those that promote muscular activity.

Herbal laxatives must be used with great care with babies and infants, as some can spark off diarrhoea. If your baby has a pale complexion and weak constitution and gets diarrhoea consult a qualified practitioner as soon as possible.

While some herbal laxatives can be habit forming this does not apply to the remedies mentioned below. Nevertheless, they should always be used for a short time only. If constipation persists, see a qualified practitioner.

Herbal Remedies

Cascara

In low to moderate dose, Cascara acts to soften the stool. Best suited to short-term use (a few days) to relieve the odd case of constipation which is not an ongoing problem.
Decoction: use ½ teaspoon of the chopped, dried bark to 1 cup of water. Simmer for 5 minutes, strain. Can be sweetened with honey or rice malt. Dilute with water if necessary.
DOSE
2-3 years: 20-30 mL (²/₃-1 fl oz) 1 to 3 times daily
4-5 years: 40-50 mL (1¹/₃-1²/₃ fl oz) 1 to 3 times daily
6-7 years: 60-70 mL (2-2¹/₃ fl oz) 1 to 3 times daily

8 years and older: 80-100 mL (2¹/₃-3 fl oz) 1 to 3 times daily

NOTE: Do not give for longer than two weeks at a time. Reduce dose if laxative effect is too strong, causing diarrhoea or abdominal pain. Give with Ginger, Chamomile or Fennel.

Licorice

A gentle laxative which softens the stools. It is for short-term use only, for example after fevers.
Decoction: use ½ teaspoon chopped Licorice root to 1 cup of water. Simmer covered for 10 minutes.
DOSE
1-2 years: 20 mL (²/₃ fl oz) 3 times daily
3-4 years: 30-50 mL (1-1²/₃ fl oz) 3 times daily
5-6 years: 60-80 mL (2-2²/₃ fl oz) 3 times daily
7 years and older: 100-120 mL (3-4 fl oz) 3 times daily

Dandelion Root

Dandelion is a wonderful liver tonic. It is a very gentle laxative, acting by increasing the secretion of bile. Bile is an excellent laxative. For constipation caused by impaired digestive function.
Decoction: use 1-2 teaspoons of chopped root to 1 cup of water, simmer covered for 5-10 minutes. Can be sweetened with honey or rice malt. Dilute with water if necessary. Suitable for a digestive cause.
DOSE
1-2 years: 15-30 mL (½-1 fl oz) 3 times daily
3-4 years: 40-60 mL (1¹/₃-2 fl oz) 3 times daily
5-6 years: 70-90 mL (2¹/₃-3 fl oz) 3 times daily
7 years and older: 100-150 mL (3-5 fl oz) 3 times daily

Chicory

The bitterness of Chicory leads to a gentle laxative effect similar to that of Dandelion described above.
Decoction: use 1-2 teaspoons of chopped root to 1 cup of water, simmer covered for 5-10 minutes, strain. Can be sweetened with honey or rice malt. Dilute with water if necessary. Suitable for a digestive cause.
DOSE
1-2 years: 15-30 mL (½-1 fl oz) 3 times daily
3-4 years: 40-60 mL (1¹/₃-2 fl oz) 3 times daily
5-6 years: 70-90 mL (2¹/₃-3 fl oz) 3 times daily

7 years and older: 100-150 mL (3-5 fl oz) 3 times daily

Chamomile

Chamomile combines relaxing properties with a gentle stimulation of the digestion. Particularly suitable when constipation is caused by emotional stress or anxiety in the child.

Infusion: use 1 teaspoon dried flowerheads to 1 cup of boiling water. Let steep for 5 minutes, strain. Can be sweetened with honey or rice malt. Dilute with water for smaller children. Suitable for stress-related constipation.

DOSE

1-2 years: 20-40 mL (²/₃-1¹/₃ fl oz) 3 to 4 times daily

3-4 years: 50-80 mL (1²/₃-2²/₃ fl oz) 3 to 4 times daily

5-6 years: 100-125 mL (3-4 fl oz) 3 to 4 times daily

7 years and older: 150-200 mL (5-6²/₃ fl oz) 3 to 4 times daily

Homoeopathic Remedies

Where the constipation is accompanied by frequent ineffectual urging, and then only a small amount of stool passes, **Nux vomica** 30C will be indicated.

If the stool is large, dry, hard and this is associated with dryness of other parts of the body such as lips and mouth, **Bryonia** 12C will be useful.

Dose: Twice daily for up to three days.

This is a chronic condition. Where dietary measures are insufficient and the above medicines do not seem appropriate it should be referred to your homoeopathic practitioner.

Chinese Remedies

1 'Heat'

Red complexion. Red lips. Dry mouth. Thirst. Red tongue with a dry yellow coating. Fingernails may be red. Pulse is rapid and more forceful than normal. There may be fever or a recent history of febrile illness. Prominent veins at the back of the ear.

DA CHENG QI TANG

2 'Food Stagnation'

Abdomen feels and may also appear to be swollen. There may be colicky pain, foul smelling belching or vomiting. Loss of appetite. There may also be mild signs of heat (red face,

lips and tongue). The tongue coating is thick and appears oily. The region between the upper lip and nose has a yellow or dark hue.

BAO HE WAN

3 'Qi Stagnation'

Very similar picture to 2 (above), i.e. food stagnation. The main differences are: the coating on the tongue is thin and appears sticky rather than oily. There is always a strong emotional component — anger, irritability, fear and insecurity, frustration, sulking, etc.

LIU MO TANG

4 'Deficiency'

Pale complexion. Pale lips. Dull eyes. Low energy. Tires easily. Speaks little. Soft, low voice. Pale fingernails. Hair may be brittle with split ends. Tongue is pale with a thin coating.

ZHI GAN CAO TANG taken together with MA ZI REN WAN

Massage

Perform this massage series for several days until there is an improvement in bowel movements. Follow up with once a day for a week, then every other day for a week, and then every three to four days to keep the system functioning freely.

1 With your child lying on her back, warm a small amount of oil in your hand (rubbing hands together briskly), bend her knees (for a baby you can hold the legs with one hand as you massage with open hands on the abdomen) and massage in downward strokes, one hand following the other across the tummy. Do this five times.

2 Massage in large circles clockwise across the abdomen: the right hand makes a full circle while the left hand follows making a half circle. Do this five times.

3 Walk with your fingertips across the tummy from left to right (clockwise), feeling for any tight or restricted areas. Press in gently and hold over these spots waiting for a release or relaxation.

4 Hold left leg up and massage in small circles just above the hip bone into the lower abdomen. Press in gently and work downward.

5 Push knees into chest and hold gently, allowing your child to relax and breathe, then release legs. Do this five times holding for ten to thirty seconds.

CONVULSIONS

Convulsions are caused by an altered electrical discharge in the nervous system, according to Alice Likowski Duncan M.D., author of *Your Healthy Child*, J. P. Tarcher, California, 1991.

Convulsions (or febrile 'fits') mainly occur in young children between the ages of six months and five years as the result of a very high fever. In Chinese medicine infantile convulsions are called *jing feng*, which literally means 'fright wind'. It is believed that children are more prone to convulsions because their bodies are weak and their spirits can be easily disturbed, startled or 'frightened'.

A sudden rise in body temperature irritates the brain, and due to the brain's instability in some infants it can send out abnormal or irregular messages to the nerves. This can result in sudden and acute infantile convulsions, always accompanied by a high fever.

In the Chinese tradition, acute infantile convulsions are usually set off by overeating (leading to food stagnation) or high fever. Chronic, rather than acute, infantile convulsions are usually caused by poor digestion. They usually come after diarrhoea and vomiting and they are milder, with little or no fever at all.

In older children, convulsions are believed to be mainly caused by emotional factors. Emotional stress can weaken the immune system and give rise to viral illness, thus paving the way for the possibility of a rapid rise in temperature and high fever, which can lead to a convulsion.

In orthodox medicine, convulsions are usually regarded as being preceded by an upper viral respiratory tract infection.

Symptoms of Acute Convulsions

The symptoms are sudden in onset and may be accompanied by the following:
- rolling upwards of the eyes
- neck rigidity
- spasms of the limbs
- high fever
- salivation (possibly frothy)
- rattling sound of phlegm in the throat
- lockjaw
- coma
- hands and feet start to twitch and the twitching spreads throughout the whole body — whole body eventually goes rigid
- loss of consciousness

Symptoms of Chronic Convulsions

These are gradual in onset and can include:
- listlessness
- cold, clammy limbs
- shallow breathing
- slightly bluish complexion
- slow, intermittent spasms of the limbs
- mental apathy
- low grade fever or none at all
- unclosed eyes during sleep

Chronic convulsions may not be obvious to the naked eye and the condition is almost the opposite of acute convulsions. The body temperature is cooler with perhaps just a low grade fever. The convulsion itself will usually last a minute or so at the most. It is best treated with herbs and diet.

Additional Factors

Convulsions are not usually dangerous. About one child in twenty-five has a fit at some time or another, and although they may be frightening to observe, they will not harm the child unless they last more than ten minutes or occur once every couple of days. In this case the fits can cause permanent brain damage, because oxygen to the brain will have been cut off for too long.

The tendency to convulsions often runs in families. One convulsion is usually not dangerous; however, you should always seek medical help immediately afterwards. Often the child is admitted to hospital for observation. About 30 per cent of children who have had one febrile convulsion will most likely have another. The best thing to do is to treat the fever as soon as possible.

Emergency Treatment for an Acute Convulsion

- It can be frightening for the parent, but don't panic.
- Put the child on the floor in the recovery position (see page 156).
- Stay with her in case she injures herself.
- Call a doctor as soon as possible.
- Don't try to stop the convulsion.
- Quickly lower the temperature by loosening clothing and sponging her down with tepid water — do not put her in a bath.
- Don't put anything in her mouth.
- Do not give her anything to drink.

Prevention

To help prevent acute and chronic convulsions, support the digestive system by monitoring the diet — keep the intake of mucus-forming foods and foods that produce heat in the body extremely low (see Appendix 9). Also avoid exposing your child to frightening situations and loud, sudden noises.

Herbal Remedies

To *prevent* febrile convulsions use diaphoretics, which increase sweating and thereby reduce temperature:

Yarrow

Infusion: use 1 teaspoon of dried herb to 1 cup of boiling water. Let steep for 5 minutes, strain. Can be sweetened with honey or rice malt. Dilute with water if necessary.
DOSE
1-2 years: 15-30 mL (½-1 fl oz) 3 times daily
3-4 years: 40-60 mL (1⅓-2 fl oz) 3 times daily
5-6 years: 70-90 mL (2⅓-3 fl oz) 3 times daily
7 years and older: 100-150 mL (3-5 fl oz) 3 times daily

Elderflower

Infusion: use 2 teaspoons of the dried flowers to 1 cup of boiling water. Let steep for 5 minutes, strain. Can be sweetened with honey or rice malt.

DOSE
1-2 years: 15-30 mL (½-1 fl oz) 3 times daily
3-4 years: 40-60 mL (1⅓-2 fl oz) 3 times daily
5-6 years: 70-90 mL (2⅓-3 fl oz) 3 times daily
7 years and older: 100-150 mL (3-5 fl oz) 3 times daily

Peppermint

Infusion: use ½-1 teaspoon of dried herb to 1 cup of boiling water. Let steep for 5 minutes, strain. Can be sweetened with honey or rice malt. Dilute with water if necessary.
DOSE
1-2 years: 15-30 mL (½-1 fl oz) 3 times daily
3-4 years: 40-60 mL (1⅓-2 fl oz) 3 times daily
5-6 years: 70-90 mL (2⅓-3 fl oz) 3 times daily
7 years and older: 100-150 mL (3-5 fl oz) 3 times daily

Yarrow, Elderflowers and Peppermint in combination form a traditional diaphoretic tea with a pleasant taste. Use about ⅓ of each herb and give as hot as possible. Let the child drink as much of the tea as she wishes.

To prevent chronic convulsions including epilepsy, use Scullcap as an anti-spasmodic and nervous restorative.

Scullcap

Infusion: use ½-1 teaspoon of the dried herb to 1 cup of boiling water. Let steep for 5-10 minutes, strain. Sweeten with honey or rice malt. This herb has an unpleasant bitter taste and should be mixed with a suitable pleasant-tasting herb such as Fennel seed, Aniseed or Licorice root.
DOSE
1-2 years: 15-30 mL (½-1 fl oz) 3 times daily
3-4 years: 40-60 mL (1⅓-2 fl oz) 3 times daily
5-6 years: 70-90 mL (2⅓-3 fl oz) 3 times daily
7 years and older: 100-150 mL (3-5 fl oz) 3 times daily

Massage

First, follow safety precautions.

1 Cool your hands under cold water, then place one hand at the back of your child's neck and squeeze lightly. Place the other on her forehead and press in gently. Hold for two to four minutes, or until your child regains consciousness.

2 Or to regain consciousness, press hard with two fingertips on the point midway between the upper lip and nose. Hold for two minutes to increase blood supply to the brain.

COUGHS

There are many different kinds of cough. It can be loud or soft, dry and hacking, loose and wet, occasional or frequent or brassy or croupy. The loudness of a cough is only a measure of how much energy is being put into the cough.

When coughs are dry and hacking, it usually means that something is irritating the respiratory tract. Sometimes the sensory nerves in the mucous membrane lining can't determine whether the irritation that sets off a cough is caused by the presence of foreign matter or by the swelling and inflammation of the mucous membrane. Coughs that are loose and wet indicate that mucus is being produced. Mucus that is ejected from the lower respiratory tract often flips over into the oesophagus and gets swallowed. This is why so many infants with colds and other respiratory ailments can have diarrhoea and vomiting with mucus present. When the cough seems loose and rattly from the chest or upper mid back, this indicates that there is a great deal of extra mucus in the larger upper part of the breathing apparatus and there is very little to be concerned about.

In asthmatic and virus-related conditions in toddlers and infants, a wheezing sound is heard especially on the exhalation. This indicates that the lower, middle size airways are blocked (bronchioles), reducing the available space for air to pass through.

More serious conditions such as pneumonia are indicated by the deepest lung tissues being filled with fluid, giving rise to a very soft sound.

A cough may also be signalling lung infection such as bronchitis or pneumonia. More commonly there is just continuing mucus production in the throat or sinuses that irritates the main bronchi and produces a cough.

Then there is the so-called 'psychogenic' cough. This is considered to be reasonably common in children and to represent a sort of habit, nervous tic or attention-seeking device. The cough is usually dry, loud ('barking' or 'honking') and explosive, and recurrent in nature. Many of these psychogenic coughs are actually allergic in nature and respond to supplements that strengthen the mucous membranes and deal with the allergy.

Causes

The respiratory tract can become inflamed and over-produce mucus because of any of the following:
- Infections caused by bacteria or viruses, usually manifested when cold weather, snow or rain becomes more frequent.
- Immunisation or over-tiredness.
- Emotional traumas such as a new brother or sister, moving house, parents' separation or divorce or feelings of anger or hostility.

Acute Feverish, Hot Cough — Bronchitis

Symptoms

Fever, sore throat, cough or nasal discharge with thick, yellow phlegm, slight fever, a red face and child is often sweating. Cough is hard sounding, which comes on more in the night and keeps your child awake.

Treatment

Choose a remedy that will begin to soften the cough and allow your child to perspire more. This means that the body is fighting the infection. If symptoms do not change, try another remedy or seek professional advice.

As you administer the suggested medication, the fever should clear, the phlegm should loosen and be easier to cough up or leave the nasal passages. It is vitally important that you watch the symptoms closely, as this type of cough can easily progress into a more serious condition, such as pneumonia.

A Harsh and Irritating Dry Cough

Symptoms

- Very little if any phlegm is brought up. It may sound rather 'croupy' in severe cases.

Croup can be identified by the metallic gasping sound that is heard when a child breathes; then a metallic, hoarse cough and an unusual pulling in of the chest upon inhalation.

- There is an inflammation of the voicebox and windpipe which causes the phlegm to be rather thick and hard to expel.
- Your child may place her hand on her chest, and if she can describe how she feels may say that her chest is hurting or feels tight. If there is a tendency to asthma this may develop after a cold and manifest as a dry, irritating cough with no wheeze, with a tickle in the throat.
- If the cough makes the child vomit or if there is the presence of a whoop it could be something serious like whooping cough or cystic fibrosis.
- The cough eventually begins to soften and become more productive.
- General irritability.

Cough Caused by Inhaling Foreign Objects

The most commonly inhaled substances are peanuts or little bits and pieces children have picked up off the floor.

Symptoms

- The child will suddenly start coughing, although in many cases there is only wheezing. The cough may disappear, to be followed by the development of a fever and signs of infection in the lung.

Croup (Viral)

Croup is caused by inflammation and swelling of the larynx and can occur suddenly in young children because their breathing tubes are so small. It usually happens at night and is recognised by a painful hacking cough, followed by crying. As the child tries to draw in breath, she makes a kind of barking noise.

There are two types of croup:

- Acute — sudden onset with other presenting symptoms such as fever, chills, fatigue, diarrhoea, listlessness, etc.
- Chronic — persists over a period of time and usually has no other concurrent symptoms.

Treatment

- Reassure the child, who is usually distressed

by lack of breath. Crying will only make matters worse by reducing the oxygen supply.

- Take the child to a window or place her in front of the refrigerator and let her breathe in six to ten breaths of cool air, which will help reduce the swelling in the larynx.
- Then immediately take her to the bathroom and turn on the hot taps so that the room fills with steam. Stay in the steam for at least twenty minutes. If no hot water is available, boil kettles of water.
- Once the child is breathing more comfortably, settle her down in bed with bowls of steaming water or a humidifier. Keep the child supervised and call a doctor or ambulance if the breathing does not respond to the treatment.

Chronic Cough

Immunisations can cause a chronic cough anywhere up to four weeks after immunisation. Another common cause is a viral respiratory tract infection, which is treated with antibiotics. They appear to relieve the initial problem, but do not take care of the underlying condition, and weaken the child's resistance.

Chronic coughs can also be caused by emotional upset, especially when children are first learning to communicate, and can't get the words out fast enough to express what it is they want to say.

Symptoms

- Mucus is very thick.
- The cough keeps going away and then coming back again.
- The cough gets better at times and then gets worse again.
- The complexion of your child may alternate between grey and red with a bluish green tinge around the mouth.
- She may feel hungry at times, but appetite is generally poor.

Treatment

The most productive way to deal with this type of cough is to concentrate on clearing the mucus from the chest and stop its production. Make sure that your child gets plenty of fresh air, activity, rest and positive reinforcement.

Phlegmatic Cough

Phlegmatic cough comes on quite suddenly and may be caused by an infection.

Symptoms

- Cough is worse in cold weather and when lying down.
- Phlegm is thick and white (it may be yellow at times but mostly it is white) and there is a white discharge from the nose as well.
- The child may feel quite cold at times or alternate hot and cold feelings.
- This is a 'cold' condition in Chinese medicine and should be treated accordingly.

Treatment

Avoid all mucus-forming foods, getting chilled and getting wet. The cough should get better in a matter of a few days. If the cough returns or takes longer to disappear, it may very well have turned into a chronic cough. Consult a practitioner of your choice in this case.

Watery Cough

This type of cough also comes on suddenly and has much the same symptoms as a phlegmatic cough. When the symptoms begin to change, your child's mood should improve after an initial shedding of negative feelings and emotions.

Symptoms

- Sudden onset, usually during wet, cold weather.
- Clear phlegm runs out from the nose, either loose or viscous.
- Cough is worse when lying down.
- Feels cold, weak and chilled.
- Face is very pale, but sometimes cheeks become red.
- If able to cough up phlegm, usually it is clear and watery.

Treatment

See also Phlegmatic cough. Try the following tea: 1 teaspoon of Fennel and 1 teaspoon of Aniseed steeped in 1 cup of boiling water for 10 minutes covered. Sweeten if desired.

Usually a child with these symptoms has very little interest in doing anything; however, as the treatment takes effect her attitude should shift and the symptoms should gradually disappear. If after twelve to twenty-four hours there is no evident improvement, it may be advisable to seek a natural practitioner's advice.

Preventative Care

There are certain foods that are known to produce mucus and so should be avoided. Cheese, soy milk, cow's milk, roasted peanuts, bananas and sugar, butter, cream and more than one orange a week should be avoided during a cough or cold. If your child suffers from frequent coughs or colds, these foods should be avoided for three or four weeks and then introduced slowly back into her diet in small quantities. Make sure that your child is adequately dressed for the cold weather and does not get exposed to a cold wind or get easily chilled.

If you live in a cold climate it is best to keep your house relatively cool so that the transition from the hot to the cold weather does not shock the system too much.

General Care

Natural medicines may be used and steam inhalations and chest rubs are also very useful. It is important to keep the chest wall moving, so encourage breathing by getting the child (if she is not too sick) to do light physical exercise. Massage and vibration of the chest will help to loosen and remove mucus.

DEADLY SCENTS

Recently, essential oils have become a popular way of treating many common ailments. At Royal Children's Hospital in Melbourne, doctors have seen about two hundred children poisoned by them. Many households use natural eucalyptus oil as a gentle substitute for cold and cough remedies, but just one millilitre can put a child in a coma, and five millilitres of the other essential oils can be dangerous. Symptoms of essential oil poisoning include lethargy and perhaps vomiting. Keep them well out of the reach of children and do not leave bowls of the oils around to repel insects where children can reach them.

Nutritional supplements

For strengthening your child's system, try the following:
- Vitamin A — for strengthening mucous membranes. *Dose:* 5000 units for children

under three and 10 000 units for children over three years of age.

- Zinc — for increased immunity. *Dose:* 10 mg for children under three, 25 mg for those over three.

Home Remedies

- A Mustard plaster can help break up congestion (see Appendix 7: Compresses, Poultices and Baths). If the child complains of heat, take it off. This is a very effective, old-fashioned, treatment.
- Lotus root tea is good for dry cough. The exact dosage is given on the packet. (Use ¼ of the recommended dosage for 1-2 year olds, ⅓ for 3-4 year olds, ½ for 5-7 year olds and ¾ for 8-12 year olds.)
- Inhalation of the aromatic oils lemon and eucalyptus used in a humidifier or just inhaling the vapours in a bowl of hot steaming water can be effective to stop cough. If signs of infection are present, add Thyme oil and Tea-Tree oil. (Use ¼-½ recommended dosage for 3-4 year olds.)
- For a phlegmatic cough use a Garlic poultice. Crush a small piece of Garlic on a paper bag with a little cooking oil until pasty. Place this about a third to half-way down on the sole of the foot. Bind with a cloth or bandage and leave on overnight. Change the poultice every night. Continue for several nights to see if the poultice is helping.
- Dip an absorbent cloth into castor oil and apply to the chest. Cover with at least two layers of towel and then warm with a hot water bottle.
- For over three year olds: add 3 drops Tea-Tree oil to bath; rub pure Tea-Tree oil into chest and back;

sprinkle on pillow before sleeping; use one drop of pure Tea-Tree oil in a teaspoon of honey and sip slowly.

- Chamomile or Thyme baths may also be useful for phlegmatic cough (see Appendix 7: Compresses, Poultices and Baths).

Herbal Remedies for Dry Cough

Marshmallow

The root is prepared as a decoction: use 1-1½ teaspoons of chopped root to 1 cup of water, simmer covered for 5-10 minutes.

The leaf is prepared as an infusion: use 2 teaspoons of dried leaf to 1 cup of boiling water, let steep for 10 minutes. Can be diluted with water.

DOSE
½-1 year: 15-30 mL (½-1 fl oz) 3 times daily
2-3 years: 40-50 mL (1⅓-1⅔ fl oz) 3 times daily
4-5 years: 60-80 mL (2-2⅔ fl oz) 3 times daily
6 years and older: 80-120 mL (2⅔-3⅔ fl oz) 3 times daily

Licorice

Decoction: use ½ teaspoon chopped Licorice root to 1 cup of water. Simmer covered for 10 minutes.

DOSE
1-2 years: 20 mL (⅔ fl oz) 3 times daily
3-4 years: 30-50 mL (1-1⅔ fl oz) 3 times daily
5-6 years: 60-80 mL (2-2⅔ fl oz) 3 times daily
7 years and older: 100-120 mL (3-4 fl oz) 3 times daily

Mullein

Infusion: use 2 teaspoons of the dried leaves or ½ teaspoon of the dried flowers to 1 cup of boiling water. Let steep for 5-10 minutes, strain. Can be sweetened with honey or rice malt.

DOSE
1-2 years: 15-30 mL (½-1 fl oz) 3 times daily
3-4 years: 40-60 mL (1⅓-2 fl oz) 3 times daily
5-6 years: 70-90 mL (2⅓-3 fl oz) 3 times daily
7 years and older: 100-150 mL (3-5 fl oz) 3 times daily

Ribwort

Infusion: use 1-1½ teaspoons of the dried herb or 4-5 teaspoons of the chopped, fresh herb to 1 cup of boiling water. Let steep for 5-10 minutes, strain. Can be sweetened with honey or rice malt.

CAUTION

Seek professional advice if the following occurs:

- **A fever gets to 39°C (103°F).**
- **The child has difficulty in breathing.**
- **The child complains of pains in the chest for more than 12-24 hours.**

Seek medical attention immediately if your child's condition seems worse after she has been awake for 15-20 minutes, if she spends most of her time trying to suck in air or if her colour deepens and starts turning a little bluish.

DOSE

1-2 years: 15-30 mL (½-1 fl oz) 3 times daily
3-4 years: 40-60 mL (1⅓-2 fl oz) 3 times daily
5-6 years: 70-90 mL (2⅓-3 fl oz) 3 times daily
7 years and older: 100-150 mL (3-5 fl oz) 3 times daily

NOTE: Ribwort is a very common weed in urban areas. If you pick it yourself, make sure you do it in an area that is free from various types of pollution.

Herbal Remedies for Wet, Mucus-producing Cough

White Horehound

Infusion: use ½-1 teaspoon of the dried herb to 1 cup of boiling water. Let steep for 5-10 minutes, strain. Sweeten with honey or rice malt. This herb has an unpleasant bitter taste and should be mixed with a pleasant-tasting expectorant herb such as Fennel seed, Aniseed or Licorice root.

DOSE

1-2 years: 15-30 mL (½-1 fl oz) 3 times daily
3-4 years: 40-60 mL (1⅓-2 fl oz) 3 times daily
5-6 years: 70-90 mL (2⅓-3 fl oz) 3 times daily
7 years and older: 100-150 mL (3-5 fl oz) 3 times daily

Elecampane

Decoction: use 1-1½ teaspoons of chopped root to 1 cup of water, simmer covered for 5-10 minutes.

DOSE

1-2 years: 15-30 mL (½-1 fl oz) 3 times daily
3-4 years: 40-60 mL (1⅓-2 fl oz) 3 times daily
5-6 years: 70-90 mL (2⅓-3 fl oz) 3 times daily
7 years and older: 100-150 mL (3-5 fl oz) 3 times daily

Heartsease (Wild Pansy)

Infusion: use 1-1½ teaspoons of the dried herb to 1 cup of boiling water. Let steep for 5-10 minutes, strain. Can be sweetened with honey or rice malt.

DOSE

1-2 years: 15-30 mL (½-1 fl oz) 3 times daily
3-4 years: 40-60 mL (1⅓-2 fl oz) 3 times daily
5-6 years: 70-90 mL (2⅓-3 fl oz) 3 times daily
7 years and older: 100-150 mL (3-5 fl oz) 3 times daily

Herbal Remedies for Spasmodic Cough

Thyme

Infusion: use 1 teaspoon of dried herb to 1 cup of boiling water. Let steep for 5 minutes, strain. Can be sweetened with honey or rice malt. Dilute with water if necessary.

DOSE

1-2 years: 15-30 mL (½-1 fl oz) 3 times daily
3-4 years: 40-60 mL (1⅓-2 fl oz) 3 times daily
5-6 years: 70-90 mL (2⅓-3 fl oz) 3 times daily
7 years and older: 100-150 mL (3-5 fl oz) 3 times daily

Licorice

Decoction: use ½ teaspoon chopped Licorice root to 1 cup of water. Simmer covered for 10 minutes.

DOSE

1-2 years: 20 mL (⅔ fl oz) 3 times daily
3-4 years: 30-50 mL (1-1⅔ fl oz) 3 times daily
5-6 years: 60-80 mL (2-2⅔ fl oz) 3 times daily
7 years and older: 100-120 mL (3-4 fl oz) 3 times daily

Aniseed

Infusion: use ½ teaspoon of whole or freshly crushed seeds to 1 cup of boiling water. Let steep for 5 minutes, strain.

DOSE

1-2 years: 15-30 mL (½-1 fl oz) 3 times daily
3-4 years: 40-60 mL (1⅓-2 fl oz) 3 times daily
5-6 years: 70-90 mL (2⅓-3 fl oz) 3 times daily
7 years and older: 100-150 mL (3-5 fl oz) 3 times daily

Herbal Remedies for Croup

Licorice is a soothing anti-inflammatory, Aniseed is a relaxing expectorant, Thyme and Hyssop are relaxing and antiseptic expectorants and Eyebright and Elderflowers are anti-inflammatories.

Licorice

Decoction: use ½ teaspoon chopped Licorice root to 1 cup of water. Simmer covered for 10 minutes.

DOSE

1-2 years: 20 mL (⅔ fl oz) 3 times daily
3-4 years: 30-50 mL (1-1⅔ fl oz) 3 times daily
5-6 years: 60-80 mL (2-2⅓ fl oz) 3 times daily
7 years and older: 100-120 mL (3-4 fl oz) 3 times daily

Aniseed

Infusion: use ½ teaspoon of whole or freshly crushed seeds to 1 cup of boiling water. Let steep for 5 minutes, strain.

DOSE
1-2 years: 15-30 mL (½-1 fl oz) 3 times daily
3-4 years: 40-60 mL (1⅓-2 fl oz) 3 times daily
5-6 years: 70-90 mL (2⅓-3 fl oz) 3 times daily
7 years and older: 100-150 mL (3-5 fl oz) 3 times daily

Thyme

Infusion: use 1 teaspoon of dried herb to 1 cup of boiling water. Let steep for 5 minutes, strain. Can be sweetened with honey or rice malt. Dilute with water if necessary.

DOSE
1-2 years: 15-30 mL (½-1 fl oz) 3 times daily
3-4 years: 40-60 mL (1⅓-2 fl oz) 3 times daily
5-6 years: 70-90 mL (2⅓-3 fl oz) 3 times daily
7 years and older: 100-150 mL (3-5 fl oz) 3 times daily

Eyebright

Infusion: Use 1 teaspoon of dried herb to 1 cup of boiling water. Let steep for 5 minutes, strain. Can be sweetened with honey or rice malt. Dilute with water if necessary.

DOSE
1-2 years: 15-30 mL (½-1 fl oz) 3 times daily
3-4 years: 40-60 mL (1⅓-2 fl oz) 3 times daily
5-6 years: 70-90 mL (2⅓-3 fl oz) 3 times daily
7 years and older: 100-150 mL (3-5 fl oz) 3 times daily

Elderflower

Infusion: use 2 teaspoons of the dried flowers to 1 cup of boiling water. Let steep for 5 minutes, strain. Can be sweetened with honey or rice malt.

DOSE
1-2 years: 15-30 mL (½-1 fl oz) 3 times daily
3-4 years: 40-60 mL (1⅓-2 fl oz) 3 times daily
5-6 years: 70-90 mL (2⅓-3 fl oz) 3 times daily
7 years and older: 100-150 mL (3-5 fl oz) 3 times daily

Hyssop

Infusion: use 1-1½ teaspoons of the dried herb to 1 cup of boiling water. Let steep for 5 minutes, strain. Can be sweetened with honey or rice malt.

DOSE
1-2 years: 15-30 mL (½-1 fl oz) 3 times daily
3-4 years: 40-60 mL (1⅓-2 fl oz) 3 times daily

5-6 years: 70-90 mL (2⅓-3 fl oz) 3 times daily
7 years and older: 100-150 mL (3-5 fl oz) 3 times daily

Eucalyptus oil

A few drops of the essential oil can be put in an oil-burner or in a saucepan with hot water and placed in the room. Another good way of administering Eucalyptus oil is to put a few (2-4) drops in the child's bath.

CAUTION

Never give Eucalyptus oil internally to a child and do not apply it directly to the skin.

Homoeopathic Remedies

Bronchitis

Sudden onset from cold and dry weather indicates **Aconite** 30C. The cough is short, dry, hard and painful and the child may grasp the larynx on coughing. Restlessness and fear is often associated.

Ant-tart 12C is most indicated when there is a coarse rattling of mucus but no phlegm is raised. The child is often drowsy, covered with a cold sweat and looks bluish.

If the cough or the pain in the chest is worse for any movement and the child makes every effort to keep still, use **Bryonia** 12C. In the Bryonia case the cough is dry and will often cause pain in the head and chest. Your child may wish to hold the chest during coughing.

Ipecac 12C is indicated in bronchitis when there is a large amount of mucus, suffocative cough and nausea.

The sense of a weight on the chest, pains in the left chest and yellow blood-streaked mucus point to **Phosphorus** 12C. This child usually wants company and has a thirst for cold drinks.

Also see Arsenicum, Belladonna, Carb-veg, Hepar sulph, Kali-carb, Mercurius, Pulsatilla and Sulphur if the above medicines do not properly exhibit the symptoms.

Dose: One dose every few hours if the symptoms are intense or three times daily if less severe.

Cough

Aconite 30C aids a short, dry cough and is a major remedy for croup. There may be a feeling of suffocation. It often arises from a change to cold weather.

Antimonium tartaricum 12C has a cough with rattling of mucus in the chest and difficult or no expectoration. The child may also be very drowsy.

Bryonia 12C has a hard dry cough which often brings on pain in the chest or head. The child wants to hold the affected part. Any movement seems to aggravate the cough.

Drosera 30C has fits of coughing brought on tickling in the larynx. The Drosera cough may lead to retching or be associated with laryngitis. The cough is often better in the open air. Drosera is a great medicine in whooping cough.

Hepar sulph 30C is a remedy which is used in croupy cough brought on by the cold, dry air even in the form of a slight draught or taking off the clothes in cold weather. The cough is loose with wheezing and rattling or may be suffocative, forcing the child to sit up and bend the head backward.

Spongia 30C is particularly useful when the child rouses out of sleep with a suffocating feeling. There is panting and difficult breathing. The cough is dry and is better for eating and warm drinks.

Many other medicines may be indicated in cough, including Antimonium crudum, Arsenicum, Belladonna, Ferrum-phos, Gelsemium, Ipecac, Mag-phos, Nux vomica, Phosphorus, Pulsatilla, Rhus-tox and Veratrum.

Dose: Three times daily for up to three days.

Where this is a chronic condition, it should be referred to your homoeopathic practitioner.

Chinese Remedies

1 'Cold' — Exterior

Dull or muffled sounding cough with clear or opaque white mucus. Nasal congestion. Aversion to cold and desire for warmth. Complexion is dark. Fingernails are red. Red vein at 'San Guan'. Tongue is normal colour with a thin white coating.

XING SU SAN
XIAO QING LONG TANG copious amounts of mucus

2 'Heat' in Lungs

Develops from 1 (above) if resistance is inadequate and disease is not treated appropriately. Red complexion. Dry throat. Cough is sharper and clearer sounding than the above. Mucus is thick, yellow and more opaque. Tongue has a thick dry coating and is darker red than normal. Pulse is rapid.

CHUAN PEI MO and FRITILLARIA AND LOQUAT COUGH SYRUP
QING FEI YI HUO TANG (severe symptoms: face scarlet red during bouts of coughing, mucus is thick and green with pus, mouth is very dry, tongue is deep red with a dry yellow coating, urine is dark and reduced in quantity, constipation.) Take together with FRITILLARIA and LOQUAT COUGH SYRUP

3 'Deficiency'

This condition is the end result of 2 (above) if left untreated. It may predispose the child to a variety of chronic respiratory disorders in later life.

Long, weak, dry cough. Shallow breathing. Difficulty in breathing. Coughing is worse on exertion. Perspires easily on mild exertion and/or during coughing bouts. Low energy. Tires easily. Speaks little. Low quiet voice. Dull eyes. Poor appetite.

BU FEI TANG (pale tongue, pale complexion)
MAI MEN DONG TANG (red tongue, dry mouth and throat, flushed face, rapid pulse)

4 'Heat' — Exterior

Fever and chills with no aversion to cold. Aversion to warmth. Nasal congestion with thick yellow or green-grey mucus. Coughing up similar mucus. Sore throat. Eyes are red. Complexion is red. Urine is dark and reduced in quantity. Tongue is red with a white coating initially which turns yellow as the disease progresses. Purple vein at 'San Guan'. The veins behind the ears may be prominent. The pulse is rapid.

SANG JU YIN

5 'Food Stagnation'

Rapid breathing. Cough with thick yellow or green-grey mucus. Bad breath. Foul-smelling belching. Abdomen feels and also may appear swollen. Loss of appetite. Colicky abdominal pain. There may be vomiting. Complexion, lips and tongue are red. Tongue has a thick, yellow, oily coating. The region between the upper lip and the nose has a yellow or dark hue.

BAO HE WAN as well as FRITILLARIA and LOQUAT COUGH SYRUP

6 'Cold' with 'Dampness'

This is due to drinking too much, especially cold

or iced drinks, which weaken the stomach. The complexion is yellow-white. 'Wet' cough with copious amounts of thin watery sputum. The hands, feet and abdomen may be cold. The tongue is pale with a white, oily coating. The fingernails may be red. The stools are loose or watery. The pulse is slow.

LING GUI ZHU GAN TANG

LIU JUN ZI TANG with nausea and/or vomiting If coughing is severe and not significantly relieved by the above formulas, give SAN ZI YANG QIN TANG

Massage

Cough

1 Using a small amount (about the size of a five cent piece in the palm of the hand) of warm oil (rub hands together briskly to warm oil) massage with your hands open, from back of ears along either side of neck to shoulders. Hold hands on either side of neck and direct warm loving energy into your child's throat.

2 Massage with both hands open, one on either side of chest, pressing to the sides. Do this five times.

3 Press with fingertips on sternum, feeling for tender spots, press in and hold for thirty seconds.

4 For infants (one to twelve months): rotate big toe and press with your thumb at the base of the big toe on the bottom of foot. Do this for a few minutes on each foot. Also press into the ball of each foot with your thumb and hold any tender spots for ten to twenty seconds.

Bronchitis

1 Pour oil (about the size of a five cent piece) into the palm of your hand and rub both hands together to warm oil. For children aged twelve months and older use a similar amount of Tiger Balm or Eucalyptus with the oil.

2 Have your child lying on her back in front of you. Massage with hands conforming to the shape of your child's body, starting at the base of ribcage and moving in long smooth strokes up to her shoulders. You can move upwards with your child's inhalation, letting your hands flow up the sides of the neck also.

3 Then stroke downward on her chest with your hands, letting your fingertips stroke between the ribs.

4 Place both thumbs in the centre of the diaphragm. Move your thumbs softly along the base of the ribcage, pressing just underneath the ribcage to release the diaphragm muscle. This could be very tight. Do steps 1-4 for up to ten minutes. Encourage your child to take long, slow and easy breaths.

5 Have your child turn over onto her tummy and massage up along the spine, from base of back up to neck. Use long, slow strokes with hands open and thumbs along edge of spine. Then let your hands flow down the spine with fingers making small circles along the spine.

6 Finish with both hands on either side of ribcage directing warm, loving energy into your child's lungs.

CRADLE CAP

Cradle cap (see also Eczema) appears like a scaly crust on the infant's head, roundish or oval in shape and white or yellowish in colour. It is similar to a case of severe dandruff; however, the scales are slightly greasy and difficult to remove.

It can spread to cover the whole head and eyebrows and from there also spread to the cheeks, ears and even upper torso. However, on the body it looks more like dermatitis and appears in red, inflamed, itchy patches.

It is vital to remember that cradle cap is not caused by uncleanliness and can disappear as the baby gets older. Several causes are: sensitivity of the skin; excess oil in the skin; excess dryness in the skin; and insufficient stimulation of the scalp. The problem is also frequent in infants who may later develop significant allergies.

It is important that you treat cradle cap as soon as it appears to prevent it spreading to other parts of the body. Once it reaches this second stage, it is much harder to treat.

Prevention

- Give the baby's scalp a good vigorous scrub with a warm wash-cloth and soap. Repeat several times a week.
- Use a mild shampoo, or simply wash the head with water.

General Treatment

On the head

- Pour warmed olive or walnut oil (do not use baby oil) onto a pad of cotton cloth or cotton wool. Wipe over the scaly spots and leave for twelve hours. Wash with a mild shampoo. Ease away the now softened scales from the baby's head with a comb or fingernail. Repeat if necessary.
- Mix bicarbonate of soda with water or butter until it forms a paste. Rub into the scalp. Allow to dry. Follow with a mild shampoo.

On the face/torso

- For mild cases, use either zinc cream or castor-oil cream.
- If the area looks red, sore and inflamed, contact a practitioner of your choice.

Home Remedies

Use Tea-Tree shampoo, making sure to keep it away from eyes. Mix five drops of pure Tea-Tree oil with olive oil, rub into scalp, leave five minutes and then wash hair.

Herbal Remedies

Heartsease (Wild Pansy)

To make a rinse, prepare an infusion using 2 teaspoons of dried herb to 1 cup of boiling water Let steep for 5-10 minutes, strain and let cool down. Use as a rinse on the scalp.

CRYING

Friends don't often tell you the worst parts of early parenthood, probably because they don't want to worry you too much before the fact. They console you by telling you that the rewards will make up for the mishaps.

When my son began to scream for hours upon hours at a time at about three weeks of age, with no let-up in sight, the disagreements that I had with my husband about how to stop the baby crying were nearly as bad as the crying itself.

Crying is the only way babies can communicate their needs, but when they are young it is often difficult to determine the case. In fact, 35 per cent of babies' cries stem from 'unknown causes', according to a study done at the Mayo Clinic. It is important for your sanity, especially if your baby has been crying non-stop for hours, to remember that it is not a case of you actually doing anything wrong. It takes time to learn the meaning of your baby's cries, so be kind to yourself: relax, stay calm and try to work out exactly what your baby is trying to tell you by really listening to the differences in your baby's cries.

In the beginning, it's all really quite simple. Babies are usually hungry, tired, windy or need a nappy change. Of course, there are instances, especially if they have been put down, when they just want to be held.

It is important to be compassionate with your baby. We don't withhold comfort and compassion from adults when they are crying, so why should we withhold comfort from a little baby or child? If she cries at night because she is lonely or afraid, pick her up and find out why. Take her into your bed if you want to, and the crying will probably stop. Just remember that each child is radically different when it comes to communicating her needs and that your child will develop her own system, taking into account your responses.

There is no such thing as a baby crying just to 'exercise her lungs'. The old idea that you should let a baby cry rather than pick her up and spoil her is nonsense. There is no way a baby can be spoiled by being picked up. You can never give a baby too much attention. Some babies just cry more than others and take longer to settle down to sleep. I know the case of one parent who actually carries around her infant because he only sleeps when he is being held or in contact with her body and heartbeat. This may sound silly, but just think of it for a moment. In the womb, all that a baby knows is the sound of the mother's heartbeat and the warmth of her body. After birth, the baby has to make a complete readjustment and this takes time. Some babies can do it more rapidly than others. I cannot emphasise enough that by holding, handling and loving your baby as much as you can while responding to her needs as soon as possible, you are acting naturally and laying the foundation for a more loving, caring relationship in the years to come.

As your child gets older, crying will be less of a problem because you will be more confident in distinguishing different sounds and cries. You will also begin to know what to expect at different times of the day as you become aware of her schedule (which, mind you, changes about every six to eight weeks).

Sheila Kitzinger, author of many books on natural approaches to pregnancy, birth and childrearing, believes that some babies cry more than others because they feel isolated, bored and frustrated. They also cry in response to allergies, illness, digestive disturbances and breathing problems. She says: 'In some cases, discovering why babies cry is the means to discovering ways to help them stop. In other cases, knowing why brings parents no closer to a solution but may expand their tolerance a bit while they search for one'.

When your baby's cries make you feel frightened, angry, all alone, trapped, scared, exhausted and completely useless, remember that babies do not cry because they are 'out to get' their parents or because they are spoiled. The most common reasons for crying include:

- dirty or wet nappy
- tiredness
- over-tiredness
- over-stimulated
- too hot or cold
- thirsty
- hungry
- too much noise
- too quiet
- not enough body contact
- too much light
- wind (in stomach or intestines)
- teething
- fever
- nappy pin sticking into the body
- nightmares
- need to be wrapped securely
- blankets have fallen off
- lack of a defined border (too large a bed or crib without adequate contact with the periphery)
- uncomfortable position
- colic

Of course, there will be some cries that appear to have no concrete cause. I just call it 'fussy time' and it usually occurs around five in the evening till sleep time.

Here are some guidelines to help you determine the cause of different cries:

- Distress cry — This is often a piercing, unpleasant, screeching cry that will rattle your bones and make you jump out of your skin. It could result from a physical hurt or bad dreams or whatever. It usually doesn't have any rhythm to it and psychologist Edward Tronick describes this cry as a 'long and catlike wail'. About all you can do is give plenty of cuddles, patting, stroking and lullabies.
- Hunger cry — Usually this one starts off with a few grumbles and light sounds, often accompanied by a physical searching on mother's body if the child is being breastfed. If unanswered it will turn into a cry which is loud and full-throated. The only remedy for this one is obviously food and lots of it!
- Fussing cry — Babies do often seem to fuss for no apparent reason. It may be just a whimper, or perhaps the early stages of fatigue. Picking your baby up may help immediately or perhaps walking her around, singing to her and cuddling may just be enough to send her off to sleep or at least settle her down for a while. As I mentioned before, the most popular 'fussy' time is

between the hours of five and seven when for no apparent reason babies just seem to feel uncomfortable and ill at ease. Don't worry, the time will pass rather quickly if you don't resist it.

- Pay attention cry — This cry, which may start off somewhat full, will only get increasingly vigorous and rhythmic the longer the baby goes without the attention she wants. It may even sound as if she is angry; however, what is really occurring is that she easily and quickly loses control, breathing changes, she can even start to gasp, hold her breath, arch her back, and then will be unable to regain her emotional balance for quite some time. Be patient and try to catch this cry in the early stages. Try to figure out what the problem is. Look for disturbing objects, for example, nappy pins, flies, mosquitoes or barking dogs. Singing, cuddling, rocking and walking the floor can really help.

What To Do When Your Baby Cries

There is no instant cure for babies' crying. What suits one family will most likely not suit another. There are really no hard and fast rules, and be prepared to try different approaches — what worked one night or day may not necessarily work at all the next time you try it!

Physical contact

Pat, stroke, rock, cuddle and by all means pick up your baby quickly. A study done at the University of California at Davis revealed that mothers who take longer to go to their crying babies because they were afraid of spoiling them have babies who cry more often at three months than do mothers who answer their babies' cries quickly.

Try each different way of physically comforting your baby for a few minutes before moving on to the next one. Babies need time to integrate.

Rocking

You will have to determine what the best method of rocking will be for your baby. Up and down or side to side are some of the choices, as well as using a rocking chair, which is usually the most soothing. How fast you rock may also determine how successful you will be.

Swaddling

This technique may seem inhibiting; however, keeping a baby snug in a blanket duplicates the womb-like environment. In a major study reported in the journal *Child Development*, one-month-olds who were cosily swaddled cried less, slept more, breathed more regularly and had slower heart rates than unswaddled babies. In fact, swaddling was the number one way to stop the babies' crying and help them sleep.

However, there may be certain times when swaddling doesn't work. According to Evelyn B. Thoman and Sue Browder in their book, *Born Dancing*, 'Drawbacks to swaddling are three-fold. First, a newborn baby who can't regulate his own body temperature very well, may become too hot and develop a rash. Second, some babies who lay at odd angles in the womb (bent over backward or with their legs up against their chins, for example) may find being forced into a traditional swaddling position uncomfortable. Third, babies with congenital hip dislocations should never be swaddled. (In case of doubt, ask your paediatrician.)'

Massage and warm baths

Many parents are discovering how relaxing the ancient art of massage can be for both themselves and their babies. A relaxed baby won't cry, and massage also is a wonderful time of intimacy and bonding. Try massaging when you think a crying session is imminent. You should actually use massage as a preventative measure, because it is rather difficult to massage a crying baby.

Baths are rarely necessary to clean a baby, as they hardly get dirty when they are very young. Try using it as a way of relaxation, either just before bedtime with a touch of lavender oil in the bath to help soothe and relax the baby even more, or just before 'fussy time' so that she can wind down gently and slowly.

Homoeopathic Remedies

When crying is caused by pain, Arsenicum, Belladonna and Chamomilla can be helpful. Sometimes crying is due to anger and frustration and in these cases you will notice a clear difference in the tone of the crying and associated movements. In these cases Chamomilla, Nux Vomica and Staphisagria should be studied and used where indicated.

CUTS AND GRAZES

Treating small cuts and scrapes can be a constant ritual in some families and one which is an inevitable part of childhood.

General Treatment

1 Stop the bleeding by applying direct pressure to the wound. This can be done with a clean cloth or towel or, if the cut is small, simply with clean fingers. Usually the flow of blood will be stemmed in a minute or two.

2 Clean the wound by washing it under cold water. This will do two things: remove or dilute any bacteria and remove debris such as dirt or gravel.

3 Apply an ointment such as Pawpaw ointment, Calendula herbal ointment or Tea-Tree ointment. Freshly crushed Pawpaw or Garlic could also be applied.

4 Either cover the area with a light gauze bandage, or a normal bandage will do, depending on the size of the injury. It is also important to allow the wound to 'breathe'; however, when exposed to air, cuts will form scabs which actually slow down new cell growth.

How to remove sticking plaster

- Saturate the plaster in oil to moisten the adhesive before removing.
- If the bandage is stuck on hair, remove in the direction that the hair grows.
- Remove after a good soaking in the bath.
- Using a small pair of nail scissors, cut the bandage part away from the adhesive part.

CAUTION

Seek medical advice:
- **If the wound starts to swell and go red more than a finger width beyond the cut, as an infection may be present.**
- **If the wound is large and/or gaping, as stitches may be required.**
- **If you cannot wash or remove all the debris out of the wound, especially if it is caused by glass.**

Remove this gently from the sore and then peel away the adhesive sections.
- Soak in salty water; this will soften and eventually remove the plaster.

See also Bleeding.

Home Remedies

- For minor cuts, after washing, submerge the affected area completely in cold water; or apply cayenne pepper or lemon juice to help stop the bleeding and pain as well as to prevent any swelling.
- Once the bleeding has stopped, Calendula (Marigold) lotion can be used to clean the wound. It is a good antiseptic that prevents infection and promotes rapid healing. To make the lotion, pick the flowers from your marigold plant at the end of the day. Spread them on a sheet of paper for 4-5 days to dry. Put 28 g (1 oz) of flowers in a jar and fill with Witch Hazel. Leave to mature for two weeks, then drain. You can also use Calendula cream.
- White cabbage draws pus. Dip the leaves in water and apply as a poultice to any runny or infected sores, painful boils or inflamed injuries. Replace the leaf as it gets warm.

Herbal Remedies

Calendula is a tissue healer and stops bleeding; Chickweed is also a tissue-healer and prevents scarring; and Ribwort will stop bleeding and promote healing.

Calendula (Marigold)

Compress: first make an infusion using 2-3 teaspoons of dried flowerheads to 1 cup water, let steep for 10-15 minutes, strain and let cool down. Dip a piece of cotton (such as a tea-towel) in the decoction, fold it a couple of times and apply to the affected area. Reapply a number of times. Alternatively, instead of reapplying the compress, cover it with a towel and secure it with a bandage.

Chickweed

Compress: first make up an infusion using 2 teaspoons of dried herb or 6-8 teaspoons of fresh, chopped herb to 1 cup of boiling water. Let steep for 5-10 minutes, strain. Dip a piece of cotton (such as a tea-towel) in the infusion, fold it a couple of times and apply to the affected area. Reapply a number of times, then cover with a tea-towel or handkerchief and secure with a bandage.

Fresh Chickweed: if Chickweed grows as a weed in your garden, you can use the fresh herb for minor cuts and grazes. Pick a suitable amount of the herb, avoiding the roots, rinse thoroughly under running water, chop it up into small pieces or bruise it by hand before applying to the affected area. Secure with a bandage. Leave for ½-3 hours. Remove if skin irritation occurs.

Ribwort

Compress: first make up an infusion using 2 teaspoons of dried herb or 6-8 teaspoons of fresh, chopped herb to 1 cup of boiling water. Let steep for 5-10 minutes, strain. Dip a piece of cotton (such as a tea-towel) in the infusion, fold it a couple of times and apply to the affected area. Reapply a number of times, then cover with a tea-towel or handkerchief and secure with a bandage.

Fresh Ribwort: you can use the fresh herb for minor cuts and grazes. Pick a leaf or more, rinse thoroughly under running water, chop it up into small pieces or bruise it by hand before applying to the affected area. Secure with a bandage. Leave for ½-3 hours. Remove if skin irritation occurs.

Homoeopathic Remedies

The pain of a clean incision responds to **Staphisagria** 30C. It may be given as needed in the early stages and then twice daily for a further two days to promote healing.

DEHYDRATION

Infants and children become dehydrated more quickly than adults because they have a comparatively greater need for fluids. With the loss of body fluids due to vomiting, excessive perspiration on a very hot day, high fever with accompanying conditions such as excessive perspiration, rapid respiration, coughing and runny nose, or diarrhoea, the condition can become quite serious. If the levels of body fluids, minerals and salts get too low, urination drops, the skin gets dry and the baby looks dull-eyed, unresponsive and withdrawn. If this happens, seek medical attention *immediately*, as the condition is *dangerous*.

Symptoms

- lack of wet nappies for six to eight hours, lack of urination in the older child for ten hours
- drowsiness
- rapid pulse
- rapid or slow breathing
- dryness of the mouth (when exploring with your finger)
- sunken eyes
- dry or wrinkled skin
- loss of elasticity of the skin
- doughy skin on the abdomen
- weak cry
- depression of the soft spot on the top of the head
- absence of tears

General Treatment

If any signs of dehydration begin developing, a formula that gives the child fluid, minerals and salts in the correct concentration should be given. All formulas will also contain glucose or sugar in some form as this helps the absorption of the minerals and salts.

Some commercial formulas available in chemist shops include Gastrolyte and Repalyte.

If these are not available an approximation of the correct concentration can be obtained by using flat lemonade or cordial like Ribena made up to a normal concentration with the addition of 1 teaspoon of salt to 1 litre of fluid. If signs do not improve quickly, see a doctor. (See also Diarrhoea.)

Undiluted milk, and even skim milk, are dangerous, as they are too concentrated and will worsen the dehydration.

Home Remedies

If a child is vomiting, or has a fever or diarrhoea give her as much fluids as possible in the form of water, juices, broths or anything that she will take. Try giving her an ice cube to suck on or a frozen juice paddle pop. Even if she regurgitates most of what she takes, the little bit that is being retained is better than nothing.

If she is definitely dehydrated mix together the following:
4 cups boiled water
2 tablespoons honey
¼ teaspoon sea salt
¼ teaspoon baking soda
Give small sips frequently alternating with orange juice blended with a banana.

If you are treating a breastfeeding infant give her as much milk as possible or give one of the recommended solutions in a bottle or spoon feed.

Homoeopathic Remedies

Dehydration is normally due to conditions such as vomiting, diarrhoea and fever and the relevant sections should be studied. The correct homoeopathic medicine for these conditions will usually enable the child to imbibe and assimilate fluids and so quickly ameliorate this condition. This is a potentially serious condition and should be referred to your practitioner.

DIARRHOEA

Diarrhoea, or loose stools, is a common occurrence in infants and children, both as an acute condition or chronic long-term loose stools. It's not unusual for parents of newborn babies to suspect diarrhoea when what they are actually seeing is the normally loose stool of a totally breastfed baby. Breastfed babies have the loosest stools, and very rarely have what is medically classified as diarrhoea.

Diarrhoea can also alternate with constipation where the stools are soft and runny but only occur once every three or four days. Diarrhoea is not usually a severe or lasting disorder, but can be dangerous in babies and very young children when dehydration (excessive loss of body fluids) occurs. The risk is still greater if the diarrhoea is accompanied by fever and vomiting as the fluids and the salts can be lost even more rapidly. In chronic cases, it may affect the growth and development of the child.

Diarrhoea is often one of the most common symptoms of bacterial or viral infections, because they usually affect the immature digestive system of very young children.

If there is blood in the stools, it may suggest colitis or a condition called tropical sprue. This, of course, requires the assistance of a trained health practitioner or hospitalisation.

Acute Diarrhoea

When deciding how to treat diarrhoea with natural medicine, it is important to determine exactly how your child is affected.

There are two main types of patterns of acute diarrhoea: hot and cold.

Hot acute diarrhoea

This type is caused by heat-producing foods such as oily, spicy or rich foods, over-heating, sunstroke and some bacterial or viral infections that cause heat symptoms in the body, for example, scarlet fever. The primary cause is an infection of some kind. The symptoms are:

- Fever above 39°C (102°F) with sweating
- Red face
- Bad temper
- Irritable
- Abdominal discomfort when moving bowels
- Anus may be red, sore and inflamed and cause discomfort when going to the toilet

Cold acute diarrhoea

This type is caused by cold foods, exposure to cold wind and weather, food allergies, infections, some antibiotics, undercooked foods or severe fright. The symptoms are:

- Pale face
- Little energy
- Pains in the abdominal area most of the time
- Onset of diarrhoea is quite sudden
- Body temperature is always cold and the child wants to be kept bundled up all the time
- Undigested foods appear in a loose stool
- Shows very little, if any, interest in anything
- Sleeps a lot

Causes of acute diarrhoea

- Excessive or irregular eating — This can damage a child's digestive energy. If this happens then the food passes through to the large intestine, leaving undigested food in the stool as seen in the nappy.
- Cold foods — Refrigerated and frozen foods and drinks as well as foods that are cold in nature, such as banana, apple, celery, pears, yoghurt, cucumber, melons and lettuce, to name just a few.
- Antibiotics — These are difficult for immature digestive systems to digest and can upset the digestive flora.
- Adult foods — Immature digestive systems have a hard time handling heavy, fried, greasy and spicy or 'highly flavoured' foods like too much meat. A sudden attack of diarrhoea is the way that the body gets rid of the undigested food.
- Food poisoning — Too many fast foods that are not properly cooked or under-cooked eggs

ui chicken can lead to various types of salmonella food poisoning.

- Over-heating — The craving for icy cold drinks caused by too much time in the hot summer sun can be a problem, because cold drinks can cause acute diarrhoea.
- Changes in diet — As a baby moves away from a totally milk-based diet on to a variety of different solid foods, she begins to develop a bowel flora which is mixed like that of an adult. (Breastfed babies' bowels are almost totally populated by Lactobacillus bacteria of the Bifidus type, with just some Acidophilus.) Many cases of 'transitory' diarrhoea in babies and young children are caused by fluctuation or changes in the type of bacteria in the bowel (see app. 6).
- Allergy — Allergic responses can damage the mucosa of the bowel, making it inefficient in its job of absorbing water and nutrients. An allergic reaction may also lead to a loss of the enzyme lactase that is required to break down milk sugar or lactose.
- Teething (see Teething).
- Emotional upsets.

General treatment for acute diarrhoea

Most infections of a bacterial or viral nature will take anywhere from one to five days to pass and usually come on rather suddenly. If your child is passing stools every 20-30 minutes, is in distress or is ill for more than 24 hours choose an appropriate treatment. Most cases of mild, cold-type diarrhoea will, however, heal reasonably quickly with no treatment necessary. Seek a practitioner's advice if diarrhoea persists for more than three days.

Home remedies for acute diarrhoea

- If the diarrhoea is very severe and the child does not want to eat, fast her, making sure she has plenty of clear fluids such as boiled water, vegetable juices or broths.
- Avoid all cool or cold foods (see Appendix 9) and foods that are refrigerated as well.
- Avoid junk food, all fruit juices and raw fruits as much as possible.
- Serve regular meals and try to include mashed potato, rice or some noodles.
- It is essential to replace body fluids quickly in babies and small children during acute attacks of diarrhoea. Try cooking white rice in double or triple the usual amount of water,

and then mixed with some vegetable broth. Give this first in teaspoonfuls and then increase the amount as necessary.

- If your child does not respond to natural medicines it may be entirely possible that she does not have enough internal energy to combat the infection or illness. In this instance I would not hesitate to consult a medical practitioner and combine natural and orthodox treatments.
- If there is blood in the stools, consult a natural practitioner or doctor immediately.
- For the 'cold' acute diarrhoea, roast 50 g (2 oz) uncooked rice in a frypan over medium-low heat, stirring constantly until the grains are golden in colour and grind to a powder (in blender is the quickest). Boil with some water until it becomes like porridge.
- For 'cold' acute diarrhoea, roast salt in a skillet or in the oven until hot. Use enough salt to cover the abdomen of your child. Place in a pillowcase. Place a towel on the abdomen and put the pillowcase on top. (See Appendix 7: Compresses, Poultices and Baths.)
- For 'hot' acute diarrhoea, roast 20 g ($2/3$ oz) dry lotus seeds (available from Chinese grocery stores) and grind into a powder, boil with 200 mL ($7½$ fl oz) water until it becomes like a porridge (about 150 mL/5 fl oz). Take 50 mL (2 fl oz) 3 times a day.
- For acute diarrhoea, tape mashed garlic onto the middle of both soles of the feet or on to the navel.

Naturopathic remedies for acute diarrhoea

To replace body fluids and salts lost in diarrhoea of very young babies or infants, prepare the following:

Boil 200 mL of purified water. When it cools, add 1 heaped teaspoon of sugar, $1/16$ teaspoon (0.1 g) sea salt and ⅛ teaspoon (0.2 g) bicarbonate of soda. Stir until they are well combined and give when cool.

You can also buy a ready-made electrolyte replacement powder from your chemist, or use flat lemonade.

To heal the stomach after an episode of acute diarrhoea, the following remedies are good:

- Micelle A — 0.5 mL per day
- Zinc — 10 mg per day
- 1 teaspoon of Slippery Elm powder mixed into a mashed banana twice daily (for hot conditions)
- Viral and bacterial diarrhoea may be helped

by Lactobacillus bifidus or Acidophilus powder (see Appendix 6). Diarrhoea which develops after antibiotic therapy will also respond to this: administer Lactobacillus bifidus at least two hours after antibiotic treatment.

- Garlic will help with bacterial diarrhoea, but *do not* use more than two cloves of raw garlic daily.
- Some foods are medicinal due to their ability to counter toxic bacteria in various ways or because they have astringent or healing qualities that help the bowel itself. These include low fat plain yoghurt, apples, Carob powder, Linseed meal, Slippery Elm, pomegranates, bananas.

If there is severe diarrhoea caused by infection such as gastroenteritis, it is very important to avoid milk, fatty foods, and excessive raw fruits and vegetables for at least five days (it takes five days for the gut mucosa to rebuild itself). Try a diet of small, regular meals with no snacks in between and include grain and vegetable soup, dry crackers, toast, porridge made from several grains mixed together, soaked overnight and then cooked the following morning.

Chronic Diarrhoea

Chronic diarrhoea is a recurring illness. It can last for weeks, even become progressively worse over that time.

Causes

- Teething
- Unsuitable types of milk or foods, that is, allergenic food
- Excessive or irregular eating patterns
- Not burping after feeds
- Foods which are too rich
- Foods too high in fibre
- Too much fruit juice — The concentrated sugars present in fruit juice (not necessarily added ones) hold on to fluid in the bowel and cause the stools to be watery and pass too rapidly. One litre a day or even less can cause diarrhoea. Susan Thompson, in her book, *A Healthy Start for Kids*, reports on a study that was conducted in Australia on toddlers less than two years of age. 75 per cent of these children showed evidence of poor absorption of a 10 g fructose dose. This is the amount in 170 mL of pear or apple juice or 350 mL

of orange juice. Sorbitol, which has a laxative effect, is also found to be naturally occurring in apple and pear juice. If your child is prone to diarrhoea, you should try watering down juices or avoiding them altogether until she is older.

- Irregular appetite
- Too much fluid — According to Susan Thompson, intakes of around 200 mL per kilogram of body weight have been associated with diarrhoea, which resolved, on reducing intake, to 90 mL per kilogram of body weight per day. To check your child's intake, divide the total amount she drinks in a day (in mL) by her body weight.
- Weak digestion due to overall weakness in newborns, or immunisation, antibiotics, allergy or food intolerance.
- Not enough fat in the diet.
- Immature bowel — It is not unusual for children to move food through their system at a more rapid pace than necessary. Their bowel movements will be more frequent and a little looser than normal. This should resolve itself around the age of three.

Toddlers very often get diarrhoea for no apparent reason. There are several possible avenues worth exploring if the condition persists for too long:

- Food intolerance — commonly wheat, cow's milk, oranges, soy products, peanuts, eggs and yeast
- Sensitivity to chemicals or dust, etc. (see Allergies, Food Intolerance and Chemical Sensitivity)
- Low hydrochloric acid in the stomach
- Weak pancreatic function

CAUTION

Diarrhoea can be a serious and even life-threatening condition, especially for infants and small children. If the complaint does not quickly respond to treatment, if the child appears dehydrated or if blood appears in the stool, *seek professional help without delay*.

Herbal Remedies for Acute Diarrhoea

Any of the herbs mentioned below will be helpful — use what you have available.

Agrimony

Agrimony is indicated in a wide range of gastro-intestinal complaints and is very well suited to children, especially when diarrhoea is caused by inflammation or infection of the bowel.

Infusion: use 2 teaspoons of dried herb to 1 cup of boiling water. Let steep for 5-10 minutes, strain. Can be sweetened with honey or rice malt. Dilute with water if necessary.

DOSE

1-2 years: 15-30 mL (½-1 fl oz) 3 to 4 times daily
3-4 years: 40-60 mL (1⅓-2 fl oz) 3 to 4 times daily
5-6 years: 70-90 mL (2⅓-3 fl oz) 3 to 4 times daily
7 years and older: 100-150 mL (3-5 fl oz) 3 to 4 times daily

Tormentil

A strong-acting astringent which in full doses will control most cases of diarrhoea. Make sure that the cause of the problem is eliminated.

Decoction: use 1-2 teaspoons of chopped rhizome to 1 cup of water, simmer under lid for 5-10 minutes, strain. Can be sweetened with honey or rice malt. Dilute with water if necessary.

DOSE

1-2 years: 15-30 mL (½-1 fl oz) 3 to 4 times daily
3-4 years: 40-60 mL (1⅓-2 fl oz) 3 to 4 times daily
5-6 years: 70-90 mL (2⅓-3 fl oz) 3 to 4 times daily
7 years and older: 100-150 mL (3-5 fl oz) 3 to 4 times daily

Golden Seal

Golden Seal has astringent and healing actions and also promotes liver function, bile secretion and overall digestive function. It is useful in all types of diarrhoea, but in particular, those cases which are caused by food sensitivity or allergy.

Decoction: use ½ teaspoon of chopped root and rhizome to 1 cup of water, simmer covered for 5-10 minutes, strain. Can be sweetened with honey or rice malt. Dilute with water if necessary.

DOSE

2-3 years: 15-20 mL (½-⅔ fl oz) 3 to 4 times daily
4-5 years: 30-40 mL (1-1⅓ fl oz) 3 to 4 times daily
6-7 years: 50-60 mL (1⅔-2 fl oz) 3 to 4 times daily
8 years and older: 80-100 mL (2⅔-3 fl oz) 3 to 4 times daily

Chamomile

The 'cure-all' for gastrointestinal problems in children. It combines relaxing, calming, anti-inflammatory and astringent actions with a gentle stimulating effect on the digestion. Highly recommended.

Infusion: use 1 teaspoon dried flowerheads to 1 cup of boiling water. Let steep for 5 minutes, strain. Can be sweetened with honey or rice malt. Dilute with water for smaller children.

DOSE

1-2 years: 20-40 mL (⅔-1⅓ fl oz) 3 to 4 times daily
3-4 years: 50-80 mL (1⅔-2⅔ fl oz) 3 to 4 times daily
5-6 years: 100-125 mL (3-4 fl oz) 3 to 4 times daily
7 years and older: 150-200 mL (5-6⅔ fl oz) 3 to 4 times daily

Marshmallow

A soothing mucilagenous herb which is indicated when there is inflammation of the digestive tract.

The root is prepared as a decoction: use 1-1½ teaspoons of chopped root to 1 cup of water, simmer covered for 5-10 minutes.

The leaf is prepared as an infusion: use 2 teaspoons of dried leaf to 1 cup of boiling water, let steep for 10 minutes. Can be diluted with water.

DOSE

½-1 year: 15-30 mL (½-1 fl oz) 3 times daily
2-3 years: 40-50 mL (1⅓-1⅔ fl oz) 3 times daily
4-5 years: 60-80 mL (2-2⅔ fl oz) 3 times daily
6 years and older: 80-120 mL (2⅔-4 fl oz) 3 times daily

Slippery Elm bark

Slippery Elm bark is soothing and slightly astringent, indicated in inflammatory bowel conditions. It has considerable nutritive value.

Use 2-3 teaspoons of powdered bark to ½ cup of hot water; this will form a paste that can be sweetened with honey or rice malt or mixed with fruit, porridge, etc.

DOSE

½-1 year: 2-4 teaspoons of the paste 3 to 4 times daily
2-3 years: 2-3 tablespoons 3 to 4 times daily
4-6 years: 4-6 tablespoons 3 times daily
7 years and older: 6-8 tablespoons 3 times daily

NOTE: Do not give the dried powder internally!

Black tea

Black tea is an astringent anti-diarrhoeal.

Prepare a strong cup of normal, black tea, sweeten with honey or rice malt *but do not add milk or soy milk.*

Fennel

Fennel is especially good for small children. It is anti-inflammatory.

Infusion: use ½-1 teaspoon of the dried seeds (best lightly crushed in a mortar) to 1 cup of boiling water. Let steep for 5 minutes, strain. Can be sweetened with honey or rice malt. Dilute with water if necessary.

DOSE

1-2 years: 15-30 mL (½-1 fl oz) 3 times daily
3-4 years: 40-60 mL (1⅓-2 fl oz) 3 times daily
5-6 years: 70-90 mL (2⅓-3 fl oz) 3 times daily
7 years and older: 100-150 mL (3-5 fl oz) 3 times daily

Herbal Remedies for Chronic Diarrhoea

Golden Seal

Golden Seal has astringent and healing actions and also promotes liver function, bile secretion and overall digestive function. It is useful in all types of diarrhoea, but in particular, those cases which are caused by food sensitivity or allergy.
Decoction: use ½ teaspoon of chopped root and rhizome to 1 cup of water, simmer covered for 5-10 minutes, strain. Can be sweetened with honey or rice malt. Dilute with water if necessary.

DOSE

2-3 years: 15-20 mL (½-⅔ fl oz) 3 to 4 times daily
4-5 years: 30-40 mL (1-1⅓ fl oz) 3 to 4 times daily
6-7 years: 50-60 mL (1⅔-2 fl oz) 3 to 4 times daily
8 years and older: 80-100 mL (2⅔-3 fl oz) 3 to 4 times daily

Calendula (Marigold)

Calendula has healing, anti-inflammatory and astringent properties. It does not contain tannins.
Infusion: use 2 teaspoons of the dried flower-heads to 1 cup of boiling water. Let steep for 5 minutes, strain. Can be sweetened with honey or rice malt. Dilute with water if necessary.

DOSE

1-2 years: 15-30 mL (½-1 fl oz) 3 times daily
3-4 years: 40-60 mL (1⅓-2 fl oz) 3 times daily

5-6 years: 70-90 mL (2⅓-3 fl oz) 3 times daily
7 years and older: 100-150 mL (3-5 fl oz) 3 times daily

Also Chamomile, Marshmallow, Slippery Elm (see under *Acute Diarrhoea*)

Homoeopathic Remedies

Arsenicum 12C may be used where the diarrhoea is from bad food or excess fruit and the child is restless or weak. The stools are usually foul smelling, watery and brown.

Chamomilla 30C is a great remedy for diarrhoea during teething. The stools are mostly greenish and slimy or with white and yellow mucus. The child is often impatient, restless and irritable.

Colocynthis 12C is indicated for diarrhoea with cramping which comes on directly after eating. It is often associated with anger.

Rheum in the 12C potency, or Rhubarb, as it is commonly known, is very useful for diarrhoea during teething. The diarrhoea is usually accompanied by screaming. The stool and body smell may be sour.

Veratrum album 30C is indicated when the diarrhoea is associated with great weakness, vomiting and cold sweat. There may be a thirst for cold water.

Other medicine: Antimonium crudum.

Dose: Administer one dose three times daily or every two hours if it is severe.

Chinese Remedies

1 'Deficiency'

Pale complexion. Pale lips. Pale tongue. Runny nose with clear watery or white mucus (no signs of a head cold or cough). A blue vein or blue tint in the area between the eyebrows above the bridge of the nose. There may also be poor appetite, nausea and vomiting.

QIAN SHI BAI ZHU SAN
LI ZHONG WAN (cold hands and/or feet and/or abdomen)
SHEN LING BAI ZHU SAN (severe diarrhoea, weight loss, poor appetite, low energy, severe flatulence after administering the previous formula)

2 'Heat'

Usually this is due to the child eating an excessive amount of rich, oily or fatty food.

Red lips. The complexion may also be red.

Purple vein at 'San Guan' (see app. 8). The tongue is red with a yellow coating. Tiredness. Irritability or depression. Diarrhoea is usually yellow with a strong smell.

SHAO YAO TANG

Since there is usually an underlying weakness associated with this condition, once the acute symptoms have subsided the digestive system should be strengthened by careful attention to diet and with the appropriate herbal formula:

SI JUN ZI TANG

XIANG SHA LIU JUN ZI TANG (child is prone to mucus)

HUANG QI JIAN ZHONG TANG (cold hands and feet, overly sensitive to the cold)

3 'Food Stagnation'

Accumulation of undigested or partially digested food in the stomach and intestines can also cause diarrhoea. See Abdominal Pain for symptom picture and treatment. As with 2 (above) there is usually an underlying weakness and appropriate steps should be taken to improve the child's digestive functions.

HUO XIANG ZHENG QI TANG

Massage

Treating diarrhoea is the one time you could massage counter clockwise on the abdomen. If there is cramping, use a warm water bottle on the abdomen to relax, first.

1 Turn child on to the right side. Lift left leg and massage in small circles from hip bone toward the navel.

2 Gently press with fingertips into the abdomen; if you feel a tight and constricted spot, hold for thirty seconds, and have child breathe into belly.

3 Turn the child on to her back. Massage the abdomen with hands open and relaxed, moving from left to right across the stomach.

or, on the bottom of each foot press in with thumb from the heel to the middle of foot. Work gently into this soft area, as it could be tender.

4 Use the palm or four fingers to rub the abdominal region for 5 minutes.

5 Put your thumb and index finger on either side of the navel (about 2.5 cm/1 inch away on either side) and gently vibrate for about two minutes.

6 Place one hand on lower back and one hand on the stomach and hold, directing warm, loving energy into the child's abdomen. Relax and breathe.

EARACHES

Earaches are among the most common of childhood ailments. According to Paul Bergner, reporting in the *East-West Journal* of November-December 1991, 'Minor ear infections are the most common medical problem in children under six years of age in the U.S. — about nine out of ten will have at least one infection annually.' If your child complains of an earache, you should look for any other accompanying symptoms such as fever and tenderness of the ear and the surrounding area to determine if there may be an infection requiring medical attention. In babies accompanying symptoms of infection can also include irritability, runny nose, cough, diarrhoea, loss of appetite, poor weight gain and persistent crying.

The most common ear complaint is otitis media, an inflammation of the middle ear which is usually caused by a viral infection with a secondary bacterial infection. It often appears with a cold or sore throat, because such an infection can easily travel from the back of the throat along the Eustachian tube which connects the pharynx with the middle ear.

Many children suffer from recurrent middle ear infections. One factor is the age of the child. Between the ages of four and eight is when the incidence of middle ear infections is greatest. This is the time when adenoid and tonsil tissues grow most rapidly. When mucus builds up in the middle ear it can be accompanied by swollen glands, cough and a runny nose.

To complicate matters, your child could exhibit a slight hearing loss in between bouts. In cases of 'glue ear' the fluid in the middle ear becomes thick or gluey. This causes severe hearing loss and needs to be dealt with professionally.

Sometimes the skin of the outer ear can become infected as well by bacteria. This is called otitis externa and is commonly caused by a foreign object being put into the ear to stop an itch or clear out impacted wax, or from swimming in unclean water where fungus seeps inside of the skin in the ear canal, or

water just gets trapped inside the ear after swimming. It can be painful and itchy, perhaps even red and swollen. If inflamed consult a practitioner immediately.

CAUTION

If your child has put something into her ear, take her to the doctor at once. It's dangerous for you to try to remove the object.

If an earache persists for longer than 48 hours, seek medical attention.

Allergies, especially to cow's milk, dust, animal hair and pollen, are among the most common causes of earaches in children. They cause swelling of the mucous membranes, which interferes with the drainage of secretions through the Eustachian tube, thus resulting in infection. The Eustachian tube can also become blocked with water (after swimming) or impacted ear wax.

Other causes of earache include:
- Diet too high in fatty, greasy, oily and spicy foods
- Over-excitement
- Over-tiredness
- Sudden change in the weather (usually hot to cold)
- Emotional upset

Excess fluid can remain in the middle ear and continue to cause recurring earache even after the infection has cleared. If this is the case, do not continue giving antibiotics but rather administer treatment which will reduce the fluid production and drain the ears. This is a common problem with two-thirds of children with ear infections continuing to have effusion one week after the infection is gone, one-third continuing to have effusion four weeks after the infection is gone and 10 per cent having the effusion three months after the infection cleared.

General Care

If your child wakes up in the middle of the night with an earache, the best thing to do is to stay with your child, prop them up, apply warm water compresses and administer a natural remedy. A hot water bottle behind the ear will sometimes suffice. The neck and throat area should be kept warm as well. Alternating hot and cold packs may also help relieve pain. If possible keep the ears covered with a hat or ear muffs.

CAUTION
Most acute ear infections are self-limiting and can therefore be treated safely at home. However, if there is a fever over 38°C (101°F), a discharge from the ear, or if the symptoms persist for more than 48 hours or are unusually severe, seek medical attention immediately.

If an allergy exists this must be dealt with (see Allergies, Food Intolerance and Chemical Sensitivity).

Do what you can to decongest the nasal area. Eucalyptus oil and Tea-Tree oil inhalations can be used. I have had great success using warm oil to massage the sinus, throat and neck area. Warmth and massage help to circulate the blood and lymph and will help resolve congestion in the area.

Eliminate all dairy foods, sugar and high protein foods like peanut butter. Increase vitamin C foods. Dilute all fruit juices (1:3) with water, as undiluted fruit juice increases mucus production.

Home Remedies

- Grate an onion and apply as a poultice on the back of the ears and side of the neck. Re-apply frequently (see app. 7).
- Two drops of heated (not hot) garlic oil: press 4 cloves of peeled garlic and combine with ¼ cup olive oil in a glass jar. Cover and set aside at room temperature or in the sun 1–2 days. Strain and discard the garlic, making sure that no garlic is left in the oil. Store until needed — it will last 6 months. Warm the oil and test on your wrist to a comfortable temperature. Have your child tilt her head to one side and put 2 drops in each ear even if only one is affected. Put a cotton ball in each ear to keep the oil from dripping out. Repeat twice daily for no longer than four days. If it does not improve consult a practitioner of your choice. Garlic oil, however, may aggravate ear pain. If it does, discontinue use.
- A few drops of Witch Hazel, dropped in the ear, can control pain and inflammation.
- For outer ear infections (Otitis Externa), dilute 1 part Echinacea tincture (Pi5) with three parts boiled water and dip a piece of cotton in it. Place it in the ear and leave it there 4–6 hours. Then remove the cotton, and discard it. Prepare a fresh solution and clean the ear with a piece of cotton dipped into the Echinacea several times daily.
- Peel and grate an onion. Squeeze out juice. Warm the juice and apply 2–3 drops in ear with an eye dropper or cotton wool. Works immediately!
- Apply two drops of heated (but not hot) olive oil into the ear with a dropper or dip some cotton wool into the oil and put it into the ear. Leave the cotton wool in for a while and change it frequently.
- Place the palm of the hand over the afflicted ear.
- Apply a poultice of mashed up greens (parsley, watercress or spinach) or tofu, directly behind the ear to take away the heat and ease the pain (see Appendix 7: Compresses, Poultices and Baths).
- Chamomile tea will have a soothing effect and help the child sleep.
- Roast ½ cup salt in oven or skillet until warm. Place in a cotton sock and hold on the ear. The salt must be applied warm. If it is too hot, cover the ear with a cloth and then apply.
- To shrink swollen mucous membranes, combine 2 teaspoons sea salt and 2 teaspoons lemon juice with 1 cup warm boiled water (or quantities to taste). Gargle 3 times daily (4 years and older).
- Drink as much water as possible to keep mucus secretions thin. A vaporiser also helps.
- To remove ear wax, providing the ear is not infected, apply a few drops of olive oil in each ear 3 times a day for 7–10 days. Place a cotton ball in each ear afterwards, for a few minutes, to stop the oil from coming out. If not successful see a practitioner who may have to irrigate the ear to remove the wax.

Orthodox Medical Treatment

There is some evidence that using antibiotics to treat children's infections does not improve the chances of avoiding the serious results of ear infection — hearing loss, spread of infection or mastoiditis. Antibiotics may slightly shorten the duration of pain and infection, but they will also reduce the body's natural immune response, increasing the risk of developing a new infection.

Herbal Remedies

Mullein

Mullein is a decongestant and anti-inflammatory. An oil in which the flowers have steeped can be applied topically: drop 1-3 drops of warm (*not hot*) Mullein oil into the ear. This gives relief from the pain.
Infusion: use 2 teaspoons of the dried leaves or ½ teaspoon of the dried flowers to 1 cup of boiling water. Let steep for 5-10 minutes, strain. Can be sweetened with honey or rice malt.
DOSE
1-2 years: 15-30 mL (½-1 fl oz) 3 times daily
3-4 years: 40-60 mL (1⅓-2 fl oz) 3 times daily
5-6 years: 70-90 mL (2⅓-3 fl oz) 3 times daily
7 years and older: 100-150 mL (3-5 fl oz) 3 times daily

Fenugreek

Fenugreek is an anti-inflammatory and decongestant which removes mucus.
Decoction: use 1 teaspoon of the crushed seeds to 1 cup of water. Simmer for 5 minutes, strain. Can be sweetened with honey or rice malt. Dilute with water if necessary.
DOSE
1-2 years: 15-30 mL (½-1 fl oz) 3 times daily
3-4 years: 40-60 mL (1⅓-2 fl oz) 3 times daily
5-6 years: 70-90 mL (2⅓-3 fl oz) 3 times daily
7 years and older: 100-150 mL (3-5 fl oz) 3 times daily

Eyebright

This herb is anti-catarrhal and anti-inflammatory.
Infusion: use 1 teaspoon of dried herb to 1 cup of boiling water. Let steep for 5 minutes, strain. Can be sweetened with honey or rice malt. Dilute with water if necessary.
DOSE
1-2 years: 15-30 mL (½-1 fl oz) 3 times daily
3-4 years: 40-60 mL (1⅓-2 fl oz) 3 times daily

5-6 years: 70-90 mL (2⅓-3 fl oz) 3 times daily
7 years and older: 100-150 mL (3-5 fl oz) 3 times daily

Golden Rod

Golden Rod is also anti-catarrhal and anti-inflammatory.
Infusion: use 1 teaspoon of dried herb to 1 cup of boiling water. Let steep for 5 minutes, strain. Can be sweetened with honey or rice malt. Dilute with water if necessary.
DOSE
1-2 years: 10-20 mL (⅓-⅔ fl oz) 3 times daily
3-4 years: 30-40 mL (1-1⅓ fl oz) 3 times daily
5-6 years: 50-60 mL (1⅔-2 fl oz) 3 times daily
7 years and older: 70-100 mL (2⅓-3 fl oz) 3 times daily

Elderflower

Elderflower is anti-catarrhal and anti-inflammatory. It also reduces fever.
Infusion: use 2 teaspoons of the dried flowers to 1 cup of boiling water. Let steep for 5 minutes, strain. Can be sweetened with honey or rice malt.
DOSE
1-2 years: 15-30 mL (½-1 fl oz) 3 times daily
3-4 years: 40-60 mL (1⅓-2 fl oz) 3 times daily
5-6 years: 70-90 mL (2⅓-3 fl oz) 3 times daily
7 years and older: 100-150 mL (3-5 fl oz) 3 times daily

Catmint

Catmint is a decongestant with calming and relaxing properties.
Infusion: Use 1 teaspoon of dried herb to 1 cup of boiling water. Let steep for 5 minutes, strain. Can be sweetened with honey or rice malt. Dilute with water if necessary.
DOSE
1-2 years: 15-30 mL (½-1 fl oz) 3 times daily
3-4 years: 40-60 mL (1⅓-2 fl oz) 3 times daily
5-6 years: 70-90 mL (2⅓-3 fl oz) 3 times daily
7 years and older: 100-150 mL (3-5 fl oz) 3 times daily

Homoeopathic Remedies

A sudden earache which appears after a chill and is better for warmth calls for **Aconite** 30C.

Belladonna 30C also has a sudden onset and has a special affinity for the right ear. The pain is usually throbbing and worse for jarring. It may accompany fever with dry skin and thirstlessness.

When the child becomes extremely irritable with the pain and one cheek is red and hot and the other is pale and cold, **Chamomilla** 30C is called for.

The outstanding feature of **Hepar sulph** 12C is that the ear is sensitive to slight touch or the slightest draught of cold air. This child will want the ear wrapped up and may also be extremely irritable.

For earaches which are worse at night and have infection in the middle ear with intense pain, **Mercurius** 30C is the choice. This is often associated with profuse sweat or salivation and bad breath.

When the ear is inflamed and the pains are worse for warmth and in the evening, **Pulsatilla** 12C should be given. The child is usually weepy, wants company and the fresh air.

Dose: One dose every fifteen minutes if the pain is severe or three times daily if the condition is mild.

Chinese Remedies

Usually difficult to diagnose in a young child who has not started speaking. If you suspect an ear infection, have a practitioner inspect the ear with an otoscope.

1 Early Stage (No Discharge)

Fever and chills. Crying. Restlessness. Child may pull or rub the ear. (On inspection the ear drum is red and does not reflect light.) There may be diarrhoea and/or vomiting.

XIAO CHAI HU TANG
TUO LI XIAO DU YIN (weak constitution or weakness after a prolonged febrile illness)

2 After Rupture of Ear Drum

HUANG QI JIAN ZHONG TANG
LING GUI WEI GAN TANG (diarrhoea, cough, red complexion)
QIAN JIN NEI TUO SAN (weak constitution or weakness after prolonged febrile illness)

Massage

1 Massage down either side of neck, hands open; press firmly, from top to bottom.
2 Massage by stroking down with fingertip behind ear, along the line of head. Use only as much pressure as the child can tolerate.
3 Gently hold each ear with thumb inside ridge of ear, and index finger outside and behind ear. Lightly stretch and pull the ear. Do this for two minutes, maintaining light, even pressure.

4 For infants or ears too tender to touch, press at base of second, third, fourth and fifth toe on each foot on the bottom of the foot with thumb or finger. Do this on each foot, feeling for tender spots, and hold for thirty seconds.

GLUE EAR

Glue ear describes the presence of a sticky fluid in the ear. The child may have earache, degrees of deafness, feeling of fullness in the ear or popping sensations in the ear. Glue ear is a common cause of poor school performance because of the associated loss of the hearing and the possible 'spaced out' feeling in the child. Glue ear can also cause slight balance problems leading to poor motor co-ordination. Laser acupuncture is very successfully used in the treatment of chronic glue ear.

Causes

Glue ear can follow on from an ear infection or it can have a slow, insidious onset. Children who develop glue ear often have a history of frequent upper respiratory infection and usually have the physical appearance of the allergic child (see Allergies, Food Intolerance and Chemical Sensitivity). Allergies to food, chemicals and airborne substances play a very significant role in the development of glue ear, so it is important to identify and treat any underlying allergy.

Home Remedies

The treatments described for earache are also applicable here; however, as this is a chronic condition, long-term therapy is necessary.

- Regular warm massages to the neck and head area with warm oil containing aromatic oils such as Eucalyptus, Cajuput, Tea-Tree and Thyme will help to increase the circulation of the blood and lymph assisting the body's ability to heal itself.
- Onion poultices described for earache can be used on a regular basis and are very helpful in terms of aiding circulation and clearing fluid from the ears (see page 247).
- Herbs and supplements — Those used for earache are also good for glue ear; however, they need to be taken for a longer period.

Homoeopathic Remedies

Glue ear is a chronic condition that is often benefited by homoeopathy and should be referred to your professional practitioner.

ECZEMA

Skin rashes are very common childhood complaints. Like asthma, the incidence of eczema has been on the increase over the last few years, and orthodox medicine has been hard pressed to treat it adequately. The best that orthodox medicine can do is arrest the symptoms with cortisone and other steroid creams and ointments. Natural medicine, on the other hand, usually has more success attacking the actual cause of the eczema.

Eczema is the skin's most common manifestation of allergic responses.

Food sensitivities can be contributing factors and some of the more common foods that may lead to eczema include: corn, eggs, shellfish, wheat, chocolate, beef, milk, oranges and other dairy products, soy bean products, potatoes, fish, peanuts and greasy foods. When these foods are eliminated from your child's diet very often improvement is seen rather quickly.

Sometimes environmental changes, such as central heating in the home in winter, pollen in the air or a pet introduced into the household, can also set off a skin rash.

Sometimes when a child is not able to express herself, digestion is affected, the stomach becomes upset, and eczema can be the result. Usually this occurs in children over the age of seven, as when they are younger expression is very rarely a problem — if anything, over-expression is! If parents do not allow natural expression to take place very often a child will begin to repress her innermost feelings and not express them.

There are four different types of eczema: itching, dry, wet, and a combination of all three. They can vary in size and shape and can change in colour, size and shape from day to day.

In infants and children eczema is most likely to occur on the cheeks, the belly button or under the nappy as a flat, red, shiny, rather patchy rash that usually itches and comes up inflamed. Sometimes eczema can have a rather elongated appearance around the back of your baby's legs, under the edge of the nappy, across the abdomen or in the groin. If your baby scratches it continuously it will weep, then when it is finally allowed to dry, scabs will usually form (see also Nappy Rash).

Itching Eczema

The skin is very itchy and your child will want to scratch non-stop. This produces a very sore, broken and bleeding surface, which then has to be carefully watched so that infection does not set in. In traditional Chinese medicine it is believed that this type of skin condition is due to poisons and toxins that are trapped underneath the skin and may be accompanied by constipation.

Dry Eczema

Many children suffer from dry skin during winter, but with eczema the skin may become so dry that it scales, and although skin creams and ointments do help somewhat nothing seems to cure this condition. When the skin is rubbed, scale-like pieces begin to flake off and the skin underneath is red and in severe cases can sometimes bleed. According to traditional Chinese medicine, this type of eczema is caused by digestive disturbances that respond by an accumulation of mucus in the tissues under the skin.

Wet Eczema

This type of eczema looks completely different from the dry or itching kind, with the skin being shiny and wet. When scratched, the fluid collected under the skin can sometimes ooze out. This type of eczema is often accompanied by diarrhoea or loose stools and, again, according to Chinese medicine is caused by an imbalance in the digestive system.

Diet
Babies

• Give your baby regular feeds and not too much at one time. Basically, *do not over-feed*.

- Burp your baby after each feed and wait two hours between each feed when possible.
- If you are breastfeeding, try avoiding those foods that may cause eczema (see above) and also spicy foods.
- If you are bottle feeding your baby, it is entirely possible that she may have an allergy to cow's milk. In this instance, change to goat's, rice (see Appendix 2) or soy bean milk if child is over 12 months.
- To make milk more digestible, try simmering the milk for 15 minutes with half an onion.

Weaned babies and toddlers

- Follow the guidelines listed above for babies and if your child drinks a lot of milk use soy bean, goat's or almond milk.
- Try the elimination diet (see Allergies) if these suggestions are not working for your child as she may have an allergy to another food.

ECZEMA BREAKTHROUGH

Studies recently conducted in Italy and England have found an association between atopic eczema in children and low levels of gamma linolenic acid (GLA) which is found only in human breast milk and in evening primrose oil.

A study reported in *Lancet* in 1982 showed that in an experimental controlled scientific trial with 60 adults and 39 children, there was significant improvement of eczema after they had received evening primrose oil. Both low and high doses of the oil were administered. The severity of eczema improved by 30 per cent in the low dose group and by 43 per cent in the high dose group.

General Care

- Keep all the affected areas clean and, if worried about scratching or infection, bandaged.
- Keep all fingernails short, smooth and well scrubbed.
- Check that your child is not sensitive to the washing detergents that you may be using.
- Check that your child is not sensitive to synthetic clothing.
- Do not put wool clothing next to your child's skin. Try a cotton shirt under the wool garment.

Steps To Recovery

- It is not at all uncommon, when eczema is being treated with natural remedies, that it gets worse before it gets better. So do not be disheartened, because the condition will eventually improve.

Home Remedies

- For dry eczema, cover the child from head to toe before bedtime with a thin layer of olive oil, lanolin-based cream with vitamins A and E, Aloe Vera gel or Calendula cream once or twice a week.
- For dry eczema, bathe your child only once or twice a week before bedtime with some sesame oil in the bath.
- Wrap 3-4 cups (15-20 oz) of oatmeal, rice or oat bran in a piece of cheesecloth, muslin or a sock. Add this to the bath water (see Appendix 7: Compresses, Poultices and Baths).
- To relieve itching and discomfort, add 2-3 drops of Bach Rescue Remedy to the bath water (see Appendix 7: Compresses, Poultices and Baths).
- For itching skin without a rash, Witch Hazel will provide instant relief. However, it is only temporary and as it has astringent properties it should not be used on rashes. Aloe Vera gel will also temporarily relieve itching. Try a cooked potato poultice (see Appendix 7: Compresses, Poultices and Baths).
- Prickly heat — all babies suffer from prickly heat; which comes out as tiny little red spots. Don't over-dress your baby and only use loose cotton clothing or none at all. Apply Calamine lotion or add 1-2 cups (4-8 oz) of Cornflour or Arrowroot powder to her bath water.

Herbal Remedies
Burdock

This herb promotes the cleansing of tissues of metabolic waste products and accumulated toxins. Indicated in a range of skin diseases, in particular dry eczema.

Decoction: use 1 teaspoon of the chopped root to 1 cup of water. Simmer for 10-15 minutes covered, strain. Can be sweetened with honey or rice malt. Dilute with water if necessary.

DOSE
4-5 years: 20-30 mL (²/₃-1 fl oz) 3 times daily
6-7 years: 40-50 mL (1¹/₃-1²/₃ fl oz) 3 times daily

8 years and older: 60-80 mL (2-2⅔ fl oz) 3 times daily

NOTE: This herb may lead to an initial worsening of symptoms. Start with a low dose, gradually building up to the dose indicated above. Not suitable for small children; give Red Clover instead.

Yellow (Curled) Dock

Another 'blood purifying' herb, Yellow Dock acts as a mild laxative. Indicated in chronic eczema, especially when there is weak digestive function. It is rich in iron.

Decoction: use 1-1½ teaspoons of chopped root to 1 cup of water, simmer covered for 5-10 minutes. Can be sweetened with honey or rice malt. Dilute with water if necessary.

DOSE

1-2 years: 15-30 mL (½-1 fl oz) 3 times daily
3-4 years: 40-60 mL (1⅓-2 fl oz) 3 times daily
5-6 years: 70-90 mL (2⅓-3 fl oz) 3 times daily
7 years and older: 100-150 mL (3-5 fl oz) 3 times daily

NOTE: Do not give for longer than two weeks at a time. Reduce dose if diarrhoea occurs.

Red Clover

Red Clover is somewhat similar in action to Burdock (see above) but milder and therefore generally better suited to children. The tea can also be applied externally to dry and scaly skin conditions.

Infusion: use 3 teaspoons of dried flowers to 1 cup of boiling water. Let steep for 5 minutes, strain. Can be sweetened with honey or rice malt. Dilute with water if necessary.

DOSE

1-2 years: 15-30 mL (½-1 fl oz) 3 times daily
3-4 years: 40-60 mL (1⅓-2 fl oz) 3 times daily
5-6 years: 70-90 mL (2⅓-3 fl oz) 3 times daily
7 years and older: 100-150 mL (3-5 fl oz) 3 times daily

Dandelion root

This herb is for skin conditions caused by digestive malfunction.

Decoction: use 1-2 teaspoons of chopped root to 1 cup of water, simmer covered for 5-10 minutes. Can be sweetened with honey or rice malt. Dilute with water if necessary.

DOSE

1-2 years: 15-30 mL (½-1 fl oz) 3 times daily
3-4 years: 40-60 mL (1⅓-2 fl oz) 3 times daily
5-6 years: 70-90 mL (2⅓-3 fl oz) 3 times daily

7 years and older: 100-150 mL (3-5 fl oz) 3 times daily

Stinging Nettle

For allergic skin conditions in particular. Stinging Nettle is rich in minerals.

Infusion: use 1½-2 teaspoons of the dried herb to 1 cup of boiling water. Let steep for 5 minutes, strain. Can be sweetened with honey or rice malt. dilute with water if necessary.

DOSE

1-2 years: 15-30 mL (½-1 fl oz) 3 times daily
3-4 years: 40-60 mL (1⅓-2 fl oz) 3 times daily
5-6 years: 70-90 mL (2⅓-3 fl oz) 3 times daily
7 years and older: 100-150 mL (3-5 fl oz) 3 times daily

Heartsease (Wild Pansy)

Heartsease can be used as an anti-inflammatory in weeping eczema, especially where the child also has bronchial problems such as asthma.

Infusion: use 1-1½ teaspoons of the dried herb to 1 cup of boiling water. Let steep for 5 minutes, strain. Can be sweetened with honey or rice malt.

DOSE

1-2 years: 15-30 mL (½-1 fl oz) 3 times daily
3-4 years: 40-60 mL (1⅓-2 fl oz) 3 times daily
5-6 years: 70-90 mL (2⅓-3 fl oz) 3 times daily
7 years and older: 100-150 mL (3-5 fl oz) 3 times daily

Also try the following:
● Evening Primrose oil: 2-4 capsules a day
● Lactobacillus Bifidus powder to control abnormal bowel flora.

DOSE

0-2 years: ¼ teaspoon twice daily
2-5 years: ⅓ teaspoon twice daily
Over 5 years: ½ teaspoon twice daily

The following ointments to give some symptomatic relief from dryness and itching: Calendula, Chickweed and Nettle.

Homoeopathic Remedies

Eczema is a chronic condition that is often benefited by homoeopathy and should be referred to your professional homoeopathic practitioner.

Chinese Remedies

1 'Excess'

Strong constitution. Normally good health, strength and energy. Tongue is red with a yellow coating. There may be constipation. Complexion is red.

ZHI TOU CHUANG YI FANG

2 'Deficiency'

Weak constitution. Low energy. Poor appetite. Easily tired. Quiet and withdrawn. Pale complexion, lips and tongue (face, lips and tongue may become red during the attack of eczema, but normally they are pale).

XIAO CHAI HU TANG

3 'Dampness'

Small blister-like lesions which ooze a yellowish liquid. Tongue has a thick, moist coating.

WU LING SAN (taken together with one of the above formulas)

EMERGENCIES

Artificial Resuscitation

If oxygen is denied to the brain for more than three to four minutes, brain damage can result, and death can follow shortly afterwards. The aim of any form of artificial resuscitation is to clear the airways and restart breathing to restore the circulation. The most effective technique is mouth-to-mouth resuscitation. It should be continued until natural breathing starts or medical help arrives. The first practice session should not be on your unconscious child, so prepare yourself for an emergency by learning the technique as part of the first aid courses run by organisations such as St John's Ambulance Brigade or the Red Cross Society.

Procedure

1 Check your child's breath by placing your cheek next to her nose, looking for the rise and fall of her chest. If she is not breathing, commence resuscitation.
2 Lay your child on her back and check her airways for obstructions.
3 Tilt back her head to open her airways.
4 Pinch her nose with your fingers and make a seal over her mouth with your mouth.
5 Give 5 breaths. Watch your child's chest as you do so to see if it is rising and falling. Your exhalation will have enough oxygen in it to maintain your child's circulation. If your child's chest does not rise and fall, check for obstructions again. Breathe gently into your child's lungs. If a baby, only puff from your cheeks.
6 Continue mouth-to-mouth resuscitation, checking your child's chest frequently to see if her own breathing has started.
7 If the child's breathing has stopped due to drowning, position her head and chest lower than her hips while resuscitating to try and drain her lungs.

Cardiac Massage

Cardiac massage should only be used in situations where your child's heart has stopped beating or there is no pulse, for example, after electric shock, drowning or a major accident.

Like artificial resuscitation, this technique should be *professionally* learnt.

Checking the pulse

To check the pulse of your child, feel for the carotid artery on the neck just under the jaw next to the cartilage covering the throat. You can also check the pulse by placing two fingers on the inside of a baby's arm between shoulder and elbow. Practise on your child so that in the event of an emergency, you can check the pulse easily. If there is no pulse start cardiac compression immediately.

Cardiac compression

Compress the lower half of the breast bone using the heel of your hand covering an area about 20-40 mm (1-2 in). Press down at the rate of eighty times per minute. For an infant, use two fingers in the centre of the breast bone at the rate of 100 times per minute.

Continue mouth-to-mouth resuscitation at the rate of two breaths to every fifteen cardiac compressions. Never stop cardiac compressions for more than five seconds at a time, and continue until professional help arrives, or until the pulse returns.

CAUTION

If cardiac massage is applied to a child whose heart is still beating or if it is applied incorrectly, it may cause death or irreparable damage. It should also be used in conjunction with mouth-to-mouth resuscitation until help arrives.

The Recovery Position

1 After having made sure that the airway is clear, turn the child on her side and make sure that her head is pointing slightly downwards.
2 The uppermost arm should be bent across the body so that the elbow is in line with the shoulder. The bottom arm should be straight by the child's side.
3 The uppermost leg should be bent across the body with the knee in line with hip.
4 Check that the airway is still clear.

FEVER

Fever is not a disease. Fever is one of the body's most powerful defences against the invasion of viruses and bacteria. This is why, when you phone your doctor looking for advice he is not as interested in how high the temperature is as in any other symptoms that may be present.

If you turn to aspirin or paracetamol at the first sign of a fever, you will be depriving the body of one of its best defences. Fever comes about because pyrogens, the fever-producing substances, appear in the blood and affect the temperature control in the brain, calling for more heat. Pyrogens also stimulate white blood cells to destroy viruses and bacteria.

The common cold and flu are the most common sources of elevated body temperatures in children of all ages. Too much greasy, fried or oily food, sugar or spices can also bring on a fever, as can a sudden change in weather from cold to hot. Fevers of up to even 38.5°C (102°F) are not dangerous. The danger comes from dehydration caused by accompanying conditions such as excessive perspiration, rapid respiration, coughing, runny nose, vomiting and diarrhoea. Just make sure that your child gets plenty of fluids, around ½ cup every hour, and treat the source of the infection (ear, chest, gastroenteritis and so on) using treatments that stimulate the immune system.

For a relatively small number of children, fevers can be serious, since there may be a risk of fits, so observe the facts in the 'Caution' box. Convulsions are not related to the height of your child's temperature but to how *rapidly* the temperature rises. (See also Convulsions.)

Symptoms of Fever

- Irritability
- Clinginess
- Feels either too cold or too hot
- Face may become flushed and forehead feels hot to the touch
- Dryness in the mouth
- Bitter taste in the mouth
- Bad breath

- Possible dry, uncomfortable feeling in the throat
- Possible headache with a feeling of heaviness in the head (flu-like symptom).

In addition to the symptoms listed above, fevers may be further differentiated as follows:

- Cold — There are feelings of cold and chills, with possible teeth chattering and shivering. Face is pale and your child isn't able to wear enough clothing to get warm, especially hands and feet.
- Hot — Your child will complain of feeling too hot, wanting to take off her clothes and throw off her blankets. Face is flushed, feels irritable and may also feel chilled at times.

Some children with minimal illness will present a high temperature, while a very sick child may only have a degree or less of fever. Therefore, the temperature of a child does not always determine the seriousness of a child's illness. The accompanying symptoms will tell the tale.

Temperature readings will vary according to

CAUTION

- **If your newborn has a fever during the first few months of her life, take her to a doctor. The fever may be a symptom of an infection that is related to the delivery or perhaps even prenatal in origin.**
- **Consult your doctor immediately if your child is having behavioural symptoms such as twitching or other strange movements, has a major change in appearance, loses consciousness, is having difficulty in breathing or cannot stop vomiting.**
- **Sometimes the fever can be the result of poisoning or too much sun and heat, and if you think that this might be the case, seek medical attention immediately. If there is no doctor available, take your child to the nearest hospital emergency room.**

how the temperature is taken. Rectal temperatures in older children are usually about a degree higher than those taken orally, and underarm temperatures are usually about a degree lower.

The use of aspirin may cause a child to experience irritation and bleeding of the lining of the gastrointestinal tract and has also been associated with serious complications when given to a child with chickenpox or flu, according to Morris A. Wessel, M.D., in his book, *Parents Book, or, Raising a Healthy Child.*

General Care

- Try to expel the fever by having your child sweat it out if possible.
- Encourage her to rest as much as possible: however, if your child insists on moving about, a little fresh air and sunshine will do her no harm. Babies will sleep as long as they need to, but older children may need to be encouraged to do so.

Diet

It is best to feed your child as little as possible during the first twenty-four hours of a fever, as fasting can have a stimulating effect on the immune system, which helps to combat the illness. However, do as your child dictates. If your child doesn't have much of an appetite, just give her plenty of liquids.

Light soups, broths and stews from vegetables are best during and after an illness. Avoid heavy, rich foods. Small amounts of food are best when recovering from the fever. Start off with broths, very diluted tea, milk or diluted fruit juice, working your way to porridge and toast. Feed your child frequently with small amounts and if your child feels very weak, try serving chicken soup or beef broth.

There is a tendency for constipation to occur during fevers, and the added toxicity from the bowel continues to stimulate the fever. In naturopathic and herbal medicine some gentle purging of the bowel is recommended to help bring down the fever. Do not over-use laxatives as this will weaken the child too much.

Home Remedies

- A tepid (not cold) sponge bath is good for high temperatures, especially around the hands, head and feet.

- Lots to drink.
- Try a tofu or tofu and green vegetable compress to take some of the heat from the body (see Appendix 7: Compresses, Poultices and Baths).
- A cabbage leaf on the forehead can lower the temperature. If your child refuses this, try a cool, damp face cloth.
- A cottage cheese compress can be a very effective way to remove heat (see Appendix 7).
- For the chills of fever try a hot salt poultice (see Appendix 7).

Herbal Remedies

Elderflower, Peppermint, Yarrow and Linden all reduce fever by increasing sweating. The tea should be given hot at frequent intervals. All four herbs can be mixed to form a pleasant tasting tea.

Elderflowers

Infusion: use 2 teaspoons of the dried flowers to 1 cup of boiling water. Let steep for 5 minutes, strain. Can be sweetened with honey or rice malt.
DOSE
1-2 years: 15-30 mL (½-1 fl oz) 3 times daily
3-4 years: 40-60 mL (1⅓-2 fl oz) 3 times daily
5-6 years: 70-90 mL (2⅓-3 fl oz) 3 times daily
7 years and older: 100-150 mL (3-5 fl oz) 3 times daily

Peppermint

Infusion: use ½-1 teaspoon of dried herb to 1 cup of boiling water. Let steep for 5 minutes, strain. Can be sweetened with honey or rice malt. Dilute with water if necessary.
DOSE
1-2 years: 15-30 mL (½-1 fl oz) 3 times daily
3-4 years: 40-60 mL (1⅓-2 fl oz) 3 times daily
5-6 years: 70-90 mL (2⅓-3 fl oz) 3 times daily
7 years and older: 100-150 mL (3-5 fl oz) 3 times daily

Yarrow

Infusion: use 1 teaspoon of dried herb to 1 cup of boiling water. Let steep for 5 minutes, strain. Can be sweetened with honey or rice malt. Dilute with water if necessary.
DOSE
1-2 years: 15-30 mL (½-1 fl oz) 3 times daily
3-4 years: 40-60 mL (1⅓-2 fl oz) 3 times daily
5-6 years: 70-90 mL (2⅓-3 fl oz) 3 times daily

7 years and older: 100-150 mL (3-5 fl oz) 3 times daily

Linden (Lime flowers)

Use 1-1½ teaspoons of dried herb to 1 cup of boiling water. Let steep for 5 minutes, strain. Can be sweetened with honey or rice malt. Dilute with water if necessary.

DOSE

1-2 years: 15-30 mL (½-1 fl oz) 3 times daily
3-4 years: 40-60 mL (1⅓-2 fl oz) 3 times daily
5-6 years: 70-90 mL (2⅓-3 fl oz) 3 times daily
7 years and older: 100-150 mL (3-5 fl oz) 3 times daily

Catmint

Catmint lowers fever without increasing sweating.
Infusion: Use 1 teaspoon of dried herb to 1 cup of boiling water. Let steep for 5 minutes, strain. Can be sweetened with honey or rice malt. Dilute with water if necessary.

DOSE

1-2 years: 15-30 mL (½-1 fl oz) 3 times daily
3-4 years: 40-60 mL (1⅓-2 fl oz) 3 times daily
5-6 years: 70-90 mL (2⅓-3 fl oz) 3 times daily
7 years and older: 100-150 mL (3-5 fl oz) 3 times daily

Cascara

Cascara can be given if constipation is present.
Decoction: use ½ teaspoon of the chopped, dried bark to 1 cup of water. Simmer for 5 minutes, strain. Can be sweetened with honey or rice malt. Dilute with water if necessary.

DOSE

2-3 years: 20-30 mL (⅔-1 fl oz) 1 to 3 times daily
4-5 years: 40-50 mL (1⅓-1⅔ fl oz) 1 to 3 times daily
6-7 years: 60-70 mL (2-2⅓ fl oz) 1 to 3 times daily
8 years and older: 80-100 mL (2⅔-3 fl oz) 1 to 3 times daily

NOTE: Do not give for longer than two weeks at a time. Reduce dose if laxative effect is too strong, causing diarrhoea or abdominal pain. Give with Ginger, Chamomile or Fennel.

Homoeopathic Remedies

When there is a rapid onset of the symptoms and your child is thirsty, restless and fearful, the remedy will be **Aconite** 30C. These children often become intolerant of warmth and throw off the bed covers.

Belladonna 30C is also indicated for sudden onset, but exhibits dilated pupils, red, hot skin, and an aggravation from uncovering as there may be chills. Children needing Belladonna will often have a hot head while the rest of the body is cold. It is a great remedy when there is delirium with the fever.

Ferrum-phos 6C is beneficial in the beginning stages of fever where there is also chill with the desire to stretch.

Nux vomica 30C has great heat but feels chilled with the least movement or uncovering.

The **Pulsatilla** 12C fever is characterised by a lack of thirst which is uncommon in fevers.

Dose: Every hour in a high fever. For a mild fever one dose three times daily for up to two days.

When one of the above remedies is not clearly indicated you should read the other indications in the Materia Medica section. Medicines such as Apis, Arnica, Arsenicum, Bryonia, Chamomilla, Gelsemium, Phosphorus, Rhus-tox, Sulphur and Veratrum may also be indicated in fevers.

Massage

1 Rotate the big toe, moving it in both directions.
2 Press across the tip of the big toe with thumb or index finger and all around the big toe; press and hold on any tender spots.
3 Press at the base of the big toe and into the pad (or ball of foot) just below the big toe.
4 With child 2 years and older. have her imagine a cool stream of water running down her spine.

FIRST AID

The most important thing in a situation requiring first aid is to stay calm. Panicking not only impairs your ability to deal with the accident, but also affects your child. So stay outwardly calm at least, assess the situation quickly, decide on an appropriate course of action, then explain what you are going to do, while continuing to reassure your child.

It is very important to be familiar with life-saving techniques such as artificial resuscitation. St John's Ambulance, the Red Cross, or your local hospital can give you details of where first-aid course are held. You should always keep a current book of first-aid techniques with your first-aid supplies.

Emergency first-aid procedures are described in the relevant sections, as indicated below.

Abdominal Thrust, see Choking, page 110

Artificial Resuscitation, see Emergencies, page 156

Burn Procedures, see Burns and Scalds, page 106

Cardiac Massage, see Emergencies, page 156

Clearing the Oesophagus/Trachea, see Choking, page 110

Poisoning Procedures, see Poisoning, page 194

Pressure and Immobilisation, see Bleeding, page 100 and Bites and Stings, page 96

Recovery Position, see Emergencies, page 156

Splinting and Immobilisation, see Fractures and Dislocations, page 161

Foreign Bodies

Children have an amazing capacity for placing objects in any openings they can — mouth, ears, nose or just for a change, their sibling's eye.

To help remove a foreign body from any part of the head area, wrap the child in a blanket or any other large cloth. It will immobilise her, making it easier to try and remove the object and will also help calm the child by making her feel more secure.

In the eye

If something gets in the child's eye, the eye will water, or the child will cry, both of which are the body's natural flushing actions. If the object remains in the eye, try licking the eye — your tongue is very sensitive and will usually find the object and remove it. In addition, your tongue is wet and slippery and will not damage the eye in the way a corner of a handkerchief could. If there is still discomfort, bathe the eye in warm, salty water, or an eye bath, and if this doesn't help, cover the eye with a pad and take your child to a doctor or the nearest hospital for further treatment.

Any chemicals or other artificial substances should be flushed out of the eye. Hold the child's head under a running tap (not full pressure), or under the shower, injured eye downwards to avoid the chemical being washed into the other eye, and flush the eye for at least ten minutes. Bathe every part of the eye by opening the lids with your fingers. If there is any injury to the eyeball itself, take the child to the doctor immediately.

In the ear

Do not try and remove any object lodged in the ear as you may do irreparable damage. The object must be taken out at the first attempt with the right equipment. This is best done by a doctor or at the hospital.

In the nose

Try to get the child to blow out the object by covering the other nostril with your finger or while the nostril is covered blow into her mouth. If you can see the object, try to gently remove it with tweezers. Otherwise, take your child to a doctor or hospital.

If the object is swallowed

Many objects will be simply passed in the stools in four to five days and cause no problems. Large coins and buttons may get stuck in the stomach or food pipe. Watch the child for five to six days and if the object is not passed in the stools, surgery may be necessary.

With items that are sharp, like pins or needles, and also batteries, which do contain a small amount of mercury, more care needs to be taken. Though they are normally passed in bowel motions, medical attention is essential. While laxatives or any special diet are not recommended, large quantities of bananas are said to have been of some help. See also Choking.

Fractures and Dislocations

Both of these injuries, especially in toddlers, are mainly caused by falls and in these cases prevention is the best cure. This can be done by careful planning, safety measures and education (see section on Safety). However, even with all precautions taken, it is possible for a child to sustain a fracture or dislocation.

Treatment

- Keep the child calm if you suspect a broken or dislocated limb, and seek medical help immediately.
- While transporting the child or waiting for help to arrive, immobilise the limb. If the arm is affected, bind it to the chest; if the leg is affected, bind it to the other leg. If possible, raise the limb slightly. Splints can be used if you have something suitable on hand.
- If the bone is protruding, cover the area with a sterile dressing or clean material.
- Do not move the child if a spinal or head injury is suspected. Call an ambulance.
- Do not give the child anything to eat or drink, in case an anaesthetic may be necessary.

Homoeopathic Remedies

Symphytum 6C is an excellent remedy to promote the healing of a fracture. It should be given three times daily for ten days, although this period can be extended where necessary.

FLATULENCE

Flatulence or 'wind', as it is most commonly known, is an everyday bodily occurrence that usually has no painful symptoms. It is often blamed as the major cause for crying babies. While a large bubble of gas in the stomach is likely to cause a minor amount of discomfort, this is very unlikely to happen after every feed. However, a cuddle with the baby held upright and a few pats on the back are all that's needed if you feel it is better for your baby to burp.

Flatulence is not usually a problem for breastfed babies. Any tummy discomfort that may be caused by gulping, can be avoided by expressing a little milk at the beginning of the feed when your milk 'lets down'.

Wind may be a slight problem when bottle feeding if the hole in the nipple is too small or too large. Nipples that you buy from a druggist will have the correct age imprinted on them. Use this as a guide and, if all else fails, simply experiment until your baby's drinking pattern is smooth and regular.

Chronic Flatulence

Chronic flatulence can be caused by the following:

- Food intolerance — In a baby it may be Lactose intolerance but food allergy of any type may play a role.
- Abnormal bowel flora — This may be due to a weak immune system or may follow antibiotic therapy.
- Inflammation of the gastrointestinal tract — This may follow gastroenteritis, food allergy or abnormal flora.
- Weak secretion of digestive juices — This can occur from both the stomach and the pancreas.

If any of the above causes exist, they must be treated.

Food allergies must be excluded (see Allergies).

Bowel flora can be normalised with Lacto-bacillus, Acidophilus or Bifidus, available from health food stores, the health food section of large supermarkets, or your naturopath.

DOSE

0-2 years: ¼ teaspoon twice daily
2-5 years: ⅓ teaspoon twice daily
5-7 years: ½ teaspoon twice daily
Over 7 years: ½ to ¾ teaspoon twice daily
See also Colic.

For chronic flatulence you should consult a practitioner of your choice.

Herbal Remedies

The following herbs can be used to relieve flatulence. They all have carminative action and act by relaxing the intestinal muscles, especially sphincters.

Chamomile

Infusion: use 1 teaspoon dried flowerheads to 1 cup of boiling water. Let steep for 5 minutes, strain. Dilute with water for smaller children.

DOSE

1-2 years: 20-40 mL (⅔-1⅓ fl oz) 3 to 4 times daily
3-4 years: 50-80 mL (1⅔-2⅔ fl oz) 3 to 4 times daily
5-6 years: 100-125 mL (3-4 fl oz) 3 to 4 times daily
7 years and older: 150-200 mL (5-6⅔ fl oz) 3 to 4 times daily

Ginger

Infusion: use 3 slices (2-3 cm/1 inch in diameter and 2-3 mm/⅛ inch thick) of fresh Ginger to 1 cup of boiling water. Let steep for 5 minutes. Sweeten with honey or rice malt. Dilute with water for small children.

DOSE

2-3 years: 20 mL (⅔ fl oz) 2 to 3 times daily
4-5 years: 30-50 mL (1-1⅔ fl oz) 2 to 3 times daily
6 years and older: 60-80 mL (2-2⅔ fl oz) 2 to 3 times daily

Peppermint

Peppermint relaxes the gut.

Infusion: use ½-1 teaspoon of dried herb to 1 cup of boiling water. Let steep for 5 minutes, strain. Dilute with water if necessary.

DOSE

1-2 years: 15-30 mL (½-1 fl oz) 3 times daily
3-4 years: 40-60 mL (1⅓-2 fl oz) 3 times daily
5-6 years: 70-90 mL (2⅓-3 fl oz) 3 times daily
7 years and older: 100-150 mL (3-5 fl oz) 3 times daily

Dill

Infusion: use ½-1 teaspoon of the dried seeds (best lightly crushed in a mortar) to 1 cup of boiling water. Let steep for 5 minutes, strain. Can be sweetened with honey or rice malt. Dilute with water if necessary.

DOSE

1-2 years: 15-30 mL (½-1 fl oz) 3 times daily
3-4 years: 40-60 mL (1⅓-2 fl oz) 3 times daily
5-6 years: 70-90 mL (2⅓-3 fl oz) 3 times daily
7 years and older: 100-150 mL (3-5 fl oz) 3 times daily

Fennel

Infusion: use ½-1 teaspoon of the dried seeds (best lightly crushed in a mortar) to 1 cup of boiling water. Let steep for 5 minutes, strain. Dilute with water if necessary.

DOSE

1-2 years: 15-30 mL (½-1 fl oz) 3 times daily
3-4 years: 40-60 mL (1⅓-2 fl oz) 3 times daily
5-6 years: 70-90 mL (2⅓-3 fl oz) 3 times daily
7 years and older: 100-150 mL (3-5 fl oz) 3 times daily

Caraway

Infusion: use ½-1 teaspoon of the dried seeds (best lightly crushed in a mortar) to 1 cup of boiling water. Let steep for 5 minutes, strain. Can be sweetened with honey or rice malt. Dilute with water if necessary.

DOSE

1-2 years: 15-30 mL (½-1 fl oz) 3 times daily
3-4 years: 40-60 mL (1⅓-2 fl oz) 3 times daily
5-6 years: 70-90 mL (2⅓-3 fl oz) 3 times daily
7 years and older: 100-150 mL (3-5 fl oz) 3 times daily

Cinnamon

Infusion: use ½ teaspoon of the crushed, dried bark quills to 1 cup of boiling water. Let steep for 5 minutes, strain. Can be sweetened with honey or rice malt. Dilute with water if necessary.

DOSE

1-2 years: 15-30 mL (½-1 fl oz) 3 times daily
3-4 years: 40-60 mL (1⅓-2 fl oz) 3 times daily
5-6 years: 70-90 mL (2⅓-3 fl oz) 3 times daily
7 years and older: 100-150 mL (3-5 fl oz) 3 times daily

Aniseed

Infusion: use ½ teaspoon of whole or freshly crushed seeds to 1 cup of boiling water. Let steep for 5 minutes, strain.

DOSE

1-2 years: 15-30 mL (½-1 fl oz) 3 times daily
3-4 years: 40-60 mL (1⅓-2 fl oz) 3 times daily
5-6 years: 70-90 mL (2⅓-3 fl oz) 3 times daily
7 years and older: 100-150 mL (3-5 fl oz) 3 times daily

Meadowsweet

Meadowsweet is a soothing, anti-inflammatory herb for the stomach in cases of acute stomach upset, excess acidity and inflammation of the gut.

Infusion: use 1½-2 teaspoons of dried herb to 1 cup of boiling water. Let steep for 5 minutes, strain. Can be sweetened with honey or rice malt. Dilute with water if necessary.

DOSE

1-2 years: 15-30 mL (½-1 fl oz) 3 times daily
3-4 years: 40-60 mL (1⅓-2 fl oz) 3 times daily
5-6 years: 70-90 mL (2⅓-3 fl oz) 3 times daily
7 years and older: 100-150 mL (3-5 fl oz) 3 times daily

Homoeopathic Remedies

If associated with pain refer to the colic section. If not, then you should administer **Carb-veg** 12C twice daily for three days. If this is not effective, seek the advice of your homoeopathic practitioner.

Chinese Remedies

1 'Deficiency'

Pale or yellowish complexion. Pale lips. Poor appetite. Blue vein or dark tint in the region between the eyebrows at the bridge of the nose. Child may sleep with eyes slightly open. The tongue is pale with a thin white coating. Tends to be quiet with low energy. Often has a runny nose. Frequent diarrhoea or loose stools.

XIANG SHA YANG WEI TANG
SHEN LING BAI ZHU TANG (diarrhoea or loose
stools)
XIANG SHA LIU JUN ZI TANG (frequent
discharge of mucus from nose and/or throat)

2 'Excess'

Normally good health, strength, energy and
appetite
YUE JU WAN (mild to moderate symptoms)
MU XIANG SHUN QI SAN (thick coating on
the tongue, more severe symptoms)

Massage

See Abdominal Pain. Add two more steps:

1 Walk with your fingertips clockwise across
abdomen, feeling for bubbles.
2 Grasp child's ankles, straighten legs, pulling
them toward you, then bending at knees push
child's legs into abdomen slowly, so that knees
touch her chest. Hold for ten to thirty seconds
while she breathes slowly. Do this five times.
and/or turn child on left side and place a warm
(wrist temperature) hot-water bottle on child's
tummy.

GERMAN MEASLES (RUBELLA)

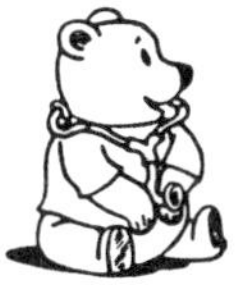

German measles is a mild infection, less serious and shorter-lived than ordinary measles. It often comes and goes unnoticed. Highly infectious, it normally has an incubation period of two to three weeks.

CAUTION

It is especially important that any woman who is pregnant be kept far away from any child with suspected German measles, especially during the first four months of pregnancy, because if she contracts rubella during this vital time of her pregnancy, there is a very high risk that her child will be born with eye or brain damage.

The infection is usually characterised by fever and a red rash consisting of small spots covering the body. It may simply look like a skin rash; however, very soon after the rash appears the glands in the back of the neck begin to swell, there may be diarrhoea, vomiting, irritability and phlegm in the chest and nose, with a cough and a slight fever. In very serious cases the fever may reach 39C (102F) and the child may exhibit signs of feeling restless and uncomfortable.

The rash and fever will continue two to three days after which time the symptoms will disappear as quickly as they appeared.

General Care

The best way to ease your child through this condition is to encourage plenty of rest, sleep, liquids and luke-warm sponge baths, especially around the head, hands and feet if the fever is high.

Homoeopathy is especially useful at this time. Consult a homoeopathic practitioner for the best results or see the Homoepathic Remedies following.

If complications occur, such as nausea, vomiting, aches in the head or neck or confusion, consult a medical practitioner at once.

Avoid foods that affect mucus production: meat, fatty food, fried food, too much salt, cream, butter, cow's milk, cheese, roasted peanuts, excessive sugar, bananas, oranges (one or two per week is not considered harmful).

Herbal Remedies

Echinacea will support the immune system. If the child has a high fever, give one or more of the following: Yarrow, Elderflower, Peppermint, Catmint and/or Linden.

Echinacea

Decoction: use 1 teaspoon of dried root and rhizome to 1 cup of water, simmer covered for 5 minutes. Dilute with water if necessary. Can be sweetened with honey or rice malt.
DOSE
1-2 years: 10-15 mL (⅓-½ fl oz) 3 times daily
3-4 years: 20-30 mL (⅔-1 fl oz) 3 times daily
5-6 years: 40-50 mL (1⅓-1⅔ fl oz) 3 times daily
7 years and older: 60-100 mL (2-3 fl oz) 3 times daily

Elderflower

Infusion: use 2 teaspoons of the dried flowers to 1 cup of boiling water. Let steep for 5 minutes, strain. Can be sweetened with honey or rice malt.
DOSE
1-2 years: 15-30 mL (½-1 fl oz) 3 times daily
3-4 years: 40-60 mL (1⅓-2 fl oz) 3 times daily
5-6 years: 70-90 mL (2⅓-3 fl oz) 3 times daily
7 years and older: 100-150 mL (3-5 fl oz) 3 times daily

Peppermint

Infusion: use ½-1 teaspoon of dried herb to 1 cup of boiling water. Let steep for 5 minutes, strain. Can be sweetened with honey or rice malt. Dilute with water if necessary.
DOSE
1-2 years: 15-30 mL (½-1 fl oz) 3 times daily
3-4 years: 40-60 mL (1⅓-2 fl oz) 3 times daily
5-6 years: 70-90 mL (2⅓-3 fl oz) 3 times daily

7 years and older: 100-150 mL (3-5 fl oz) 3 times daily

Yarrow

Infusion: use 1 teaspoon of dried herb to 1 cup of boiling water. Let steep for 5 minutes, strain. Can be sweetened with honey or rice malt. Dilute with water if necessary.

DOSE

1-2 years: 15-30 mL (½-1 fl oz) 3 times daily
3-4 years: 40-60 mL (1⅓-2 fl oz) 3 times daily
5-6 years: 70-90 mL (2⅓-3 fl oz) 3 times daily
7 years and older: 100-150 mL (3-5 fl oz) 3 times daily

Catmint

Infusion: Use 1 teaspoon of dried herb to 1 cup of boiling water. Let steep for 5 minutes, strain. Can be sweetened with honey or rice malt. Dilute with water if necessary.

DOSE

1-2 years: 15-30 mL (½-1 fl oz) 3 times daily
3-4 years: 40-60 mL (1⅓-2 fl oz) 3 times daily
5-6 years: 70-90 mL (2⅓-3 fl oz) 3 times daily
7 years and older: 100-150 mL (3-5 fl oz) 3 times daily

Linden (Lime flowers)

Infusion: use 1-1½ teaspoons of dried herb to 1 cup of boiling water. Let steep for 5 minutes, strain. Can be sweetened with honey or rice malt. Dilute with water if necessary.

DOSE

1-2 years: 15-30 mL (½-1 fl oz) 3 times daily
3-4 years: 40-60 mL (1⅓-2 fl oz) 3 times daily
5-6 years: 70-90 mL (2⅓-3 fl oz) 3 times daily
7 years and older: 100-150 mL (3-5 fl oz) 3 times daily

Homoeopathic Remedies

The medicines that apply for the measles (the common type) or those for fever will also suit German measles where the characteristic symptoms apply (see Fever and Measles).

The remedy **Rubella nosode** 30C is a beneficial prescription for women who are pregnant or who are planning pregnancy, to minimise the possibility of acquiring German measles. See your homoeopath about this.

Chinese Remedies

Similar to measles (see Measles), the symptoms are considered to be due to 'heat' and 'toxins'.

YIN QIAO SAN

HEADACHES

Headaches, surprisingly, are quite a common occurrence in children. Often they are hard to detect in smaller children; however, statistics show that over 20 per cent of school-age children suffer from headache complaints. Rather than reaching for the over-the-counter remedies that relieve only the symptomatic sensations, it is much better for your child's health to find, and then appropriately deal with, the underlying cause.

Headaches can be separated into two categories: the migraine and other types. Migraines may only occur once or twice in a lifetime or as frequently as once a week or twice a month. In most cases they seem to have a connection with food allergy (see Allergies, Food Intolerance and Chemical Sensitivity). The childhood migraine is not uncommon, though it is usually more common where there is a family history of migraine.

Symptoms

There is a wide variety of symptoms accompanying headaches. Often these are dependent on the specific cause or causes. It is also important to note that often headaches will accompany other illnesses such as colds or sinusitis. Childhood migraine can be identified by the presence of symptoms such as nausea, vomiting, abdominal pain, pale stools and fever.

Other general headache symptoms may be throbbing of the child's temples, red and hot face, dilated pupils, general tiredness, rapid pulse, thirst with desire for cold drinks or poor appetite.

Causes

Many headaches among children are caused by some dietary excess. However, hopefully, you should have a good idea of what your child is consuming and therefore be able to rule out imbalance in the diet reasonably quickly. Commonly, headaches are a response to stress or anxiety, such as an insecure or unpleasant situation which the child would rather avoid. They may also occur with simple over-excitement.

Fevers and many other childhood illnesses, such as infected sinuses, are often accompanied by a headache.

Recurring headaches can stem from straining of the eye-muscles and can thus indicate a need for glasses. Just as easily, dental cavities may also be a cause.

Muscle tension headaches are usually associated with a mechanical problem such as poor posture, lack of proper neck movement, vertebral subluxation or general spinal problems.

Finally, ordinary headaches or migraines may be caused by an allergy, side effects of medication, food intolerance, pesticides or chemical sensitivity (car exhaust fumes, city air with lead carbon monoxide from factories). Accompanying food intolerance headaches are often signs of weakness in the liver and digestive system.

CAUTION

It is imperative that you seek the opinion of a qualified medical practitioner if:
- **The headaches are frequent and recurring.**
- **There are signs that the child is unwell, apart from the headache.**
- **The child is unwell between attacks.**
- **The child is showing signs of unusual tiredness, loss of weight and poor appetite.**
- **The child becomes clumsy or shows signs of personality change.**

General Treatment

There are many treatments that are relatively simple. In addition to treatment aimed at bringing relief from the immediate symptoms, the underlying causes should be sought out and treated.

Sometimes encouraging the child to sleep or

just lying the child down in a darkened, well-aired room with a cool cloth on the forehead and a cup or bottle of a soothing, relaxing herbal tea (see below) will help.

Massage can also be extremely helpful. Try adding a drop or two of essential oil of Lavender or Rosemary to the massage oil and rubbing the feet as well as the head and neck. A bath with a few drops of these oils may also help. For sinusitis or head-cold related headaches, steam inhalation may be useful (see below).

Treatment for Recurrent Headaches

For mechanical headaches it is best to consult an osteopath or chiropractor for assessment of the spine, muscles and posture. Treatment and individual advice can then be successfully given. Also supplementation with B complex vitamins and the minerals calcium, magnesium and potassium can sometimes be helpful.

For headaches caused by allergy or food intolerance, an elimination diet should be carried out to identify the problem food if it is not already known (see section on Allergies). You should also be aware that the offending substance may take up to forty-eight hours to produce the headache.

Children and adults prone to migraines have been found to have an increased tendency for the blood platelets to clot. Substances such as Ginger, Garlic, fish oil and vitamin B3 (Niacin) will help to counteract this problem.

With all headaches, however, reassuring and caring interaction with your child will be highly beneficial.

Prevention

Regular exercise, clean air and a healthy, balanced diet are perhaps the most important preventative measures. Many headaches are caused by food high in sugar, saturated fat and spices.

Home Remedies

- For a headache caused by a head cold, catarrh or sinusitis, use Catmint tea with Chamomile and Thyme as an inhalant. Take a medium-sized saucepan and fill to one-third with water, bring to boil, take off stove and put in a handful of Chamomile flowers and one to two pinches of Thyme. Immediately cover with tight lid, let it stand for five to ten minutes, then take off the lid and let your child (with a towel over her head to guide the steam) inhale the hot steam, being careful not to burn her face.
- For infected sinuses, use above recipe and add one to two drops of water soluble Tea-Tree oil. A bath with five drops of Eucalyptus oil in it will also help.
- For headaches caused by stress and tension, give Chamomile, Valerian or Lemon Balm teas.
- For pain in the front or the sides of the head, including migraine headaches, cold applications, for example a cold, wet towel, should be applied to the forehead or top and sides of the head. Apply repeatedly for ten to fifteen minutes.
- For tension headaches in the back of and deep inside the head, warm applications, for example, warm towels, should be applied to the back of the head and neck. Or simply wrap a warm towel around the neck. Apply repeatedly for ten to fifteen minutes.
- Try a teaspoon or two of honey which may stop an early migraine.
- Place the child's feet in a bucket of very warm to hot water and at the same time have someone hold an ice pack on the back of her neck.

Herbal Remedies
Linden (Lime flowers)

Linden is relaxing and is particularly suited to headaches caused by anxiety or emotional or mental stress.

Infusion: use 1-1½ teaspoons of dried herb to 1 cup of boiling water. Let steep for 5 minutes, strain. Can be sweetened with honey or rice malt. Dilute with water if necessary.

DOSE

1-2 years: 15-30 mL (½-1 fl oz) 3 times daily
3-4 years: 40-60 mL (1⅓-2 fl oz) 3 times daily
5-6 years: 70-90 mL (2⅓-3 fl oz) 3 times daily
7 years and older: 100-150 mL (3-5 fl oz) 3 times daily

Catmint

Catmint is good for headaches caused by stress or anxiety, sinus trouble and colds.

Infusion: Use 1 teaspoon of dried herb to 1 cup of boiling water. Let steep for 5 minutes, strain. Can be sweetened with honey or rice malt. Dilute with water if necessary.

DOSE

1-2 years: 15-30 mL (½-1 fl oz) 3 times daily
3-4 years: 40-60 mL (1⅓-2 fl oz) 3 times daily
5-6 years: 70-90 mL (2⅓-3 fl oz) 3 times daily
7 years and older: 100-150 mL (3-5 fl oz) 3 times daily

Chamomile

Chamomile is indicated for similar types of headaches as Catmint (see above) but also where digestive upset or food allergy may be the cause.

Infusion: use 1 teaspoon dried flowerheads to 1 cup of boiling water. Let steep for 5 minutes, strain. Can be sweetened with honey or rice malt. Dilute with water for smaller children.

DOSE

1-2 years: 20-40 mL (⅔-1⅓ fl oz) 3 to 4 times daily
3-4 years: 50-80 mL (1⅔-2⅔ fl oz) 3 to 4 times daily
5-6 years: 100-125 mL (3-4 fl oz) 3 to 4 times daily
7 years and older: 150-200 mL (5-6⅔ fl oz) 3 to 4 times daily

Peppermint

Peppermint is for headache caused by nasal and/or sinus congestion as well as headache caused by impaired gall bladder function (intolerance of fats).

Infusion: use ½-1 teaspoon of dried herb to 1 cup of boiling water. Let steep for 5 minutes, strain. Can be sweetened with honey or rice malt. Dilute with water if necessary.

DOSE

1-2 years: 15-30 mL (½-1 fl oz) 3 times daily
3-4 years: 40-60 mL (1⅓-2 fl oz) 3 times daily
5-6 years: 70-90 mL (2⅓-3 fl oz) 3 times daily
7 years and older: 100-150 mL (3-5 fl oz) 3 times daily

Vervain

Vervain is indicated for tension headaches and headaches caused by poor digestive function.

Infusion: use 1-1½ teaspoons of dried herb to 1 cup of boiling water. Let steep for 5 minutes, strain. Can be sweetened with honey or rice malt. Dilute with water if necessary.

DOSE

1-2 years: 15-30 mL (½-1 fl oz) 3 times daily
3-4 years: 40-60 mL (1⅓-2 fl oz) 3 times daily
5-6 years: 70-90 mL (2⅓-3 fl oz) 3 times daily
7 years and older: 100-150 mL (3-5 fl oz) 3 times daily

Lemon Balm

Lemon Balm is a refreshing and pleasant tasting herb for headaches caused by nervous tension or stress.

Infusion: use 1-1½ teaspoons of dried herb to 1 cup of boiling water. Let steep for 5 minutes, strain. Can be sweetened with honey or rice malt. Dilute with water if necessary.

DOSE

1-2 years: 15-30 mL (½-1 fl oz) 3 times daily
3-4 years: 40-60 mL (1⅓-2 fl oz) 3 times daily
5-6 years: 70-90 mL (2⅓-3 fl oz) 3 times daily
7 years and older: 100-150 mL (3-5 fl oz) 3 times daily

Feverfew fresh leaf

If you grow Feverfew in the garden you can use it to reduce the frequency and severity of migraine attacks. Let the child eat ¼-½ fresh leaf daily (put it in a sandwich or salad). Certain individuals are sensitive to this plant and may develop symptoms such as soreness or ulcers of the mouth. Discontinue treatment if side-effects develop.

Ginger

For congestive headaches and headaches caused by heavy, fatty food, Ginger is indicated.

Infusion: use 3 slices (2-3 cm/1 inch in diameter and 2-3 mm/⅛ inch thick) of fresh Ginger to 1 cup of boiling water. Let steep for 5 minutes. Sweeten with honey or rice malt. Dilute with water for small children.

DOSE

2-3 years: 20 mL (⅔ fl oz) 2 to 3 times daily
4-5 years: 30-50 mL (1-1⅔ fl oz) 2 to 3 times daily
6 years and older: 60-80 mL (2-2⅔ fl oz) 2 to 3 times daily

Dandelion Root

Dandelion stimulates the digestive function in general and the liver in particular. It is suitable for headache caused by overeating, especially fatty foods.

Decoction: use 1-2 teaspoons of chopped root to 1 cup of water, simmer covered for 5-10 minutes. Can be sweetened with honey or rice malt. Dilute with water if necessary.

DOSE

1-2 years: 15-30 mL (½-1 fl oz) 3 times daily
3-4 years: 40-60 mL (1⅓-2 fl oz) 3 times daily
5-6 years: 70-90 mL (2⅓-3 fl oz) 3 times daily
7 years and older: 100-150 mL (3-5 fl oz) 3 times daily

Homoeopathic Remedies

Many homoeopathic medicines are used for headaches and all have their own particular indications. The following are the most commonly indicated:

Belladonna 30C is indicated where the headache is bursting and throbbing and the child's face is red and hot with dilated pupils. Pain comes on suddenly and is worse for the least jar, movement, stooping or lying. It is often ameliorated by firm pressure.

Bryonia 12C headaches are characterised by being worse for the slightest movement and being better for lying perfectly still with firm pressure on the painful part.

Gelsemium 30C is useful for headaches which are specially located at the back of the head and are associated with great heaviness and tiredness of the body. It is an excellent remedy for headaches brought on by excitement and anxiety.

Dose: Hourly during a severe headache or every three hours if the headache is milder.

For other medicines see the Materia Medica for: Aconite, Antimonium crudum, Arsenicum, Hepar sulph, Ignatia, Mag-phos, Nat-mur, Nux-vomica, Rhus-tox, Ruta grav, Pulsatilla, Staphisagria.

Chinese Remedies

In addition to treatment aimed at bringing relief from the immediate symptoms, any underlying causes should be sought and treated.

Headache often accompanies the common cold. See under Colds for different types and treatments.

1 'Deficiency'

Pale or yellowish complexion, lips and tongue. Low energy. Tires easily. Poor appetite. Speaks little, quiet voice. The hair may be brittle with many split ends. Hands and feet may be cold.

HUANG QI JIAN ZHONG TANG
QIAN SHI BAI ZHU SAN (poor digestion, frequent diarrhoea or vomiting)
XIANG SHA LIU JUN ZI TANG (discharge of clear or white mucus from nose or throat)

2 'Heat'

Red complexion, lips and tongue. The tip of the nose may become red, as may the eyes. The child may grind the teeth while sleeping. Fingernails are purple. Vein at 'San Guan' is purple. The tongue may develop a yellow coating. Dry mouth and throat. Thirst with desire for cold drinks. Urine is dark and reduced in quantity. The pulse is rapid.

QING WEI SAN
LONG DAN XIE GAN TANG (severe symptoms as described above)

NOTE: These two formulas are very cooling and should only be given as long as the child fits the above symptom picture. Prolonged use may result in weakening the child's digestive system.

Massage

For infants and children up to two years of age if you think they might have a headache:
1 Rotate the big toes and press across the top of each big toe and all the toes with thumb or fingertips.
2 With your thumb or index finger press up and down big toe and also at base of big toe on the bottom of the foot.

For all ages (older children can find this point and work it themselves):
Find the point on the top of the hand between the thumb and index finger in the soft webbing of tissue and press in and hold. This point can be quite tender, but it works very quickly in releasing headache pain.

For children three years and older:
1 With the child lying on her back and you sitting behind her head, press at the base of her skull with your fingertips, holding tender points for 30 seconds or longer.
2 Place your thumbs in centre of the child's forehead and press evenly across the forehead towards ears, then when you reach the temple make small light circles with your fingertips.
3 There are points just below the eyebrow (close to the nose) on the socket of eye. Also just above the eyebrow, centred above the eye and in the centre of the forehead between the eyes. Hold these points also for thirty seconds to one minute, pressing with even moderate pressure, until any tenderness disappears.

HEAD INJURIES

Most head injuries are merely bumps and bruises and are not serious. If your child seems dazed and shaky, lay her down, cover her with a light blanket and read her a story or otherwise entertain her for a while. For an hour or so after the bump, watch out to see if she vomits, seems irrational with blurred speech, bleeds from the ears, nose or mouth, and check the pupils for uneven dilation. If any of these signs is present, or you feel your child is not acting reasonably normal, contact your doctor or the nearest hospital immediately as there may be injury to the skull.

Homoeopathic Remedies

Arnica 30C is a useful first aid medicine for the effects of head injuries. Give hourly if the effect is severe or three times daily for two days if the effects are mild.

CAUTION
If there is a loss of consciousness or you suspect it may occur, contact a medical practitioner immediately.

HEAD LICE

Schools are full of children with lice and my son was no exception. A friend passed this remedy on to me and after using it one time they were gone!

Combine ½ teaspoon each of Rosemary, Eucalyptus and Pennyroyal oil. Then add 2½ tablespoons pure olive oil. Drop some onto your skin and make sure that it doesn't burn. If so add more olive oil. After washing your child's hair with very hot water, comb the oil through it with a regular comb. Then using the flea comb, comb out any nits or eggs. Tie a cotton scarf around her head and leave on overnight. It may tingle, but if it burns wash it out immediately, dilute the mixture and try again. The next morning, wash the hair with shampoo. This should suffice, however if necessary repeat the treatment again.

Preventative Treatment

Rub Tea-Tree or Sassafras oil into the scalp when lice have been reported in your area.

HYPERACTIVITY

'I just can't seem to get him to stay still, he runs around constantly and often is violent. He doesn't do well at school, not even sports, which I thought he would be great at with all his excess energy. He can't seem to relate to his peers, has about a two minute concentration span coupled with erratic swings in behaviour. The only peace we seem to get is when he is asleep.'

This is a typical description of a hyperactive or hyperkinetic child. Most children, at some stage, will show one or even several of these characteristics. This does not necessarily mean that they are 'hyperactive'. The truly hyperactive child is often quite difficult to diagnose.

Because some experts believe that hyperactivity is simply a consequence of emotional, organic or social circumstances, parents who have hyperactive children are often labelled as 'bad parents' who are not providing their child with a warm, loving and caring environment. This is untrue and places unnecessary guilt upon the very people who are trying to help their child.

It is true, however, that many children suffering from hyperactivity are very susceptible to the effects of various foods and chemicals. An early pioneer in the work on food, chemicals and behaviour was Dr Ben Feingold (see Box). People still think of the Feingold diet, a diet low in food additives and salicylates, as *the* approach to treating hyperactivity. Research studies done with the diet show mixed results, probably because the diet does not consider environmental chemicals or foods.

Ten times more boys than girls exhibit hyperactivity. It has been thought that many children are susceptible to the effects of various food additives, exhibiting such signs as hyperactivity, distractibility, excitability, impulsiveness, irritability (especially in classroom situations when forced to control or inhibit hyperactive behaviour). They also sleep less, and wear out shoes, clothing and toys more quickly than other children.

About half a million American children receive some form of drug to control their hyperactive behaviour in any one year. One of the problems with drug therapy is that they tend to have many side-effects, such as stomach-aches, headaches, insomnia, nausea, anorexia and depression. Other approaches have included individual psychotherapy, family therapy, behaviour modification, and special education programs. Even though hyperactivity has been somewhat controlled through these means, as these children grow up they exhibit a poor self-image, low self-esteem, a sense of failure and depression. Many depressives, sociopaths and alcoholics have histories of hyperactivity as children.

General Treatment

Each hyperactive child needs to be considered individually — what works for one child may not necessarily work for another.

The Feingold Diet still remains a good starting point, with the elimination of all preservatives, colouring, artificial flavouring and generally any chemical additives. These are found mostly in highly processed food and labels on cans and packages should be scrutinised carefully. Foods which contain salicylates (chemical compounds of salts or esters derived by salicylic acid), such as tomatoes, apples, plums, grapes or raisins, oranges, strawberries, cucumbers, spearmint and peppermint should also be eliminated. As a general rule, the blander tasting fruits such as pears contain less salicylates than the stronger tasting ones such as pineapples.

Your child may also be affected by other foods. These can be found and also eliminated from the diet. (See Allergies.)

Apart from diet, children can be affected by environmental factors or 'irritants'. These are normally artificial or highly processed articles such as plastic food wrap, mothballs, chlorine in swimming pools, glue, coloured or scented paper products, oven cleaner, fabric softener, adhesive bandages, coloured or perfumed soap, dye, polyester fabric or items, vinyl wallpaper, etc. It is recommended that the most 'natural' alternative for these 'man-made' items be used whenever possible.

The third area that needs to be considered is education. Many hyperactive children have learning difficulties. Though by traditional school standards they may be considered 'slow',

---

THE FEINGOLD DIET

Dr Ben Feingold, an allergist from San Francisco and an early pioneer in the work on food additives — particularly colouring agents — alerted people that these may be associated with hyperactivity and learning difficulties. His awareness came when he was treating a woman suffering from acute hives in 1965. He withdrew artificial colours and flavours from her diet after suspecting that she was sensitive to them. Her skin condition cleared after a few days of following his suggestions. Her psychiatrist also noticed that her aggressive behaviour, hostility and difficulty in getting along with others dramatically improved.

Dr Feingold also found that some patients who reacted adversely to aspirin and other salicylates by contracting rashes also exhibited difficulty in concentrating and irritability. When they were eliminated from the diet, the symptoms disappeared. He also noticed that there was a cross-reactivity between salicylates and other unrelated chemicals of the same molecular weight, such as Tartrazine-E102 (yellow food colouring). Upon these observations, he devised a special diet for the treatment of hyperactive children. It was called the KP diet. He suggested that there were three areas of foods that had to be eliminated during the diet: artificial colours and flavours; all foods containing natural salicylates, such as almonds, apples, apricots, cherries, cider, currants, etc.; and miscellaneous items such as aspirin containing compounds and all medications with artificial colours and flavours, as well as perfumes, toothpaste and tooth powder.

He also claimed that many of the adverse reactions affected other parts of the body as well, such as the skin, gastrointestinal, skeletal, neurological and respiratory systems.

Dr Feingold alerted the Nutrition Foundation and made quite an impact with his claims and the implications for the food industry were enormous. This started off many investigations to investigate Feingold's claims. Many controlled studies were undertaken, including alternating Feingold's diet with challenge diets containing the additives. The children who were on the Feingold diet for a time, showed that they were healthier than the average hyperactive child who was not, and were thus more able to withstand the food additive challenge. Better still, more research discovered that hyperactive children placed on a diet with no junk food for six months improved greatly on scales measuring attention span, hyperactivity and irritability.

Many of the studies that were made in relationship to Feingold's work also fell short of recognising other relevant variables that were not controlled: Robert Buist, in his book *Food Chemical Sensitivity* (Harper & Row, Australia 1986), reports that Brenner in 1979 reported that artificial colourings and flavourings caused hyperactivity only in children with high blood copper levels. Another possible variable occurs when children are exposed to fluorescent lighting in classrooms, as they are more prone to hyperactive behaviour.

Some test tube studies reported that food colourings damage nerve tissue. Much of the decline in academic ability that is showing up in our young adults in Western countries is, therefore, directly attributed to the slow but steady increase in the amounts and different types of food additives being used in our foods over the last ten to fifteen years. Another study observed that 59 per cent of hyperactive children react adversely to chocolate.

Many studies since Feingold's observations and findings have been conducted and have shown that other chemicals and protein components of foods, as well as naturally occurring amines in foods, might be contributing to the problem of hyperkinetic behaviour as well as other problems in children such as rashes, headaches and gastrointestinal problems. Feingold's diet may in fact be inadequate because it only addresses naturally occurring food chemicals and chemical additives and not, for example the allergic effects of foods in general, what combination they are consumed in and how frequently in successive days. Many children also react to atmospheric pollutions, that is, the chemicals in the air around us.

HYPERACTIVITY

Hyperactivity, an emotional disturbance in children, is commonly related to the liver's inability to detoxify the chemical additives in foods and drugs such as in antibiotics. These substances remain in the child's body and act as an irritant to the nervous system. In many young children, the kidney and liver function is still not fully mature and their bodies have difficulty in detoxifying and excreting drugs and chemicals. It is of prime importance to remember that children are continuing to develop daily.

this does not mean that they are 'dumb' (in fact, in many cases, children diagnosed as hyperactive often have very high IQ levels). If you feel your child might have learning difficulties, start by speaking to the class teacher, who will have suggestions for help.

The final and often overlooked area of treatment is exercise. This may seem a little odd for a child who is continually 'on the go'; however, many children suffering from hyperactivity have poor co-ordination skills. A series of simple exercises suited to your child's age should be done daily, and should include combined arm, head and leg movements.

1 Place child on towels on a high table. Lie her on her stomach with one arm facing upwards (bent) and the other arm facing down (straight); the legs should be corresponding to the arms. Swap placement of arms and legs from left to right, with the head turning to face the bent limbs. This can be repeated many times, with one adult doing each side and a third moving the head.

2 Trampolining, dancing, gymnastics.

3 Crawling on all fours.

4 Allow the child to make herself mobile by lying her on a small cart on wheels and encouraging her to pull herself along.

Your child may need only one or all of these approaches; however, it is vital that the home environment remains as positive, loving and caring as possible — without this all other treatments will only be superficial.

Homoeopathic Remedies

Where changes in diet fail, this is usually a constitutional problem and should be referred to your homoeopath.

Massage

The trick here is getting your child to sit still long enough for you to touch her. Bedtime is often the best time.

1 Press into the centre of the big toe and hold, on each foot.

2 Press into the point just below the ball of the foot under the big toe, folding the big toe toward bottom of foot, and hold for about 30 seconds on each foot.

3 Finally, hold both feet and press with your thumb into the centre of the ball of the foot, pushing in with your thumb as you inhale together, then release your thumb and pull toes toward you, and exhale together (saying 'Let's both take a big breath, hold it, then blow out all the busyness of the day'). Do this three times. Then imagine (with her or for her) floating on a big cloud, feeling your body getting lighter and lighter. You can also use quiet music to relax.

NOISE POLLUTION

Scientists have recently found evidence to support the belief that loud noise is harmful to children. Children who are continuously exposed to more than 68 decibels (the noise level in a well-patronised restaurant) display typical signs of the beginning of a damaged nervous system. These include the circulation of blood slowing down, metabolism speeds up dramatically, and muscles become more tense. Loud noises make children tired, can contribute to hyperactivity and disrupt their attention span.

In Los Angeles children living close to the airport were compared with children living further away in much quieter surroundings. 53 per cent of the children who lived near the airport were unable to piece together a nine-piece jigsaw puzzle in the given time of four minutes. 31 per cent actually gave up before the four minutes were up. In contrast, only 36 per cent of the children from the other suburbs couldn't complete the puzzle and of those only 7 per cent gave up before the alloted time.

(Adapted from *Parents and Children Magazine*, Dec/Jan 1990)

MEASLES

Measles, also known as rubeola or English measles, is a contagious viral disease which can occur at any age. It is most common between the ages of one and five and can be contracted by contact with an infected child or by touching an object used by an infected child. It is spread through the air by sneezing or coughing. The incubation period is most often about 10 to 14 days and one bout of measles usually gives immunity for life. However, there are rare instances of children having had it two or three times.

Nowadays, measles is not considered to be dangerous in most instances; however, in developing countries, particularly where malnutrition is a widespread problem, measles continues to be a major threat to children's lives.

Even though there have been very strong immunisation campaigns (for information about immunisation see page 69) in countries like America, in Chinese medicine measles is looked upon as a beneficial disease that rids the body of accumulated poisons. After this illness you will note a change in your child's attitude, behaviour and attention. Most likely your child will be less irritable, less negative and healthier.

Symptoms

The first symptoms of measles usually look like a common cold: a hard, dry cough, irritated eyes sensitive to the light and a high fever with watery eyes. The fever rises and then a rash appears inside the mouth and a rash of small pink spots appears behind the ears and below the hairline. After about three to four days the rash spreads downward to cover the whole body. In mild cases there might only be a few scattered red spots, while children with severe cases can be almost completely blanketed with red spots and very distressed and irritable, with swollen or very red eyes.

After the rash takes full hold, additional symptoms such as listlessness, a higher fever and a red tongue with yellow coating may appear. Eventually the temperature goes down, the rash changes colour from red to a purple-red and over a week or so the rash completely fades away.

Measles is contagious for seven or eight days beginning three to four days before the rash comes out.

A child who has had a serious bout of measles may suffer nightmares, skin rashes and/or impaired vision after the rash has cleared. If this happens to your child, you should give treatment to strengthen the immune system and seek medical attention if the symptoms don't start to clear.

Possible Complications

Although uncommon, measles can cause an accumulation of mucus in the lungs. This allows bacteria to grow and can cause a secondary infection which invades the bronchi. This is serious if it results in bronchopneumonia — the bronchi become inflamed, breathing becomes shallow and asthma can develop. If this condition should occur, seek medical attention immediately.

Another possible complication of measles is encephalitis (inflammation of the brain tissue). Although much less common than it was many years ago, it is a very serious and possibly fatal condition. If your child becomes delirious or comatose, seek immediate medical attention.

General Treatment

Allow your child to take as much time as she needs to recover. Don't be in a hurry to send your child back to school. Measles requires plenty of bed rest, sleep and fluids.

Keep your child's room reasonably dark even though she may not have obvious symptoms of eye sensitivity and don't allow her to watch television or read.

When her appetite returns, simple foods in

small quantities are best. Porridge, soft grains such as rice or barley soup are helpful for assisting the digestive system to cope with foods after a period of not eating.

Home Remedies

- Bathe the eyes with weak tea or mildly salty water.
- A soothing eyebath can be prepared with Chamomile or Eyebright (1 teaspoon herb to 1 cup of water — bring to the boil, cover and simmer for a couple of minutes).
- Give plenty of fluids.
- Simmer ½ cup (3 oz) barley in 4-5 cups of water with a small piece of lemon peel until barley is cooked, then strain. Add a little honey to sweeten the soup after cooking and give every two waking hours.
- The rash can be soothed by giving warm baths with Sage tea, cornflour or arrowroot, or using calamine lotion.
- Cough can be treated with a decoction of Marshmallow or Licorice root (1 teaspoon per cup of water, cover, simmer for ten minutes and strain) or tea of Aniseed or Thyme (½ teaspoon per cup of boiling water, let steep five to ten minutes covered, strain and serve).

Herbal Remedies

Elderflower, Peppermint and Yarrow can be used singly or in combination to control fever. Give the tea hot at frequent intervals.

Elderflower

Infusion: use 2 teaspoons of the dried flowers to 1 cup of boiling water. Let steep for 5 minutes, strain. Can be sweetened with honey or rice malt.
DOSE
1-2 years: 15-30 mL (½-1 fl oz) 3 times daily
3-4 years: 40-60 mL (1⅓-2 fl oz) 3 times daily
5-6 years: 70-90 mL (2⅓-3 fl oz) 3 times daily
7 years and older: 100-150 mL (3-5 fl oz) 3 times daily

Peppermint

Infusion: use ½-1 teaspoon of dried herb to 1 cup of boiling water. Let steep for 5 minutes, strain. Can be sweetened with honey or rice malt. Dilute with water if necessary.
DOSE
1-2 years: 15-30 mL (½-1 fl oz) 3 times daily
3-4 years: 40-60 mL (1⅓-2 fl oz) 3 times daily

5-6 years: 70-90 mL (2⅓-3 fl oz) 3 times daily
7 years and older: 100-150 mL (3-5 fl oz) 3 times daily

Yarrow

This is a good treatment for the early stage of measles.
Infusion: use 1 teaspoon of dried herb to 1 cup of boiling water. Let steep for 5 minutes, strain. Can be sweetened with honey or rice malt. Dilute with water if necessary.
DOSE
1-2 years: 15-30 mL (½-1 fl oz) 3 times daily
3-4 years: 40-60 mL (1⅓-2 fl oz) 3 times daily
5-6 years: 70-90 mL (2⅓-3 fl oz) 3 times daily
7 years and older: 100-150 mL (3-5 fl oz) 3 times daily

Marshmallow

Use this for treating a measles cough.
Decoction: use 1-1½ teaspoons of chopped root to 1 cup of water, simmer covered for 5-10 minutes.
Infusion: use 2 teaspoons of dried leaf to 1 cup of boiling water, let steep for 10 minutes. Can be diluted with water.
DOSE
½-1 year: 15-30 mL (½-1 fl oz) 3 times daily
2-3 years: 40-50 mL (1⅓-1⅔ fl oz) 3 times daily
4-5 years: 60-80 mL (2-2⅔ fl oz) 3 times daily
6 years and older: 80-120 mL (2⅔-4 fl oz) 3 times daily

Licorice

Another good treatment for a measles cough.
Decoction: use ½ teaspoon chopped Licorice root to 1 cup of water. Simmer covered for 10 minutes.
DOSE
1-2 years: 20 mL (⅔ fl oz) 3 times daily
3-4 years: 30-50 mL (1-1⅔ fl oz) 3 times daily
5-6 years: 60-80 mL (2-2⅔ fl oz) 3 times daily
7 years and older: 100-120 mL (3-4 fl oz) 3 times daily

Aniseed

Aniseed is a relaxing expectorant with a sweet taste very popular with children and useful for coughs. Fennel seed can be used as a substitute.
Infusion: use ½ teaspoon of whole or freshly crushed seeds to 1 cup of boiling water. Let steep for 5 minutes, strain.
DOSE
1-2 years: 15-30 mL (½-1 fl oz) 3 times daily
3-4 years: 40-60 mL (1⅓-2 fl oz) 3 times daily

5-6 years: 70-90 mL (2⅓-3 fl oz) 3 times daily
7 years and older: 100-150 mL (3-5 fl oz) 3 times daily

Thyme

Thyme is another excellent relaxing expectorant, useful for treating coughs.
Infusion: use 1 teaspoon of dried herb to 1 cup of boiling water. Let steep for 5 minutes, strain. Can be sweetened with honey or rice malt. Dilute with water if necessary.

DOSE

1-2 years: 15-30 mL (½-1 fl oz) 3 times daily
3-4 years: 40-60 mL (1⅓-2 fl oz) 3 times daily
5-6 years: 70-90 mL (2⅓-3 fl oz) 3 times daily
7 years and older: 100-150 mL (3-5 fl oz) 3 times daily

Echinacea

Echinacea stimulates the immune system and will support the body in dealing with the infection quickly and effectively, thus reducing the risk of complications developing.
Decoction: use 1 teaspoon of dried root and rhizome to 1 cup of water, simmer covered for 5 minutes. Dilute with water if necessary. Can be sweetened with honey or rice malt.

DOSE

1-2 years: 10-15 mL (⅓-½ fl oz) 3 times daily
3-4 years: 20-30 mL (⅔-1 fl oz) 3 times daily
5-6 years: 40-50 mL (1⅓-1⅔ fl oz) 3 times daily
7 years and older: 60-100 mL (2-3 fl oz) 3 times daily

Homoeopathic Remedies

Aconite 30C is indicated in the early stages when the child is restless, the eyes and nose are streaming and the eyes are sensitive to light. There may be a hard, croupy cough.

Euphrasia 12C is indicated where the eyes are sensitive to light, red and swollen with streaming tears which irritate the cheeks. There may be a watery nasal discharge which does not irritate. A dry cough with throbbing headache is often associated.

Pulsatilla 12C should be given if the child wants company and sympathy, is inclined to be weepy and wanting to be in the open air. Catarrhal symptoms predominate, like thick yellow discharge from the nose or from the eyes. There may be a loose cough.
Dose: One dose twice daily for up to five days.

Other medicines such as Aconite, Apis, Arsenicum, Belladonna, Bryonia, Ferrum-phos, Phosphorus, Gelsemium, Mercurius or Sulphur should be referred to if the above medicines are not indicated.

Chinese Remedies

1 First Stage

Before skin eruptions appear. Fever and chills. Cough. Runny nose. Sneezing. Nasal congestion. Frequent yawning. Red eyes. Restlessness. If the other children at your child's school or kindergarten are coming down with measles and your child develops these symptoms, you can strongly suspect measles.

Treatment at this stage is aimed at assisting the discharge of 'Foetal Toxins' to help bring out the rash and avoid complications.

SHENG MA GE GEN TANG (weak or delicate constitution)
XUAN DU FA BIAO TANG

2 Second Stage

Skin eruptions start to appear (initially behind ears and around the neck) and spread over the whole body. Fever and cough worsen. Loss of appetite. Tongue is red with a yellow coating. Pulse is rapid. Purple vein at 'San Guan'.

YIN QIAO SAN (with cough, sore throat, nasal congestion)
TENG HUA BAI DU SAN (fully erupted skin rash with mild upper respiratory tract symptoms)

3 Third Stage

Convalescent stage. The rash begins to disappear. Fever comes down.

SHA SHEN MAI MEN DONG TANG

4 Complications

If your child has symptoms which are different from the descriptions presented here, it is strongly advised that you seek professional help.

MOTION SICKNESS

Causes

- Physical: weak muscular activity in the stomach where digestion slows or ceases.
- Functional: sense of balance is not working properly, affecting the nervous system. There is an irregularity between messages from the eyes and the balance mechanism in the inner ears. The brain then receives the wrong information about the environment.

General Treatment
Chronic motion sickness

- 'Travel Calm Ginger': This product contains 400 mg of ginger, and comes in a tablet form. It is available from health food stores. It must be taken before leaving and repeated every two hours. It doesn't taste good, so try crushing up the tablet in a spoon and adding honey or jam. Please also consult a practitioner of your choice, to work out the correct dosage for your child. Ginger absorbs acid and blocks nausea in the gastrointestinal tract.
- Take a train: This seems like an odd treatment, but I found it worked perfectly with my child. One adult would take our daughter on the train, while the other would drive. We would then meet at the train station and the short drive to wherever we were going was normally not a problem. A bus isn't quite as good, but it is still better than a car.
- Travel at night: Thankfully most children sleep at night, and the short times of wakefulness do not seem to be a problem. Because they cannot see the motion, their balance is less likely to be affected.

Periodic travel sickness

Some of these treatments can also be used for children who suffer regularly from travel sickness.
- Ensure that your child has good posture.
- Discourage reading, playing games or looking down.

- Keep a window open — fresh air works wonders.
- Try to distract your child — you can sing, play her favourite tape or tell a story.
- Avoid all bad odours, especially petrol fumes. When stopping at a petrol station, roll up all the windows and close the doors before you fill up the petrol tank.
- Have light, healthy meals before leaving and during your trip. Stay away from fatty, greasy foods. Let your child eat dry biscuits or salty foods such as light crisps or rice crackers.
- Avoid too much liquid and give only cooled boiled water.
- Ensure that your child is wearing loose clothing, especially around the waist.
- Acupressure may also be of some help. Apply pressure to a point on the wrist found by measuring two of the child's finger widths from the base of the hand. Then find the point between the two tendons running up the wrist. Apply pressure to this point by pressing upwards towards the hand. A special wristband can be bought that will do this job for you. It has a bead sewn in the correct position known as the Neiguan.
- If it is too late to prevent your child from being sick, make a ginger tea by simmering 1 teaspoon of dried ginger powder in two cups of water for 20-30 minutes. this will help to settle the child's stomach.
- The homoeopathic remedy Nux vomica may also be of some help and can be obtained from your homoeopath.
- A tip from an American doctor, C. Northrup, is to fasten an aspirin tablet (it must be aspirin), onto your child's navel, keeping it in place with a bandage or bandaid. This can be made into a fun exercise and could become a novelty with your children!
- Encouraging your child to suck on a slice of lemon during the trip may be helpful, but because most children are averse to the taste, this may only work for some.

- Rubbing your hand on the child's stomach in a counter-clockwise direction can be soothing.
- Rubbing Chamomile oil on the stomach for relief of tummy pain may be helpful.
- Allow the child to sit in the front passenger seat. This can help, but remember that it is not as safe in the front.

See also sections on Nausea and Vomiting.

Herbal Remedies

Ginger

Ginger tea, as a preventative, needs to be taken about half an hour before the travel commences. Peppermint and Chamomile may be used in the same way.

Infusion: use 3 slices (2-3 cm/1 inch in diameter and 2-3 mm/⅛ inch thick) of fresh Ginger to 1 cup of boiling water. Let steep for 5 minutes. Sweeten with honey or rice malt. Dilute with water for small children.

DOSE

2-3 years: 20 mL (⅔ fl oz) 2 to 3 times daily
4-5 years: 30-50 mL (1-1⅔ fl oz) 2 to 3 times daily
6 years and older: 60-80 mL (2-2⅔ fl oz) 2 to 3 times daily

Chamomile

Infusion: use 1 teaspoon dried flowerheads to 1 cup of boiling water. Let steep for 5 minutes, strain. Can be sweetened with honey or rice malt. Dilute with water for smaller children.

DOSE

1-2 years: 20-40 mL (⅔-1⅓ fl oz) 3 to 4 times daily
3-4 years: 50-80 mL (1⅔-2⅔ fl oz) 3 to 4 times daily
5-6 years: 100-125 mL (3-4 fl oz) 3 to 4 times daily
7 years and older: 150-200 mL (5-6⅔ fl oz) 3 to 4 times daily

Peppermint

Infusion: use ½-1 teaspoon of dried herb to 1 cup of boiling water. Let steep for 5 minutes, strain. Can be sweetened with honey or rice malt. Dilute with water if necessary.

DOSE

1-2 years: 15-30 mL (½-1 fl oz) 3 times daily
3-4 years: 40-60 mL (1⅓-2 fl oz) 3 times daily
5-6 years: 70-90 mL (2⅓-3 fl oz) 3 times daily
7 years and older: 100-150 mL (3-5 fl oz) 3 times daily

Homoeopathic Remedies

Cocculus 30C is particularly indicated where the nausea and vomiting are associated with the thought, sight or smell of food.

Tabacum 30C is a most valuable medicine where there is nausea, giddiness, coldness and weakness. Tobacco smoke will make all the symptoms worse.

Nux vomica 30C is used where there is nausea with retching often associated with headache.

Dose: the appropriate remedy should be taken twice the day before starting the trip and may be repeated where necessary. The 30C potency is recommended.

Massage

1 Press at base of second, third and fourth toes on both feet. Hold beneath each one for thirty to sixty seconds.
2 Place the index finger (an older child can do this one herself) inside the bottom of ear and thumb behind ear, then simultaneously pull the hollows of each ear outwardly. Do this for one or two minutes or until sickness eases.
3 Press across on the bottom of the left foot from the middle of the foot up to the ball of the foot. Press into any tender points and hold for ten to thirty seconds.

MOUTH ULCERS

Causes

- Food allergies, especially wheat, but can also be associated with milk, cheese, tomato, vinegar, pineapple and mustard.
- Nutritional deficiencies: noted associations have been with Iron, B12, Folic Acid and Zinc

General Treatment

- Test and eliminate food allergies. See section on Allergies.
- Supplement with Iron, B12, Folic Acid or Zinc. Test for specific deficiency by either trial or elimination. Alternatively, use multiple supplements. If these don't help, you can try Quercetin, a bioflavinoid found in food that contains vitamin C. This is best taken in a tablet form (150 mg per day). Consult a practitioner.
- Herbal treatments: rinse the mouth with a tincture made from 1 teaspoon Oak Bark, 1 teaspoon Cider Vinegar and 1 cup of water. An application for placing directly on the ulcer can be made from 1 teaspoon Myrrh, ½ teaspoon Golden Seal and ½ cup Honey.

Home Remedies

- Place baking soda on the ulcer. It will fizz in the mouth, which may shock or delight your child, but the taste is not unpleasant and it has a good healthy effect.
- Increase the child's intake of green vegetables for chronic ulcers.
- Use salt water as a mouthwash.

Herbal Remedies

If you can get hold of it, Tincture of Propolis is good for topical applications. Use mouth rinses with antiseptic herbs such as Calendula, Thyme, Sage, preferably mixed with an astringent herb such as Tormentil or Agrimony. Echinacea can be used internally to strengthen the immune system and prevent infection of the ulcer.

Thyme

Gargle and/or mouthwash: prepare as an infusion using 1-2 teaspoons of dried herb or 5-6 teaspoons of chopped, fresh leaf to 1 cup of boiling water. Let steep for 10 minutes, strain. Do not sweeten or dilute.

Calendula (Marigold)

Gargle and/or mouthwash: prepare as an infusion using 3-4 teaspoons of dried flowers to 1 cup of boiling water. Let steep for 10 minutes, strain. Do not sweeten or dilute.

Sage

Gargle and/or mouthwash: prepare as an infusion using 1-2 teaspoons of dried herb or 5-6 teaspoons of chopped, fresh leaf to 1 cup of boiling water. Let steep for 10 minutes, strain. Do not sweeten or dilute.

Golden Seal

Gargle and/or mouthwash: prepare as a decoction, using ½-1 teaspoon of dried roots and rhizome to 1 cup of water. Simmer covered for 10 minutes, strain. Do not sweeten or dilute.

Agrimony

Gargle and/or mouthwash: prepare as an infusion, using 1-2 teaspoons of dried herb to 1 cup of boiling water. Let steep for 10 minutes, strain. Do not sweeten or dilute.

Tormentil

Decoction: use 1-2 teaspoons of chopped rhizome to 1 cup of water, simmer covered for 5-10 minutes, strain.

Echinacea

Decoction: use 1 teaspoon of dried root and rhizome to 1 cup of water, simmer covered for 5 minutes. Dilute with water. Can be sweetened with honey or rice malt.

DOSE

1-2 years: 10-15 mL (⅓-½ fl oz) 2 times daily
3-4 years: 20-30 mL (⅔-1 fl oz) 3 times daily

5-6 years: 40-50 mL (1⅓-1⅔ fl oz) 3 times daily
7 years and older: 60-100 mL (2-3 fl oz) 3 times
daily

Homoeopathic Remedies

Infants with mouth ulcers which are tiny or
appear after painful vesicular eruptions (small
bubbles) often require **Borax** 6C. They usually
appear on the tongue or the inner surface of
the cheeks. The baby refuses the breast. Give
Borax three times daily for three days.

Where this medicine is not effective the
condition should be referred to your homoeopathic practitioner.

Chinese Remedies

1 'Heat'

Thirst. Tongue is dry. Frequent constipation or
hard dry stools.

SAN HUANG XIE XIN TANG

2 'Heat' and 'Deficiency'

Abdominal swelling or hardness in the upper
region, immediately below the ribs. Loss of
appetite. Nausea. There may be diarrhoea.

BAN XIA XIE XIN TANG

MUMPS

Mumps is a viral infection usually common between the ages of three and ten years. This disease causes swelling of one or both of the parotids which are two of the six salivary glands located just below and in front of the ears.

A child will be infectious from just prior to the first signs of discomfort until the gland returns to its normal size. After the infection, a child will have a lifetime immunity.

Symptoms

The symptoms usually begin with a fever, fatigue, headache, loss of appetite and back pain. Within two days after some discomfort in one of the two parotid glands, the gland swells and most children feel irritable and out of sorts. The jaw may feel somewhat stiff and it can be difficult to swallow and open the mouth. After about two or three days, and usually not longer than six or seven days, the swelling disappears. It is not uncommon for only one gland to be affected at a time. The second one may appear swollen ten or twelve days later with all of the associated symptoms.

Possible Complications

The most dangerous complication that can occur from having mumps is orchitis, a condition which affects the testicles. In rare instances this can produce sterility. Mumps can also lead to swelling of the ovaries (oophoritis), the pancreas or, very rarely, the brain. However, these complications are more likely to occur after puberty. This is why it is best that children be exposed to mumps while still young (after the age of three) so that they can acquire immunity against a serious bout after puberty. It is not known whether the mumps vaccine confers a lifetime immunity. There is no proof that immunisation against mumps at 15 months will protect your child against a serious bout of mumps after puberty with graver consequences.

General Treatment

Mumps does not require orthodox medical treatment. It is a good idea, however, to keep your child in bed for at least two or three days in a warm, quiet atmosphere. A soft diet excluding heavy animal proteins, eggs and sugar, but with plenty of fluids is best and you can apply ice packs to relieve the swelling.

Home Remedy

Dandelion Tea

Boil 15 g (½ oz) of Dandelion root in two cups of water until it is reduced to one cup. Strain. Sip it throughout the day, but not more than 2 cups.

Herbal Remedies

Mullein is used as a traditional remedy, Calendula, Clivers, and Red Clover as eliminative and lymphatic agents, Echinacea as a systemic anti-infective and Thyme as a mouthwash and gargle. To manage high fever use diaphoretics such as Elderflower, Yarrow, Peppermint and/or Linden (see Fever).

Mullein

Infusion: use 2 teaspoons of the dried leaves or ½ teaspoon of the dried flowers to 1 cup of boiling water. Let steep for 5-10 minutes, strain. Can be sweetened with honey or rice malt.
DOSE
1-2 years: 15-30 mL (½-1 fl oz) 3 times daily
3-4 years: 40-60 mL (1⅓-2 fl oz) 3 times daily
5-6 years: 70-90 mL (2⅓-3 fl oz) 3 times daily
7 years and older: 100-150 mL (3-5 fl oz) 3 times daily

Echinacea

Decoction: use 1 teaspoon of dried root and rhizome to 1 cup of water, simmer covered for 5 minutes. Dilute with water. Can be sweetened with honey or rice malt.

DOSE

1-2 years: 10-15 mL (⅓-½ fl oz) 2 times daily
3-4 years: 20-30 mL (⅔-1 fl oz) 3 times daily
5-6 years: 40-50 mL (1⅓-1⅔ fl oz) 3 times daily
7 years and older: 60-100 mL (2-3 fl oz) 3 times daily

Red Clover

Infusion: use 3 teaspoons of dried flowers to 1 cup of boiling water. Let steep for 5 minutes, strain. Can be sweetened with honey or rice malt. Dilute with water if necessary.

DOSE

1-2 years: 15-30 mL (½-1 fl oz) 3 times daily
3-4 years: 40-60 mL (1⅓-2 fl oz) 3 times daily
5-6 years: 70-90 mL (2⅓-3 fl oz) 3 times daily
7 years and older: 100-150 mL (3-5 fl oz) 3 times daily

Calendula (Marigold)

Infusion: use 2 teaspoons of the dried flower-heads to 1 cup of boiling water. Let steep for 5 minutes, strain. Can be sweetened with honey or rice malt. Dilute with water if necessary.

DOSE

1-2 years: 15-30 mL (½-1 fl oz) 3 times daily
3-4 years: 40-60 mL (1⅓-2 fl oz) 3 times daily
5-6 years: 70-90 mL (2⅓-3 fl oz) 3 times daily
7 years and older: 100-150 mL (3-5 fl oz) 3 times daily

Thyme

Gargle and/or mouthwash: prepare as an infusion using 1-2 teaspoons of dried herb or 5-6 teaspoons of chopped, fresh leaf to 1 cup of boiling water. Let steep for 10 minutes, strain. Do not sweeten or dilute.

Clivers (Cleavers)

Infusion: use 2 teaspoons of dried herb to 1 cup of boiling water. Let steep for 5 minutes, strain. Can be sweetened with honey or rice malt. Dilute with water if necessary.

DOSE

1-2 years: 15-30 mL (½-1 fl oz) 3 times daily
3-4 years: 40-60 mL (1⅓-2 fl oz) 3 times daily
5-6 years: 70-90 mL (2⅓-3 fl oz) 3 times daily
7 years and older: 100-150 mL (3-5 fl oz) 3 times daily

Homoeopathic Remedies

Belladonna 30C is often needed when there is high fever associated and the face is hot, dry and red.

If there is a lot of saliva, swollen tongue and profuse sweating with the swollen glands then the child will require **Mercurius** 12C.

Pulsatilla 12C is indicated when the inflammation and swelling spread to the reproductive organs or when the ears are also affected. The child is usually thirstless and desiring company.

Rhus-tox 12C may be used when there is a great enlargement of the glands and is usually worse on the left side. You may note that the tongue is coated except for the tip.

Dose: Three times daily for up to three days.

Chinese Remedies

1 Early stage

First two to three days. Fever and chills. Headache.

GE GEN TANG

2 Fully-developed symptoms

Swollen, painful parotid glands. High fever, usually alternating with chills. Loss of appetite.

XIAO CHAI HU TANG

3 Complications

Any abnormal or unusual symptoms in addition to those described here require prompt professional treatment.

NAPPY (DIAPER) RASH

Nearly all babies suffer nappy rash at least once before their first birthday and at any one time one in three will have it. It is usually concentrated around the anal and genital areas and easily spreads down the legs and up the abdomen. Because all babies have soft and delicate skin, which is easily irritated, especially when moist so much of the time, some babies with sensitive skin seem to have constant nappy rash!

Nappy rash is caused by a combination of wetness, acidic urine and reactions to certain natural chemicals in urine and stool, with wetness the most important single factor. A newborn baby urinates up to 20 times a day and even when they are a year old they are still doing it seven to ten times a day, so it's quite impossible to keep them dry for very long. Poor digestion is also a factor because the stool becomes even more acidic, and so is hot weather with the urine becoming more concentrated because of the loss of body fluids through perspiration.

Teething, diarrhoea, illness such as colds or generally just feeling out of sorts can produce nappy rashes quite easily too, as can allergies to soaps or chemicals used in detergents.

Sometimes the rash is complicated by a secondary bacterial or fungal infection. The most common culprit is thrush (candida), which is often present in babies' stools and causes a typical spotty nappy rash. Some experts believe that nappy rash lasting for three days or more will become infected.

Prevention

- Wipe your baby's bottom well each time you change a nappy. Use a moist cotton cloth and avoid rubbing.
- When fitting a nappy allow a little airflow around the waist and legs.
- Choose clothing that does not hug the body too tightly.
- If your baby has a tendency to develop nappy rashes, avoid baby bouncers or slings which hug too tightly.
- Change nappies frequently and leave them off when possible; just make sure you're prepared to wipe up after her.
- Try to avoid using plastic pants.
- Rinse nappies in a weak vinegar solution of 15 mL (½ fl oz) to 6 L (10 pt) of water.
- Avoid talc as it can irritate the skin when it gets wet.
- Use soft cloth nappies and if you dry them out in the sun, make sure that you use a fabric softener.
- Avoid disposable nappies.
- Wash nappies in pure soap or environmentally friendly detergent.

Home Remedies

- Apply dry bicarbonate of soda directly to the affected area.
- Apply cornflour or arrowroot powder to the affected area.
- Use a special cream with a water repellent base such as zinc or Calendula cream.
- Pawpaw ointment is very successful although the ointment itself is quite greasy and may not suit some babies whose rash has a moist appearance. Calendula cream can be used if the pawpaw is too greasy.

FACTS ABOUT DISPOSABLE NAPPIES

- They are 99 per cent unbiodegradeable.
- They are bleached and contain the lethal chemical dioxin (as do tampons).
- The average baby uses 9000 disposable nappies compared to 36 cloth ones.
- In the U.S. 3.5 million tonnes of nappies are dumped each year. They do not break down (they just turn into sludge).
- Excrement from disposable nappies also poses a health risk to garbage disposal workers.

- Castor oil cream will also help in many cases.
- Sunshine will dry out the affected area.
- Ensure that your child is drinking enough fluids.
- Sometimes nappy rash is as a result of a change in diet. Eliminate for two weeks any food that has only been recently introduced into your child's diet, to see whether it may be causing the rash.
- Soothe with Tea-Tree antiseptic cream
- If the child has a really stubborn rash, cover the genital area with yoghurt. This will help if the rash is caused by thrush.

NAUSEA

Nausea is very common in infants and children, but it is not so much a condition as a symptom. It can have any one of a number of causes, including smells that a child may be sensitive to. Sometimes vomiting will end nausea, but if vomiting persists for any length of time, make sure that you consult a practitioner of your choice.

Home Remedies

- Mild miso soup is good for restoring the system's balance.
- Rice water (the strained water from cooked rice) is easy to digest and good for settling the upset tummy.
- Herbs such as Chamomile, Peppermint and Fennel can be helpful.
- For older children, Ginger tea made by simmering two slices of root ginger in water for 5 minutes and sweetening with a little honey is good.
- See also Vomiting.

Homoeopathic Remedies

Where there is constant nausea or nausea with vomiting, pale face and a clean tongue **Ipecac** 12C is your medicine. It is the remedy of choice where the vomiting is brought on by over-eating.

   Nux vomica 30C is indicated for nausea with the constant desire to vomit but efforts to do so only result in retching. Nausea mostly comes on in the morning. It is indicated where there has been over-indulgence in rich food or stimulants.

Veratrum album 30C is effective when there is violent vomiting and nausea aggravated by drinking and the least motion.

   Other remedies including Aconite, Phosphorus and Pulsatilla (see the Homoeopathic Materia Medica) may be used where the character of the symptoms and the temperament of the child are indicated.

Dose: Every half-hour when the vomiting is severe. Otherwise to be taken every two hours for up to one day and stop on marked improvement.

Chinese Remedies

See Stomach-ache.

Massage

1 With the child lying on the right side hold one hand over the abdomen and massage around the left shoulder blade with the other hand. Do this for three to five minutes. Pull the hand down along the spine then around to the side (this covers the stomach area at the back). Repeat this five times.

2 Hold one hand at back of neck and the other hand on lower back, hold calmly for one to two minutes. Have child take long, slow, deep breaths and exhale together.

NOSEBLEEDS

It's almost certain that your child will suffer a nosebleed at least once. Nosebleeds are generally nothing to become alarmed about. For more information, see Bleeding.

General Treatment

1 Put your child in a sitting position leaning slightly forward, or if she feels more comfortable lying down just keep her head raised.
2 Tell her to breathe slowly through her mouth.
3 Pinch the nose closed lightly for at least five to ten minutes.
4 Hold some tissue under the nostrils to catch any blood that may drip down.
5 Tell your child to spit out any blood that may have collected in her mouth.
6 Suggest that she does not blow her nose, sniff, touch or pick at it for at least one hour after it has stopped bleeding.
7 If bleeding does not stop within thirty minutes, consult a medical practitioner immediately.

Home Remedies

- Tilt the head back and pinch the nose on the bony ridge slightly below the level of the eyes.
- Make a twist of a paper hanky, dampen it, dip it in salt and then insert into the child's nose. The salt helps the blood vessels contract.

- Place a cold cloth on the nose or the back of the neck.
- If your child suffers frequent nosebleeds, consult a practitioner of your choice.

Homoeopathic Remedies

See Bleeding.

Chinese Remedies

1 'Heat'

Red complexion. Red nose and lips. Red tongue with a yellow coating. Fingernails are purple. Child may grind teeth when sleeping. Prominent veins at back of ears. May be prone to mouth ulcers. Dry mouth. Thirst with desire for cold drinks. Dark urine in reduced quantity. Rapid pulse.

HUANG LIAN HIE DU TANG

2 'Deficiency'

Weak constitution. Poor sleep. Irritability. Dry mouth and throat. Tendency toward constipation. Pale complexion. Poor appetite. Usually underweight. Tongue is red without a coating.

ZHI GAN CAO TANG

Massage

Hold a cold washcloth at base of nose and press with finger into centre of upper lip, just below nose.

PARASITES

Most children will at some stage have a bout of worms. At about the age of two up until six or seven, children catch them easily, as they are more prone to 'experiment' with the outside world. There are many parasites that can be found both inside and outside the body and the most likely ones to be found in temperate regions are threadworms and roundworms. They like hot and humid conditions.

Children will be children and play in the dirt, then put their hands in their mouths. Infestation begins as the worms reach the intestines through the eggs that have been eaten. Another common way to transmit the eggs is through an infected cat or dog. Eggs hatch quickly, and so if the child is weak or has poor digestion they will multiply rapidly. They can be expelled in the stools if the child's digestion is strong.

Worms — General

It is not uncommon to find a small amount of blood in your child's urine after she has been treated for worms. There is very little cause for concern; however, it would be a good idea to make sure that the blood is related to the anti-worm treatment and not anything else. If the child needs worming more than twice a year, please consult a practitioner of your choice. Some general symptoms include tossing and turning in sleep, bad dreams, grinding the teeth in sleep and a dark spot that appears on the white part of the eye or a discolouration that appears on the cheek.

Tapeworm

Acquired by eating undercooked beef infected with beef tapeworm, undercooked pork containing the larval stage of pork tapeworm, or undercooked freshwater fish containing fish tapeworm. The adult ribbon-shaped worm that inhabits the intestinal tract may produce little or no intestinal upset in humans. But the knowledge of its presence, by noting segments of the worm in the faeces or on undergarments, may be quite distressing.

Roundworm

This is a large, pale-yellow worm 20-35 cm (8-14 in) long, resembling an earthworm but not segmented. They are much larger than threadworms and gain access to the mouth by contaminated fingers or food. The larvae can escape from the ova in the duodenum (first part of the large intestine) and find their way to the lungs where they develop further. They then will enter the intestines where they reach maturity.

Symptoms include irregular bowel movements, nausea, colicky abdominal pain and intestinal obstruction. Suspect worms if the child's upper lip begins to turn up and becomes darker in colour, and small white spots appear on the inside of the lips.

Threadworms

This type of worm is very common throughout the world. The eggs of threadworms come from playing in the dirt, and then placing unwashed fingers in the mouth. They develop in the small intestines, but the adult worm is found chiefly in the large intestines. Because the female worm lays fully developed ova around the anus, intense itching is one of the major symptoms. Occurring mainly at night, you can detect the worms by applying the adhesive surface of sticky tape to the perianal skin in the morning and seeing if any eggs have stuck to it.

Treatment is of utmost importance and if left unattended the infestation will eventually affect the entire constitution.

Symptoms include vomiting, nausea, poor appetite, abdominal pain, mucus-like stools, short temper, listlessness and diarrhoea.

Prevention of Most Common Parasites

1 Make sure that your child washes her hands after playing outside in the dirt, soil or petting animals.

2 Keep your child's fingernails short and clean.
3 Cook with lots of garlic, as it cleanses the blood. If your children don't like the taste, give garlic oil or tablets regularly.
4 If you suspect parasites, it might be a good idea to get the stool analysed.

Home Remedies

- Fresh carrot juice — take 1 glass on an empty stomach one to two hours before meals.
- Give your child several tablespoons of pumpkin seeds on an empty stomach and wait one hour before letting her eat anything again. Keep her eating the seeds every few hours.
- If your child can tolerate it, finely chopped garlic in a spoonful of olive oil or if your child is really keen, just give her a clove of garlic to chew two times daily.
- Garlic enema — mince 2 cloves of garlic. Add 2 cups boiling water, and strain. Use once daily for 10-14 days. (Eggs hatch every 14 days.)
- When your child is asleep, insert a thin sliver of garlic into the anus. It will come out in the stool.

Herbal Remedies

The treatment of parasites is best left to a qualified practitioner. A strong infusion of Thyme taken on an empty stomach will help to combat threadworms. Make sure the child is not constipated.

Thyme

Infusion: use 1-1½ teaspoons of dried herb to 1 cup of boiling water. Let steep for 5 minutes, strain. Can be sweetened with honey or rice malt. Dilute with water if necessary.

DOSE
1-2 years: 15-30 mL (½-1 fl oz) 3 times daily
3-4 years: 40-60 mL (1⅓-2 fl oz) 3 times daily
5-6 years: 70-90 mL (2⅓-3 fl oz) 3 times daily
7 years and older: 100-150 mL (3-5 fl oz) 3 times daily

Homoeopathic Remedies

Cina 6C is often a very useful medicine for worms. It is most useful where the child is irritable and picks the nose or bores a finger into it.

Teucrium 6C is an excellent remedy where the child is particularly restless at night in bed with itching of the anus.

Dose: These medicines should be given in the 6C potency twice daily for up to five days.

If the worms persist or persistently return, it is a chronic condition and should be referred to your homoeopathic practitioner.

Massage

See Abdominal Pains. Add:

1 On bottom of right foot press with thumb from heel in a line up towards the little toe just to the middle of foot and across the centre of foot at the midline.
2 On the left foot press with thumb or index finger from the instep down to the middle of heel. Press across the bottom of the foot from the heel to the middle of the foot. Do this on both feet. Do this for three to five minutes at least twice a day until pain ceases or until the worms have been passed.

PHLEGM/MUCUS

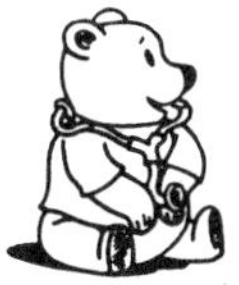

Mucus is defined as 'the slimy fluid secreted by the mucous membrane of the nose and other parts'. Phlegm on the other hand is 'the thick, slimy matter secreted in the throat, and discharged by coughing, regarded in old physiology as (cold and moist) in the four humours or bodily fluids.' (*Chalmers 20th Century Dictionary*)

Finding out the slight difference in definition doesn't really make any difference how you treat your children when they present the most predictable common childhood ailments. Frequently the production of excess mucus occurs in early childhood and infancy. Most often these terms are just part and parcel of catching colds and the flu.

Mucus is seen virtually from the time infants are totally weaned or just introduced to food. It is believed to be a factor in many illnesses, and thought to originate from poor digestion according to the Chinese doctors. If your child is too young for certain foods due to an immature digestive system; eats late at night, before going to bed; snacks too often; is tired or sick, more and more foods that affect mucus production should be avoided.

For treating complaints that have to do with mucus production or phlegm, consult each individual complaint.

Herbal Remedies

If mucus is in sinuses and discharged through the nose, anti-catarrhal herbs such as Elderflowers, Eyebright, Golden Seal, Golden Rod, Catmint or Peppermint are recommended. Fenugreek facilitates the elimination of mucus. Echinacea acts over an extended period of time (one to three months) as an immune system stimulant. If mucus or phlegm is in the lower airways (bronchi) use expectorants such as Aniseed, Elderflowers, Elecampane, Fennel, Heartsease, Mullein, Thyme and White Horehound.

Elderflower

Infusion: use 2 teaspoons of the dried flowers to 1 cup of boiling water. Let steep for 5 minutes, strain. Can be sweetened with honey or rice malt.
DOSE
1-2 years: 15-30 mL (½-1 fl oz) 3 times daily
3-4 years: 40-60 mL (1⅓-2 fl oz) 3 times daily
5-6 years: 70-90 mL (2⅓-3 fl oz) 3 times daily
7 years and older: 100-150 mL (3-5 fl oz) 3 times daily

Eyebright

Infusion: use 1 teaspoon of dried herb to 1 cup of boiling water. Let steep for 5 minutes, strain. Can be sweetened with honey or rice malt. Dilute with water if necessary.
DOSE
1-2 years: 15-30 mL (½-1 fl oz) 3 times daily
3-4 years: 40-60 mL (1⅓-2 fl oz) 3 times daily
5-6 years: 70-90 mL (2⅓-3 fl oz) 3 times daily
7 years and older: 100-150 mL (3-5 fl oz) 3 times daily

Golden Seal

Decoction: use ½ teaspoon of chopped root and rhizome to 1 cup of water, simmer covered for 5-10 minutes, strain. Can be sweetened with honey or rice malt. Dilute with water if necessary.
DOSE
2-3 years: 15-20 mL (½-⅔ fl oz) 3 times daily
4-5 years: 30-40 mL (1-1⅓ fl oz) 3 times daily
6-7 years: 50-60 mL (1⅔-2 fl oz) 3 times daily
8 years and older: 80-100 mL (2⅔-3 fl oz) 3 times daily

Golden Rod

Infusion: use 1 teaspoon of dried herb to 1 cup of boiling water. Let steep for 5 minutes, strain. Can be sweetened with honey or rice malt. Dilute with water if necessary.
DOSE
1-2 years: 10-20 mL (⅓-⅔ fl oz) 3 times daily

3-4 years: 30-40 mL (1-1⅓ fl oz) 3 times daily
5-6 years: 50-60 mL (1⅔-2 fl oz) 3 times daily
7 years and older: 70-100 mL (2⅓-3 fl oz) 3 times daily

Catmint

Infusion: use 1 teaspoon of dried herb to 1 cup of boiling water. Let steep for 5 minutes, strain. Can be sweetened with honey or rice malt. Dilute with water if necessary.
DOSE
1-2 years: 15-30 mL (½-1 fl oz) 3 times daily
3-4 years: 40-60 mL (1⅓-2 fl oz) 3 times daily
5-6 years: 70-90 mL (2⅓-3 fl oz) 3 times daily
7 years and older: 100-150 mL (3-5 fl oz) 3 times daily

Peppermint

Infusion: use ½-1 teaspoon of dried herb to 1 cup of boiling water. Let steep for 5 minutes, strain. Can be sweetened with honey or rice malt. Dilute with water if necessary.
DOSE
1-2 years: 15-30 mL (½-1 fl oz) 3 times daily
3-4 years: 40-60 mL (1⅓-2 fl oz) 3 times daily
5-6 years: 70-90 mL (2⅓-3 fl oz) 3 times daily
7 years and older: 100-150 mL (3-5 fl oz) 3 times daily

Fenugreek

Decoction: use 1 teaspoon of the crushed seeds to 1 cup of water. Simmer for 5 minutes, strain. Can be sweetened with honey or rice malt. Dilute with water if necessary.
DOSE
1-2 years: 15-30 mL (½-1 fl oz) 3 times daily
3-4 years: 40-60 mL (1⅓-2 fl oz) 3 times daily
5-6 years: 70-90 mL (2⅓-3 fl oz) 3 times daily
7 years and older: 100-150 mL (3-5 fl oz) 3 times daily

Echinacea

Decoction: use 1 teaspoon of dried root and rhizome to 1 cup of water, simmer covered for 5 minutes. Dilute with water. Can be sweetened with honey or rice malt.
DOSE
1-2 years: 10-15 mL (⅓-½ fl oz) 2 times daily
3-4 years: 20-30 mL (⅔-1 fl oz) 3 times daily
5-6 years: 40-50 mL (1⅓-1⅔ fl oz) 3 times daily
7 years and older: 60-100 mL (2-3 fl oz) 3 times daily

Aniseed

Infusion: use ½ teaspoon of whole or freshly crushed seeds to 1 cup of boiling water. Let steep for 5 minutes, strain.
DOSE
1-2 years: 15-30 mL (½-1 fl oz) 3 times daily
3-4 years: 40-60 mL (1⅓-2 fl oz) 3 times daily
5-6 years: 70-90 mL (2⅓-3 fl oz) 3 times daily
7 years and older: 100-150 mL (3-5 fl oz) 3 times daily

Elecampane

Decoction: use 1-1½ teaspoons of chopped root to 1 cup of water, simmer covered for 5-10 minutes.
DOSE
1-2 years: 15-30 mL (½-1 fl oz) 3 times daily
3-4 years: 40-60 mL (1⅓-2 fl oz) 3 times daily
5-6 years: 70-90 mL (2⅓-3 fl oz) 3 times daily
7 years and older: 100-150 mL (3-5 fl oz) 3 times daily

Fennel

Infusion: use ½-1 teaspoon of the dried seeds (best lightly crushed in a mortar) to 1 cup of boiling water. Let steep for 5 minutes, strain. Can be sweetened with honey or rice malt. Dilute with water if necessary.
DOSE
1-2 years: 15-30 mL (½-1 fl oz) 3 times daily
3-4 years: 40-60 mL (1⅓-2 fl oz) 3 times daily
5-6 years: 70-90 mL (2⅓-3 fl oz) 3 times daily
7 years and older: 100-150 mL (3-5 fl oz) 3 times daily

Heartsease (Wild Pansy)

Infusion: use 1-1½ teaspoons of the dried herb to 1 cup of boiling water. Let steep for 5 minutes, strain. Can be sweetened with honey or rice malt.
DOSE
1-2 years: 15-30 mL (½-1 fl oz) 3 times daily
3-4 years: 40-60 mL (1⅓-2 fl oz) 3 times daily
5-6 years: 70-90 mL (2⅓-3 fl oz) 3 times daily
7 years and older: 100-150 mL (3-5 fl oz) 3 times daily

Thyme

Infusion: use 1 teaspoon of dried herb to 1 cup of boiling water. Let steep for 5 minutes, strain. Can be sweetened with honey or rice malt. Dilute with water if necessary.
DOSE
1-2 years: 15-30 mL (½-1 fl oz) 3 times daily
3-4 years: 40-60 mL (1⅓-2 fl oz) 3 times daily
5-6 years: 70-90 mL (2⅓-3 fl oz) 3 times daily
7 years and older: 100-150 mL (3-5 fl oz) 3 times daily

White Horehound

Infusion: use ½-1 teaspoon of the dried herb to 1 cup of boiling water. Let steep for 5-10 minutes, strain. Sweeten with honey or rice malt. This herb has an unpleasant bitter taste and should be mixed with a pleasant-tasting expectorant herb such as Fennel seed, Aniseed or Licorice Root.

DOSE
1-2 years: 15-30 mL (½-1 fl oz) 3 times daily
3-4 years: 40-60 mL (1⅓-2 fl oz) 3 times daily
5-6 years: 70-90 mL (2⅓-3 fl oz) 3 times daily
7 years and older: 100-150 mL (3-5 fl oz) 3 times daily

Homoeopathic Remedies

Phlegm is:
Frothy — **Arsenicum** 12C
Green and offensive — **Mercurius** 12C
Stringy and yellow — **Kali-bic** 12C
Watery — **Aconite** 30C, **Arsenicum** 12C, **Bryonia** 12C, **Gelsemium** 30C, **Mercurius** 2C, **Nat-mur** 6C
Watery and acrid — **Arsenicum** 12C
White — **Nat-mur** 6C
Yellow-green and bland — **Pulsatilla** 12C

Yellow, thick and offensive — **Hepar sulph** 12C

Dose: One dose of the selected medicine twice daily for up to three days.

Chinese Remedies

1 'Exterior' Disease

See Colds for the different symptom pictures and herbal treatments.

2 'Deficiency'

Usually follows after a day or two of dietary imbalance (i.e. over-eating, over-indulgence in rich, oily, fatty or sweet foods). Often accompanied by loose stools or diarrhoea. The mucus is clear or white and watery or thin. There are no signs of a cold or flu.

ER CHEN TANG
XIANG SHA LIU JUN ZI TANG (poor appetite, belching, swollen abdomen, possibly also stomach-ache or vomiting)
XIAN SHA YANG WEI TANG (poor appetite, bloated abdomen, stomach-ache, loss of taste, general weakness)

POISONING

The actual taste of things has very little effect on some children, so it is not enough to just hope that they won't like it. Prevention is the best policy (see Safety). However, poisoning still does occur and can be potentially fatal, so treatment must be quick, precise and direct. As we only cover the basic guidelines, it is imperative to keep the number of your local Poison Information Centre written next to the phone, and if possible a reference book listing a wide variety of poisonous substances and their treatments.

Treatment

Household substances

These are the most commonly swallowed substances and vary greatly in toxicity.

1 Treat the child immediately; do not wait for symptoms to develop.
2 Read the label or box as this will usually give some basic information.
3 Ring a doctor, hospital or Poisons Information Centre first, if it is possible.
4 Try to work out how much of the substance has been taken. Sometimes this can only be a guess but indicators such as how the breath smells and how long your child has been left alone will help.

For poisons where vomiting is desirable

Non-corrosive substances such as snail bait, alcohol, paracetamol, oral contraceptives, mothballs, nail polish, laxatives, iron tablets, codeine.
1 Put two fingers to the back of the child's throat and wiggle them until the child is sick. You can be quite firm, as it is more important that they vomit than that you cause discomfort or minor injury with your fingers. If she dry retches but nothing comes up, make her drink a glass of water and try again.
2 Give Ipecac syrup (available from pharmacies)

3 If Ipecac syrup isn't available, stir 2 tablespoons of salt or mustard powder in a glass of warm water and have the child drink it.
DOSE:
1 year: 15 mL (½ fl oz)
2 years: 20 mL (⅔ fl oz)
3 years: 25 mL (¾ fl oz)
Over 3 years: 30 mL (1 fl oz)

Follow with a glass of water and make the child vomit.

For poisons where vomiting is undesirable

Some poisons make vomiting very dangerous, as they will cause more problems burning the throat and gullet. These are mostly caustic, corrosive substances and petroleum distillates, for example, dry cleaning fluids, petrol, turpentine, paint thinners, garden spray, anti-rust.
1 Give the child as much milk as she will drink to dilute the poisoning and coat the lining of the stomach.
2 If she will not drink milk try ice cream, as this will have the same benefit as milk.
3 Give any liquid she will drink, i.e. water, juice.
4 Mix together a spoonful of baking soda with cool water and drink. Follow this with several tablespoons of olive oil or milk to coat the lining of the stomach. Do not force this down as you do not want the child to vomit.
5 Take your child to the nearest doctor or hospital if it is serious. Remember to also take the poison with you for identification and correct treatment.

Garden plants

It is highly unlikely that your child will die from eating poisonous plants. While many are toxic, in most cases large amounts must be consumed before severe poisoning occurs. The following is a basic list of those plants that may cause serious illness. They should ideally be removed from a garden used by young children: oleander, lantana, deadly nightshade, foxglove, angels trumpet, castor oil beans. For all of these, induce vomiting and consult a doctor or hospital.

Some other plants to be wary of are leaves of rhubarb, toadstools, laburnum pods, arum lily, daphne, lobelia.

Food poisoning

Food poisoning is easy to avoid if you are careful about what you serve your family. However, you may be caught unawares while eating out, or by food that did not appear 'off'. Several different kinds of food poisoning are found in a different variety of products.

Botulism is the best-known but also extremely rare, with most cases involving canned or home preserved food.

Salmonella is present in red and white meats and poisoning can be avoided by cooking well and refrigerating quickly after cooking.

Poisoning can also occur in foods that have been left standing for too long, such as custard or seafood that is 'old'.

Symptoms of food poisoning include vomiting, diarrhoea, abdominal cramps, temperature. Symptoms differ for botulism: weakness, difficulty in speech, headache.

General Treatment

- Give lots of fluid to prevent dehydration, preferably water or clear fluids.
- Allow child to rest.
- Keep child attended to prevent choking on vomit.
- After twenty-four to forty-eight hours re-introduce bland foods first.
- Seek medical advice for a suspected case of botulism, as it can be fatal for very young children if blood appears in diarrhoea; for persistent abdominal pain, dehydration or high fever.

Homoeopathic Remedies

The medicine of choice in food poisoning or any poisoning where there is vomiting, purging and exhaustion with restlessness requires **Arsenicum album** 12C.

Other medicines such as Aconite, Carb-veg, Nux vomica and Veratrum may be used where the character of the symptoms and the temperament of the child are indicated.

Dose: Every hour if the condition is severe or three times daily where the symptoms are not so intense.

PNEUMONIA

The very word 'pneumonia' seems to strike fear into every parent's heart. The stigma from a past time, when many children died from pneumonia, still seems to be with some of us. And, though it is a serious illness, it is by no means as threatening as we often think it is. Treatment now is remarkable and recovery is usually uncomplicated.

There are two types of pneumonia, with almost opposite levels of emergency. Though both are inflammations of the lungs, it is only *bacterial pneumonia (pneumococcal)* that needs immediate medical attention. The other kind, *viral pneumonia (bronchopneumonia)* causes no danger to the child and the body will cure itself. However, it is virtually impossible to distinguish between viral and bacterial pneumonia. Therefore, consult a practitioner of your choice immediately if you suspect that your child has pneumonia.

Bacterial Symptoms

Mild to high fever, dry hacking cough, chest pain, nausea and vomiting, weakness, difficulty in breathing and blue on fingertips and around the mouth.

Bacterial pneumonia usually comes on after a child has had a cold for several days, but it may also start without warning. It is also infectious seven days after the first symptoms occur. Your doctor should be able to detect abnormal breathing sounds with a stethoscope, which usually then need to be confirmed by a chest X-ray.

Bacterial Treatment — Orthodox

This is classed as a medical emergency and the child should see a doctor, especially if she has difficulty with breathing.

1 Antibiotics or penicillin are usually administered.
2 Give your child extra fluids.

3 Ensure rest.
4 If eating solids, keep on a light diet.
5 Moisten air in the child's room with a humidifier.

Viral Symptoms

Cold and low fever for one to two days; ability to return to normal activity, but with a persistent cough; after one week to ten days the cough becomes looser and more persistent; general tiredness.

It usually takes four weeks to clear and can only be identified medically by an X-ray. The symptoms remain mild.

Viral Treatment — Home Remedies

Viral pneumonia will run its normal course, regardless of any treatment given. Any medication will only relieve the symptoms and will actually interfere with the body's efforts to cure itself. Be sure to get a diagnosis from a practitioner of your choice before making any decisions as to how you wish to treat your child. It may also be helpful to restrict your child's activities until the pneumonia has run its course.

Homoeopathic Remedies

This condition may be dangerous and should be referred to your homoeopathic practitioner.

Massage

1 On the bottom of each foot, making thumb prints, press from the ball of the foot up to the base of the toes. Press in as deeply as your child can stand. As you press in, fold the toes toward your working thumb. You can also hold the top of the foot with one hand and, making a soft fist, press into the ball of the foot.

2 Rotate each toe (on both feet) and press into the centre of each toe (the pad of the toe).

3 Press with your thumb or index finger across the base of the ball of the foot (the ball tends to be a brighter pink colour). Do this in both directions across the whole foot.

4 Press into the centre of the ball of each foot and have your child inhale (if she is old enough to follow directions; if not, you can simply follow their breathing pattern) as you press in with your thumb, then as they exhale you release your pressure and pull the toes toward you. Do this three times. This series can be repeated every hour for five minutes or longer.

RASHES/SKIN IRRITATIONS

There is no need for grave concern every time little spots or rashes appear on your child's skin, as skin ailments are rarely life-threatening. The first condition that will usually concern you is nappy rash. Your baby's skin is very delicate and getting used to the outside world is a major chore, so don't be surprised with the little visible signs that show up on their bodies from time to time.

Part of what occurs can also be related to something that occurred inside the womb and so when your baby is born, whatever needs to come out of the body begins to make its way out via the baby's skin, (one of the primary ways in which the body releases toxins). So don't rush to your doctor's surgery too quickly. You will be able to diagnose and treat (at least the second time around) most of the common skin ailments of your child.

Your child's skin protects her from too much heat or cold, keeps body fluids in and other fluids out and protects her internal organs. In Chinese medicine the skin is considered to be the 'third lung', which simply means that what affects the skin can affect the lungs and vice versa.

Skin irritations can have a variety of causes, for example, heat, diet, stress, certain plants, nappies, chemical sensitivity to certain materials, metals, food, additives, etc. Allergic reactions often include skin symptoms. The most effective way of dealing with skin irritations is obviously to treat the causing factor, for example, remove the allergen from the diet, cool the child down, teach her not to touch stinging nettles, etc.

In all skin conditions it is vital that one rule be followed no matter what: keep the affected area clean. Infection is an ever-present hazard in any part of the body where the child has broken the skin.

If your child develops a rash and you cannot determine the cause, it would be best to consult a practitioner of natural therapies, as rashes are considered to be caused by an accumulation of poisons in the body; even though they can rarely be considered 'dangerous' rashes may in fact disturb your child's self-image and confidence.

See also Cradle Cap, Nappy Rash and Eczema.

Home Remedies

- Give your child a bath in which a muslin bag containing oatmeal is floating. The oats release into the bath a milky liquid that is soothing to irritated skin.
- A bath or rinse with 3 cups of chickweed tea (a common garden weed in many areas) is soothing and healing and is particularly good if the skin is itchy. Chickweed is also available in creams or ointment from health food stores.
- Another excellent herb for skin complaints is Calendula, available in a cream or ointment.
- Ringworm is a fungal infection. On the head it is called Tinea Capitus. In feet it is known as athlete's foot (Tinea Pedis). It responds well to Tea-Tree oil, applied directly to the affected area.

On-going skin complaints should be referred to a qualified practitioner.

Herbal Remedies

Calendula (Marigold)

One of the best herbs for rashes and the like, Marigold is a superb healing agent.
Infusion: use 3 teaspoons of the dried flowerheads to 1 cup of boiling water. Let steep for 5 minutes, strain. This infusion can be used externally as a rinse on skin complaints of various kinds.

Chickweed

Chickweed has anti-inflammatory and healing properties.
Infusion: use freshly picked Chickweed from the garden (see page 18 for identification), wash

it and chop it into 1 cm/½ inch pieces. Use 4 heaped teaspoons or more of fresh, chopped Chickweed per cup of boiling water. Let steep for 10 minutes, strain.

Apply to itchy or inflamed skin, cuts and wounds with a clean piece of cotton or by pouring the infusion on to the afflicted area. If larger areas of the body are affected, a Chickweed bath can be taken. To prepare, make a couple of litres of very strong Chickweed infusion in a saucepan, strain and add to the bath.

Homoeopathic Remedies

In homoeopathic practice, no external applications are used on the skin unless the complaint was caused by an external influence as in a burn or laceration. Chronic skin conditions must be studied individually and should be referred to your homoeopath — but where the following remedies are well indicated they will be of great benefit:

Rhus-tox 12C is the first remedy of choice for herpetic skin conditions.

Nat-mur 6C is particularly indicated where the herpes appear as singular sores on the lips.

Dose: One dose twice daily for three days.

Itchy hives that are better from heat call for **Apis** 12C. Where hives are burning and itching and have suddenly appeared, use **Rhus-tox** 12C.

Dose: One dose three times daily for up to three days.

Impetigo is a highly infective condition that should be referred to your homoeopath.

Arsenicum 12C for nappy rash, where the skin is red, burning hot and scaly in little flakes.

Dose: One dose daily for three days.

Rashes that are very itchy with an irresistible desire to scratch and worse for the heat require **Sulphur** 12C.

Dose: One dose daily for three days.

SAFETY

Most environments have many potential dangers and it is important to create a 'safety net' for your child. This should include a combination of prevention, education, common-sense and intuition.

Safety in the Home

When taking steps to make your own house 'child-proof', take the time to crawl around it on your hands and knees. It can be most informative to get your child's perspective; the world looks very different from floor level.

- Look out for the obvious hazards such as power points, and also for potential dangers from toppling tables, dangling table cloths, electric cords, reachable electronic equipment such a stereo, plastic bags stuffed at backs of cupboards, household cleaning fluids, etc.
- Never leave babies or young children unsupervised. Use a play-pen or portable cot for those times when you must leave her.
- Check your garage or storage areas and place any sharp objects or tools, including power tools, out of reach.
- Regularly check your children's toys for small pieces that may have broken off, or places where children can get fingers caught.
- Keep a list of emergency numbers near your phone. Make sure they are updated and visible in the case of an accident.
- As well as protection, educate your child as to the dangers of her environment. Let her have a kitchen cupboard or drawer filled with suitable objects for her own, and make the rest out of bounds. When you are out visiting and your child wishes to explores someone's kitchen, remind her that it is not her cupboard and so cannot be played with.
- Teach your child how to climb up and down stairs, in addition to installing safety gates. Also teach her never to play with plastic bags, pill bottles, etc., and to stay away from water and electricity.
- Encourage her not to eat plants, either in the garden or inside; many plants are toxic if

eaten by a toddler (see Poisoning). For the older child try explaining consequences — this can be a great eye-opener.

The main areas of danger to be considered are:
- Electricity — all power points and electrical appliances.
- Poisoning — from medicines, household and garden chemicals, and poisonous plants.
- Drowning — unsupervised baths, wading pools, buckets and ponds, as well as swimming pools. A child can drown in only a few inches of water.
- Burning — from open fires, heat, cooking, boiling water, etc.
- Falling — down unprotected stairs and drops.
- Crushing — over-balancing of heavy objects such as tables.
- Suffocation — from plastic bags, getting cords from blinds and curtains around necks, etc.
- Your car — It would be easy to run over a toddler, as they are not visible from the driver's seat, so never move a car near children without making sure they are well clear.
- Other people's houses!

The kitchen

This is the most dangerous room in the house, yet unfortunately it seems the most attractive. For small children it represents the ultimate in entertainment. Everything is interesting and fun to taste, touch, smell and smash. Let a child into a kitchen and she will have 'fun' for hours; she also may have a serious accident.

If it is at all possible, install a safety gate in the kitchen doorway; this will solve many problems. However, this may not be possible, or you may find it too restrictive. Even if you do install a gate, make sure you still take the following precautions.

1 Always turn the handles of cooking pots into the centre of the stove, as children often reach up and pull hot pots down on them. Never leave your child alone in the kitchen if you are frying something, as the oil can spit, or ignite. Attaching a guard rail to the stove is a wise precaution. Never carry hot items over a child's head.

2 Ensure that all household chemicals and plastic bags are securely locked away in a high cupboard. Fit child resistant latches to cupboards you wish to keep secure from your child.

3 Check your appliances — are there dangling cords? Can your child reach the appliances? Cover all unused power points with safety plugs.

4 Keep all knives and other sharp objects well out of your child's reach.

5 Be careful of anything your child could climb into and not get out of, such as a chest freezer. Keep such things locked.

6 Store breakables such as glass up high.

7 Ensure that floors have a slip-resistant surface.

8 Make sure edges on benches are rounded, or covered with pads. These are just the right height for toddlers' heads.

9 Be careful of stove knobs. Many new stoves allow them to retract when not in use. If you have an older style stove, most knobs can be removed for cleaning. Keep these in a small container near the stove and replace as you need them.

10 Make sure you empty your rubbish bin regularly as food scraps can poison a child and empty cans, etc. can give a nasty cut.

BURNS, BIKES, BITES

1990 Annual Report of The Child Safety Centre at The Children's Hospital, Camperdown.

- **4,799 children were seen in the Casualty Department during 1990.**
- **1,130 of these children were admitted for emergency in-patient care.**
- **57 per cent of injuries occurred in the child's home and most of the children were under three.**
- **Burns, injuries, dog bites and motor vehicle injuries continue to present in alarmingly high numbers.**
- **The insertion of foreign bodies is still a favoured preoccupation of the under-fives who use a variety of objects from 'healing' crystals and toy kangaroo tails to Teenage Mutant Ninja Turtle bits, sultanas and cheese.**

Bathroom

1 Never leave your child unattended in a bath, even for a few minutes. If your child has grown out of a baby bath, you can buy special supports to help them remain sitting and to stop them from slipping so easily underwater. A cheaper alternative is to put the child in a plastic laundry basket in the bath. This gives the child something to hang on to and also prevents toys floating too far away.

2 Lock up all medicines and, cleaning products in a high cupboard.

3 Make sure any electrical appliance in the bathroom such as heaters, electrical shavers, etc. is out of reach of children. Fasten them to a wall and make sure there are no electric cords trailing.

4 Make sure the child cannot lock herself in the bathroom by removing the key or making sure the lock is high enough on the door to be out of reach.

5 Make sure that the hot water is not scalding. It is worth while to turn down the temperature of the hot water and use less cold while your children are small. Safety taps can be fitted to hot water taps.

6 Use non-slip mats in the shower and bath.

7 Empty the bathtub as soon as your child finishes her bath.

Children's rooms

1 Apply the safety precautions already outlined for electricity, poisons and medicines.

2 If the windows are on the second storey or there is a reasonable drop, fit bars or safety latches that only allow the windows to be open a few inches.

3 Make sure the rooms are free of small objects that can be swallowed — the Lego, marbles and such belonging to an older child can be lethal to a baby or toddler.

4 Always block stairs both top and bottom with safety gates. Discourage older children from sliding down banisters by installing uprights at intervals to check the run.

5 Do not use pillows for children under twelve months, and in colder areas use a sleeping bag in preference to lots of blankets.

6 Do not store toys or clothes in plastic bags, as the child could be suffocated.

7 Do not let a child use an electric blanket.

8 Check the safety of the child's cot. Are the bars close enough to prevent her sticking her head through? Consider installing safety locks to drop sides.

The living room

1 Cover all unused power points with child resistant safety plugs. (Do this in all rooms.)
2 Make sure that TV, video and stereo equipment is out of reach of children and that there are no trailing power cords. Also keep records out of reach of children as their plastic inner sleeves can kill.
3 Consider padding sharp corners of furniture with tape and foam — it may look unsightly for a while but it saves your toddler from accidents.
4 If you have large glass doors, place tape in strips over the glass to remind children that it is solid.
5 Remove all breakable objects; alcohol and tobacco from your child's reach.
6 Ensure that any dangling cords from vertical blinds and curtains are out of the way, as a child can be easily strangled.
7 Watch out for things that can pinch fingers — automatically closing doors are a problem and can be fitted with springs to prevent their sudden closure. Ironing boards can be another hazard because they fold up and can crush or break a finger.
8 Tablecloths can easily be pulled off tables. Put them away in favour of place mats until your children are older.
9 Open fires, heaters, etc. should be securely screened from children. Do not leave your child alone with heaters such as paraffin stoves, which can easily be knocked over and that are filled with flammable liquid.
10 Consider investing in a play-pen. These are great for the times that you cannot supervise your child, i.e. when you are on the phone, in the garden, in the shower.
11 Do not use training walkers (movable chairs on wheels) for your baby. These are notoriously dangerous and have caused many accidents.

Outdoor areas

1 Make sure your garden is securely fenced. In addition, fence off any dangerous areas in your garden such as steps and steep drops. Use vertical slats for gates, etc. to prevent your child from climbing over.
2 Keep your gardening tools and plant fertilisers and sprays securely locked away, along with any products for your car, such as petrol and oil.

3 Discourage your child from playing in or near your car. It is easy for them to let off the handbrake, for example. Consider installing a stop such as a railway sleeper to prevent your car rolling. And **always** walk around your car before moving it to check that there are no children close by.
4 Fence off all swimming pools and cover ornamental ponds with wire mesh. Always supervise the use of paddling pools and empty them when not in use.
5 Do not let children near when you are lawnmowing or brushcutting as flying stones can be lethal.
6 Check your garden for poisonous plants and remove any.
7 Always supervise children when having a barbecue.
8 Always supervise children on a trampoline.

General safety

On the road

Studies have shown that children should not be allowed to cross roads by themselves until around eight years of age, as their spontaneity may cause them to leap without looking. Elementary road sense should be instilled in the child as soon as possible. Teach them the necessity of keeping off the road and on the curb or pavement.

In the car

It is illegal for your child to be travelling unrestrained. Restraints should be chosen according to the size and age of the child. The back of the car is safer than the front. Consider fitting safety locks to the back doors, and *never* let your child hang her head or arms out of the windows. Always check the position of children outside the car when manoeuvring near them.

Near water

Children need constant supervision near any body of water. They can drown in 2 cm (¾ in) of water.

CAUTION
In the event of any accident occurring, seek urgent medical attention; see the section on First Aid or Emergencies or under the appropriate alphabetical listing.

SLEEPING HABITS

It is not unusual for babies not to sleep through the night, especially if they are being breastfed. It has been estimated that 20 per cent of one- to two-year-olds do not sleep through the night, so if you have one of these, relax, you are not alone.

There are different stages that babies seem to go through. In the first six months it is normal for babies to wake frequently and feed day and night. A newborn baby will have long periods of sleep; however, she will wake at the smallest provocation. She may or may not be hungry, although usually she will be.

At three months of age your baby may start to sleep for longer or shorter periods. By six months another change occurs and many infants start to wake more frequently again. It may be due to dreaming but whatever the reason, there is little you can do.

Poor sleeping habits in the young child can make life very difficult for the mother, the child, the family, and the parents' relationship. There may be simple explanations.

- Is the child feeling secure and emotionally stable?
- Have there been any changes in her environment lately? Is she eating well?
- Has she been eating lollies, too much salty or spicy food or junk food, which can stimulate her behaviour or send her off balance?

Try paying attention to her diet and make sure her daily life has consistency. Put some time into 'extra attention' with her. Give Chamomile tea before bed, and during the day.

Expectations Can Be Deadly

Many so-called 'experts' see night-waking as unnatural or at least undesirable and tell parents that the best thing to do is ignore their child's cries. To leave a baby crying is quite distressing for everyone, rarely reaping a reward. We all have waking periods through the night in between light sleep and dreaming stages, before going into a deep sleep. Some babies become wide awake during the night and are unable to get back to sleep again quickly. Eventually they start to cry, and you have to attend to them. It can be very frustrating when you have tried breastfeeding, a dummy, a bottle, a nappy change, rocking, patting, singing, humming and walking around the room a hundred times over, exhausting all possibilities and your child is still awake. So get up with them and try food, a story or play, then put them back to bed. It is best to keep the room as dark as possible, as this may keep the baby from being too distracted.

How Much Sleep Do They Really Need?

No one can tell you how many hours your baby will need to sleep because all babies are different. They will develop their habits according to their own individual needs and will keep changing them as they need to for their own growth and development.

- At three months they say, the average amount of sleep is between 14 and 16 hours, with naps at almost the same time of the day every day.
- At six months the routine probably will change, sleeping more during the night and less during the day. Still, 14-15 hours is usual.
- One-year-olds tend to need less, depending upon the child. The night sleeps should start to show signs of improvement and perhaps a nap will disappear during the day.
- Two-year-olds may still wake during the night, some to cuddle up with mum and dad and more than likely just for some body heat. If they have trouble sleeping well at night, try dropping a daytime nap.
- Children who are three and over may not find the need to have a nap at all during the day. As they get older, there is more and more desire to stay up later and later and they may be very reluctant to go to bed at all.

Setting the Stage

Try setting up a routine before sleep time and follow it every day. A nice warm bath, a gentle rub, a quiet game or two, a book, some songs, whatever feels like a good routine for you and your baby. Don't be disappointed if it doesn't work right away. Remember that there will always be interruptions such as teething, wind, dreams, etc. so be flexible.

Options

1 If your baby wakes during the night, I encourage you to pick her up and cuddle her, walk her around, look at a book or play with toys, rock her and sing a lullaby or two and, if she's hungry, feed her. If this doesn't work you may wish to try controlled crying.

2 Controlled crying is a method of teaching babies how to put themselves to sleep when they wake. It should only be practised after the baby is six months old and it involves letting your baby cry, which is not easy. Here are some vital steps to follow for controlled crying:

- The baby should be in a room of her own.
- When the baby cries, go into the room and give her some comfort. Hold her for a few seconds and then put her down and leave the room. This is the hardest thing to do.
- Continue to go back and comfort her, but stretch the intervals out for longer and longer periods of time. Try five, ten and fifteen minute intervals.

  Each night there should be a rapid improvement. By the third night the crying should be minimal. If you feel that you cannot cope on your own, there are support groups that will help you with this technique.

Disturbed Sleeping Patterns

It is possible that your child wakes for no apparent reason whatsoever. Her health seems good, she is full of energy during the day, but in the night it is exactly the opposite. There is certainly consolation in knowing that this is not a life-threatening problem; however, it is positively disturbing and serious for the parents. Sleep deprivation can drive people insane, so finding the cause is of utmost importance.

The most common reason a baby wakes is to make contact with her mother; however, a baby can also wake due to an underlying cause

that needs to be attended to. There are four common patterns of insomnia:

Over-stimulation pattern

A child's sleep can be restless and disturbed and she may have difficulty in falling asleep. Her face will be pale and she will exhibit signs of weakness such as poor appetite, tiredness, sleepy during the day without too much activity. As soon as you put her to bed she wakes up and cries softly. When you attend to her she stops, but as soon as she falls asleep again she wakes disturbed.

HOME REMEDIES

- Create a calming period before bedtime by avoiding over-active play and television. This can best be achieved by keeping the lights down low, playing soft music, reading a bedtime story and giving her a warm bath with a few drops of lavender oil.
- If she wakes up frightened, give her a few drops of Bach Rescue Remedy. If fear is the cause of insomnia it may manifest itself with other symptoms such as tummy aches, pain in the lower abdomen, a rash, diarrhoea or constipation. These will disappear when the fear is released.
- Try giving her something to drink or eat when she wakes to settle her down. Sometimes this is enough and she will very happily go back to a sound sleep.

Cold pattern

Your child may wake with intestinal pain which may be similar to a pain that a baby experiences in colic. This is normally caused by too much cold energy foods or drinks (see Appendix 9). She may exhibit a lot of wind during the day; there will be a bluish-grey colour above the mouth; restless sleep with a lot of movement; she may grind her teeth; often she'll give a soft cry before waking and upon waking the cry turns into a screaming, desperate sound.

HOME REMEDIES

- Avoid the use of all cold energy foods (see Appendix 9) as well as cold in temperature.
- Use goat's milk instead of cow's.
- Try massaging your child ten to fifteen minutes before sleep as well as during the day.
- Give your child a bath with Chamomile or Lavender added to the bath water to help her relax.

Poor circulation pattern

If your child has no difficulty in going to sleep but once asleep wakes after one or two hours it is believed that the energy circulation slows down more and more and therefore the brain is deprived of its blood supply and the child wakes up. She may frequently wake up and upon waking seem happy and may go back to sleep quite easily. If no one responds to her then she will begin to speak, whimper or cry; she may be sleepy during the day; she may have very little if any appetite; she may have been ill for a long time.

HOME REMEDIES
- Avoid all rich, fatty and mucus-forming foods.
- Make sure that your child has enough to drink.
- Avoid all foods that are artificially coloured, flavoured or preserved (possible allergic reactions).
- Give Chamomile tea, Vervain tea (available in tea bags), or Valerian tea (not recommended for children under the age of two).
- Consult a practitioner of your choice if the problem persists.

Hot body patterns

Your child may have difficulty in sleeping because there is too much heat trapped inside her body. This is simply another imbalance like having a fever, but instead of the heat manifesting itself in fever, the child feels the heat in her sleep and wakes up. There are many reasons why this heat occurs, for example, it may have come from mother during pregnancy as an energy imbalance; she may have eaten too much rich, heavy or spicy food; she may have constipation; she may have had too much stimulation and excitement just before bedtime; she may have eaten too much sugar. She may want to get up and play in the middle of the night, she may wake up without crying but will make some sound to get attention, she may feel hot and want to take off her clothes and blankets, she will have difficulty in getting off to sleep and she may have red cheeks.

HOME REMEDIES
- Massage is always helpful to help a child relax and fall asleep.
- Get up and play with her for a little while and offer some food or drink.
- Try adding Chamomile or Lavender to the bath water before bedtime.

- Try Vervain tea if your child has difficulty in slowing down.
- Try Bach Rescue Remedy before bedtime.
- Try Chamomile tea if your child is teething and is very excited. If you think that the heat arises from constipation, see the Constipation section.

Herbal Remedies

Chamomile, Catmint and Valerian before bedtime to relax and calm the child.

Chamomile

Infusion: use 1 teaspoon dried flowerheads to 1 cup of boiling water. Let steep for 5 minutes, strain. Can be sweetened with honey or rice malt. Dilute with water for smaller children.
DOSE
1-2 years: 20-40 mL ($2/3$-$1\frac{1}{3}$ fl oz) 3 to 4 times daily
3-4 years: 50-80 mL ($1\frac{2}{3}$-$2\frac{2}{3}$ fl oz) 3 to 4 times daily
5-6 years: 100-125 mL (3-4 fl oz) 3 to 4 times daily
7 years and older: 150-200 mL (5-$6\frac{2}{3}$ fl oz) 3 to 4 times daily

Catmint

Infusion: use 1 teaspoon of dried herb to 1 cup of boiling water. Let steep for 5 minutes, strain. Can be sweetened with honey or rice malt. Dilute with water if necessary.
DOSE
1-2 years: 15-30 mL ($\frac{1}{2}$-1 fl oz) 3 times daily
3-4 years: 40-60 mL ($1\frac{1}{3}$-2 fl oz) 3 times daily
5-6 years: 70-90 mL ($2\frac{1}{3}$-3 fl oz) 3 times daily
7 years and older: 100-150 mL (3-5 fl oz) 3 times daily

Valerian

Decoction: use 1 teaspoon of chopped roots and rhizome to 1 cup of water, simmer covered for 5-10 minutes, strain. Can be sweetened with honey or rice malt. Dilute with water if necessary.
DOSE
1-2 years: 15-30 mL ($\frac{1}{2}$-1 fl oz) 3 times daily
3-4 years: 40-60 mL ($1\frac{1}{3}$-2 fl oz) 3 times daily
5-6 years: 70-90 mL ($2\frac{1}{3}$-3 fl oz) 3 times daily
7 years and older: 100-150 mL (3-5 fl oz) 3 times daily

NOTE: On rare occasions, Valerian may have a stimulating rather than a calming effect. If this happens, discontinue the use of this herb.

Homoeopathic Remedies

Where this is a chronic condition and does not correlate to one of the remedies below, it should be referred to your homoeopathic practitioner.

Belladonna 30C is indicated when your child wakes repeatedly in fright.

Repeated waking associated with a period of teething calls for **Chamomilla** 30C.

Coffea cruda 30C is indicated when your child cannot sleep after excitement.

Arnica 30C is indicated when your child wakes (after a shock) in fright.

Dose: one dose nightly before sleep for 3 nights.

Chinese Remedies

Disturbed sleep, in the absence of any other disease symptoms.

1 'Deficiency' with 'Heat'

Pale complexion with flushing in the malar region, irritability, tendency towards constipation. Shiny red tongue with little or no coating. Often sweats at night. May often have ulcers of the mouth and tongue. The pulse is normal to rapid.

LIU WEI DI HUANG WAN
TIAN WANG BU XIN DAN (severe symptoms)

2 'Deficiency' with 'Cold'

Pale complexion. Pale lips. Pale tongue with a thin white coating. Low energy. Tires easily. Dull eyes. Quiet voice. Speaks little. Cold hands and feet. Poor appetite. Loose stools.

GUI PI TANG
ZHI GAN CAO TANG (dry mouth and throat, absence of coating on the tongue, constipation or dry stool)

Massage

1 With your child on her back, gently press the bridge of her nose between your thumb and index finger while at the same time massaging her abdomen in a clockwise motion.

2 Press across the top of each big toe with your thumbs and also along the sides of the big toe.

SORE THROAT

Symptoms

One of the frustrations of parenthood is encountered when you know your child is sick but she is unable to tell you what is wrong, where it hurts and how she feels. Sore throats are one of these ailments, and they often go unnoticed for a while even though they are very common in children and babies. They can be identified in those too little to talk by feeling for swollen glands in the throat, difficulty in swallowing and a loss of appetite.

Causes

Sore throats most commonly are viral and may or may not be part of a flu-like illness. If they keep recurring but are not accompanied by any sort of illness they may be allergic in nature. They also can be associated with chronic ear and sinus problems, and it's a good idea to test for sensitivity to foods or things inhaled from the air like dust, mould or pollen.

Sore throats can also be due to one of the many varieties of streptococci bacteria. If this is the case your child or infant will be usually quite ill with headache, fever, a sore and spotted throat, vomiting, abdominal pain, tiredness, swollen lymph nodes on the neck or a possible fine red sandpaper rash.

If your child has chronic or recurring sore throats she may have tonsillitis. The tonsils are a very important part of the lymph system, which is similar to a filtering system for foreign organisms in the body, and it also has the very responsible job of producing the lymph cells that fight infection. If too many infections occur in the throat the tonsils themselves may become infected constantly. (see Tonsillitis)

Precautions

If the child has signs of strep throat you will need to consider antibiotics as complications may arise. Streptococcal bacteria may invade other parts of the body, particularly the kidneys. This complication requires antibiotic treatment.

Home Remedies

- Add three drops of pure Tea-Tree oil to 1 cup of warm water and gargle.
- Combine 1–2 tablespoons apple cider vinegar in half cup boiled, warm water and gargle every hour.
- Combine 1–2 teaspoons sea salt in half cup boiled, lukewarm water and gargle every hour.
- Combine 1–2 teaspoons freshly squeezed lemon juice in half cup boiled, luke warm water and gargle every hour.
- Eat lots of broths with onions, garlic and leeks.

Naturopathic Treatment

Gargles and local applications

1 Saline solution — 1 teaspoon salt in 1 cup of warm water (or to taste) can settle an itchy throat (for children over 4 years).
2 A strong tea made with 1 cup Sage or Thyme tea and 1 teaspoon of Cider vinegar and Honey is an excellent gargle.
3 Licorice, Myrrh and Golden Seal tea — gargle and drink. (As Golden Seal is very bitter, use only a pinch per cup with ½ teaspoon Licorice and ½ teaspoon Myrrh.)
4 Hot lemon drinks and barley lemon drinks help soothe.

External application

1 Mustard poultices (see Appendix 7) or continually applied hot packs are helpful.
2 Ointments containing aromatic oils such as Eucalyptus, Cajuput and Tea-Tree oil can be applied to the throat area to soothe inflammation and increase circulation.

Cold application

1 Vinegar compress — dip a cloth into vinegar

solution (1 cup vinegar to 2 cups water) and wrap it around your child's throat. Change when warm. For children 2 years and over.

2 Place cold water compress on the throat, by applying cold cloths to the throat and replacing them every ½ hour or so.

Cold can be very soothing to a sore throat. You may remember how nice it was in your childhood when you were told to eat ice cream when you had a sore throat.

- Healthy alternatives would be fresh fruit sorbets. Fruit which is naturally coloured blue contains a group of compounds which are very good anti-inflammatory agents. They also protect tissue from the damaging effects of viral infection and bacterial infection. Fruits which contain these are blueberries, cherries and blackberries. Blueberries are the best. I have made frequent use of frozen blueberries in the case of a sore throat and found them soothing and effective in controlling the throat infection.
- Ice blocks can also be made with the herb teas using fruit juice flavoured with a little Sage, Thyme and Licorice tea or other herbs which may be taken internally.

Herbal Remedies

Echinacea

This herb enhances the function of the immune system.

Decoction: use 1 teaspoon of dried root and rhizome to 1 cup of water, simmer covered for 5 minutes. Dilute with water. Can be sweetened with honey or rice malt.

DOSE

1-2 years: 10-15 mL (⅓-½ fl oz) 2 times daily
3-4 years: 20-30 mL (⅔-1 fl oz) 3 times daily
5-6 years: 40-50 mL (1⅓-1⅔ fl oz) 3 times daily
7 years and older: 60-100 mL (2-3 fl oz) 3 times daily

Elderflowers

Elderflowers are anti-catarrhal and anti-inflammatory.

Infusion: use 2 teaspoons of the dried flowers to 1 cup of boiling water. Let steep for 5 minutes, strain. Can be sweetened with honey or rice malt.

DOSE

1-2 years: 15-30 mL (½-1 fl oz) 3 times daily
3-4 years: 40-60 mL (1⅓-2 fl oz) 3 times daily
5-6 years: 70-90 mL (2⅓-3 fl oz) 3 times daily

7 years and older: 100-150 mL (3-5 fl oz) 3 times daily

Yarrow

Yarrow is astringent and anti-inflammatory. It can be used as a gargle as well as taken internally.

Infusion: use 1 teaspoon of dried herb to 1 cup of boiling water. Let steep for 5 minutes, strain. Can be sweetened with honey or rice malt. Dilute with water if necessary.

DOSE

1-2 years: 15-30 mL (½-1 fl oz) 3 times daily
3-4 years: 40-60 mL (1⅓-2 fl oz) 3 times daily
5-6 years: 70-90 mL (2⅓-3 fl oz) 3 times daily
7 years and older: 100-150 mL (3-5 fl oz) 3 times daily

Licorice

Licorice is anti-inflammatory and very soothing for a sore throat. Do not use for a prolonged period.

Decoction: use ½ teaspoon chopped Licorice root to 1 cup of water. Simmer covered for 10 minutes.

DOSE

1-2 years: 20 mL (⅔ fl oz) 3 times daily
3-4 years: 30-50 mL (1-1⅔ fl oz) 3 times daily
5-6 years: 60-80 mL (2-2⅔ fl oz) 3 times daily
7 years and older: 100-120 mL (3-4 fl oz) 3 times daily

Marshmallow

The decoction of Marshmallow is somewhat viscous and is very soothing.

Decoction: use 1-1½ teaspoons of chopped root to 1 cup of water, simmer covered for 5-10 minutes.

Infusion: use 2 teaspoons of dried leaf to 1 cup of boiling water, let steep for 10 minutes. Can be diluted with water.

Sage

Gargle: prepare as an infusion using 1-2 teaspoons of dried herb or 5-6 teaspoons of chopped, fresh leaf to 1 cup of boiling water. Let steep for 10 minutes, strain. Do not sweeten or dilute.

Thyme

Gargle: prepare as an infusion using 1-2 teaspoons of dried herb or 5-6 teaspoons of chopped, fresh leaf to 1 cup of boiling water. Let steep for 10 minutes, strain. Do not sweeten or dilute.

DOSE

*½-1 year:*15-30 mL (½-1 fl oz) 3 times daily
2-3 years: 40-50 mL (1⅓-1⅔ fl oz) 3 times daily
4-5 years: 60-80 mL (2-2⅔ fl oz) 3 times daily
6 years and older: 80-120 mL (2⅔-4 fl oz) 3 times daily

Homoeopathic Remedies

Apis 12C is indicated for burning and stinging of the throat with redness and swelling. There may be a desire for cool drinks.

Use **Belladonna** 30C where the throat is red, swallowing is painful and the pain spreads to the ear. The child is usually thirsty for cold water in this situation. It may be associated with fever and flushing of the skin.

Causticum 12C is used for rawness and soreness of the throat. There is often an associated hoarseness which is better for coughing up mucus.

The **Mercurius** 12C sore throat is usually suppurating (forming or discharging pus). This appears in the throat or on the tonsils. The tongue is often swollen with scalloped edges from the imprint of the teeth. Salivation, sweat and thirst may be increased.

Dose: To be taken three times daily for up to three days.

Massage

See Coughs. For children 1 year and older you can use a menthol rub (Tiger Balm, Eucalyptus or Olbas).

1 Massage with small circles just below ear beside the jaw (gently, as this area could be very sensitive).
2 Turn child's head to one side, grasp and knead and squeeze the relaxed (sternocleidomastoid) muscle. Do this on both sides.
3 Tap with finger tips on chest (sternum) at base of throat for thirty seconds.
4 Press at base of each big toe and rotate each toe.

SPLINTERS

Those little bits of wood that so easily slip under the skin seem like telegraph poles to some children, while to others they simply provide entertainment as they watch an adult struggle to remove the offending intruder.

Treatment

Splinters are traditionally removed with the tip of a needle, previously sterilised in the flame of a match, lighter, etc. Most children, however, are not impressed with the idea of being gouged with a needle. Soak the offending area in warm water for a few minutes. The splinter then comes out more easily, as the skin has been softened by the water. In addition, the child enjoys the involvement in fixing up the wound. If the splinter is glass or metal, and is not easily removed, take your child to a doctor.

If the splinter does not come out, you can use Tea-Tree oil to 'draw' it, combining with the body's natural methods of eliminating foreign bodies.

Herbal Remedies

Soak affected limb in warm soapy water for fifteen to thirty minutes. Then apply a drawing poultice of Slippery Elm bark, Marshmallow or Linseed.

Slippery Elm

Poultice: use 3-5 teaspoons of dried Slippery Elm powder. Gradually stir in hot water until a thick paste forms. Apply warm to affected area, cover with cling wrap and leave for ½-1 hour. Repeat if necessary.

Marshmallow

Poultice: place 2-4 teaspoons of powdered or finely chopped Marshmallow root in a bowl, gradually add hot water while stirring until a thick paste forms. Apply the poultice while still warm, cover with cling wrap and leave for ½-1 hour. Repeat if necessary.

Linseed

Poultice: use 3-5 teaspoons of ground Linseed. Gradually stir in hot water until a thick paste forms. Apply warm to affected area, cover with cling wrap and leave for ½-1 hour. Repeat if necessary.

If it is not possible to apply any of the above poultices, ointment of Marshmallow or Slippery Elm can be used instead.

STOMACH-ACHE

There can be countless reasons for a 'tummy ache'; anything from nervousness about school to worrying about something in the future. Like fevers, stomach-aches are particularly common in childhood and parents often take their children to the doctor only to find out that it really wasn't warranted in the first place. Many children complain about a tummy ache when actually the pain is somewhere else like lower down in the intestinal area. You will most likely discover with some careful detective work that the cause of discomfort was the result of eating too much or too fast; it can be the beginning of another ailment that may show up later on; perhaps emotional or psychological causes; sometimes a tummy ache shows up at the same time as leaving for school; or perhaps part of a set of symptoms caused by an allergic reaction to medication, food, chemical additives or environmental factors such as pollution.

Allergies and Stomach-aches

In this day and age, stomach-aches are frequently caused by food intolerances, cow's milk being one of the most common. See the section on Allergies to assist you in determining what foods there may be a sensitivity to.

If your child displays a number of symptoms in addition to pain, such a diarrhoea or blood in the stools or if the pain persists for longer than 3-4 hours, take your child to a medical practitioner immediately.

Herbal Remedies

When the stomach-ache is the result of anxiety or nervousness:

Chamomile

Infusion: use 1 teaspoon dried flowerheads to 1 cup of boiling water. Let steep for 5 minutes, strain. Can be sweetened with honey or rice malt. Dilute with water for smaller children.

DOSE
1-2 years: 20-40 mL (²/₃-1¹/₃ fl oz) 3 to 4 times daily
3-4 years: 50-80 mL (1²/₃-2²/₃ fl oz) 3 to 4 times daily
5-6 years: 100-125 mL (3-4 fl oz) 3 to 4 times daily
7 years and older: 150-200 mL (5-7 fl oz) 3 to 4 times daily

Scullcap

Infusion: use ½-1 teaspoon of the dried herb to 1 cup of boiling water. Let steep for 5-10 minutes, strain. Sweeten with honey or rice malt. This herb has an unpleasant bitter taste and should be mixed with a suitable pleasant-tasting herb such as Fennel seed, Aniseed or Licorice root.

DOSE
1-2 years: 15-30 mL (½-1 fl oz) 3 times daily
3-4 years: 40-60 mL (1¹/₃-2 fl oz) 3 times daily
5-6 years: 70-90 mL (2¹/₃-3 fl oz) 3 times daily
7 years and older: 100-150 mL (3-5 fl oz) 3 times daily

Linden (Lime flowers)

Infusion: Use 1-1½ teaspoons of dried herb to 1 cup of boiling water. Let steep for 5 minutes, strain. Can be sweetened with honey or rice malt. Dilute with water if necessary.

DOSE
1-2 years: 15-30 mL (½-1 fl oz) 3 times daily
3-4 years: 40-60 mL (1¹/₃-2 fl oz) 3 times daily
5-6 years: 70-90 mL (2¹/₃-3 fl oz) 3 times daily
7 years and older: 100-150 mL (3-5 fl oz) 3 times daily

Vervain

Infusion: use 1-1½ teaspoons of dried herb to 1 cup of boiling water. Let steep for 5 minutes, strain. Can be sweetened with honey or rice malt. Dilute with water if necessary.

DOSE
1-2 years: 15-30 mL (½-1 fl oz) 3 times daily

3-4 years: 40-60 mL (1⅓-2 fl oz) 3 times daily
5-6 years: 70-90 mL (2⅓-3 fl oz) 3 times daily
7 years and older: 100-150 mL (3-5 fl oz) 3 times daily

Lemon Balm

Infusion: use 1-1½ teaspoons of dried herb to 1 cup of boiling water. Let steep for 5 minutes, strain. Can be sweetened with honey or rice malt. Dilute with water if necessary.
DOSE
1-2 years: 15-30 mL (½-1 fl oz) 3 times daily
3-4 years: 40-60 mL (1⅓-2 fl oz) 3 times daily
5-6 years: 70-90 mL (2⅓-3 fl oz) 3 times daily
7 years and older: 100-150 mL (3-5 fl oz) 3 times daily

Valerian

Decoction: use 1 teaspoon of chopped roots and rhizome to 1 cup of water, simmer covered for 5-10 minutes, strain. Can be sweetened with honey or rice malt. Dilute with water if necessary.
DOSE
1-2 years: 15-30 mL (½-1 fl oz) 3 times daily
3-4 years: 40-60 mL (1⅓-2 fl oz) 3 times daily
5-6 years: 70-90 mL (2⅓-3 fl oz) 3 times daily
7 years and older: 100-150 mL (3-5 fl oz) 3 times daily

NOTE: On rare occasions, Valerian may have a stimulating rather than a calming effect. If this happens, discontinue the use of this herb.

Catmint

Infusion: Use 1 teaspoon of dried herb to 1 cup of boiling water. Let steep for 5 minutes, strain. Can be sweetened with honey or rice malt. Dilute with water if necessary.
DOSE
1-2 years: 15-30 mL (½-1 fl oz) 3 times daily
3-4 years: 40-60 mL (1⅓-2 fl oz) 3 times daily
5-6 years: 70-90 mL (2⅓-3 fl oz) 3 times daily
7 years and older: 100-150 mL (3-5 fl oz) 3 times daily

When the stomach-ache is caused by wind:

Peppermint

Infusion: use ½-1 teaspoon of dried herb to 1 cup of boiling water. Let steep for 5 minutes, strain. Can be sweetened with honey or rice malt. Dilute with water if necessary.
DOSE
1-2 years: 15-30 mL (½-1 fl oz) 3 times daily

3-4 years: 40-60 mL (1⅓-2 fl oz) 3 times daily
5-6 years: 70-90 mL (2⅓-3 fl oz) 3 times daily
7 years and older: 100-150 mL (3-5 fl oz) 3 times daily

Chamomile

Infusion: use 1 teaspoon dried flowerheads to 1 cup of boiling water. Let steep for 5 minutes, strain. Can be sweetened with honey or rice malt. Dilute with water for smaller children.
DOSE
1-2 years: 20-40 mL (⅔-1⅓ fl oz) 3 to 4 times daily
3-4 years: 50-80 mL (1⅔-2⅔ fl oz) 3 to 4 times daily
5-6 years: 100-125 mL (3-4 fl oz) 3 to 4 times daily
7 years and older: 150-200 mL (5-7 fl oz) 3 to 4 times daily

Ginger

Infusion: use 3 slices (2-3 cm/1 inch in diameter and 3 mm/⅛ inch thick) of fresh Ginger to 1 cup of boiling water. Let steep for 5 minutes. Sweeten with honey or rice malt. Dilute with water for small children.
DOSE
2-3 years: 20 mL (⅔ fl oz) 2 to 3 times daily
4-5 years: 30-50 mL (1-1⅔ fl oz) 2 to 3 times daily
6 years and older: 60-80 mL (2-2⅔ fl oz) 2 to 3 times daily

Dill

Infusion: use ½-1 teaspoon of the dried seeds (best lightly crushed in a mortar) to 1 cup of boiling water. Let steep for 5 minutes, strain. Can be sweetened with honey or rice malt. Dilute with water if necessary.
DOSE
1-2 years: 15-30 mL (½-1 fl oz) 3 times daily
3-4 years: 40-60 mL (1⅓-2 fl oz) 3 times daily
5-6 years: 70-90 mL (2⅓-3 fl oz) 3 times daily
7 years and older: 100-150 mL (3-5 fl oz) 3 times daily

Fennel

Infusion: use ½-1 teaspoon of the dried seeds (best lightly crushed in a mortar) to 1 cup of boiling water. Let steep for 5 minutes, strain. Can be sweetened with honey or rice malt. Dilute with water if necessary.
DOSE
1-2 years: 15-30 mL (½-1 fl oz) 3 times daily
3-4 years: 40-60 mL (1⅓-2 fl oz) 3 times daily

5-6 years: 70-90 mL (2⅓-3 fl oz) 3 times daily
7 years and older: 100-150 mL (3-5 fl oz) 3 times daily

Caraway

Infusion: use ½-1 teaspoon of the dried seeds (best lightly crushed in a mortar) to 1 cup of boiling water. Let steep for 5 minutes, strain. Can be sweetened with honey or rice malt. Dilute with water if necessary.

DOSE

1-2 years: 15-30 mL (½-1 fl oz) 3 times daily
3-4 years: 40-60 mL (1⅓-2 fl oz) 3 times daily
5-6 years: 70-90 mL (2⅓-3 fl oz) 3 times daily
7 years and older: 100-150 mL (3-5 fl oz) 3 times daily

Cumin

Infusion: use ½ teaspoon of the dried seeds (best lightly crushed in a mortar) to 1 cup of boiling water. Let steep for 5 minutes, strain. Can be sweetened with honey or rice malt. Dilute with water if necessary.

DOSE

1-2 years: 15-30 mL (½-1 fl oz) 3 times daily
3-4 years: 40-60 mL (1⅓-2 fl oz) 3 times daily
5-6 years: 70-90 mL (2⅓-3 fl oz) 3 times daily
7 years and older: 100-150 mL (3-5 fl oz) 3 times daily

Cinnamon

Infusion: use ½ teaspoon of the crushed, dried bark quills to 1 cup of boiling water. Let steep for 5 minutes, strain. Can be sweetened with honey or rice malt. Dilute with water if necessary.

DOSE

1-2 years: 15-30 mL (½-1 fl oz) 3 times daily
3-4 years: 40-60 mL (1⅓-2 fl oz) 3 times daily
5-6 years: 70-90 mL (2⅓-3 fl oz) 3 times daily
7 years and older: 100-150 mL (3-5 fl oz) 3 times daily

Aniseed

Infusion: use ½ teaspoon of whole or freshly crushed seeds to 1 cup of boiling water. Let steep for 5 minutes, strain.

DOSE

1-2 years: 15-30 mL (½-1 fl oz) 3 times daily
3-4 years: 40-60 mL (1⅓-2 fl oz) 3 times daily
5-6 years: 70-90 mL (2⅓-3 fl oz) 3 times daily
7 years and older: 100-150 mL (3-5 fl oz) 3 times daily

When stomach-ache is caused by poor digestion and constipation:

Golden Seal

Decoction: use ½ teaspoon of chopped root and rhizome to 1 cup of water, simmer covered for 5-10 minutes, strain. Can be sweetened with honey or rice malt. Dilute with water if necessary.

DOSE

2-3 years: 15-20 mL (½-⅔ fl oz) 3 times daily
4-5 years: 30-40 mL (1-1⅓ fl oz) 3 times daily
6-7 years: 50-60 mL (1⅔-2 fl oz) 3 times daily
8 years and older: 80-100 mL (2⅔-3 fl oz) 3 times daily

Fenugreek

Decoction: use 1 teaspoon of the crushed seeds to 1 cup of water. Simmer for 5 minutes, strain. Can be sweetened with honey or rice malt. Dilute with water if necessary.

DOSE

1-2 years: 15-30 mL (½-1 fl oz) 3 times daily
3-4 years: 40-60 mL (1⅓-2 fl oz) 3 times daily
5-6 years: 70-90 mL (2⅓-3 fl oz) 3 times daily
7 years and older: 100-150 mL (3-5 fl oz) 3 times daily

Peppermint

Infusion: use ½-1 teaspoon of dried herb to 1 cup of boiling water. Let steep for 5 minutes, strain. Can be sweetened with honey or rice malt. Dilute with water if necessary.

DOSE

1-2 years: 15-30 mL (½-1 fl oz) 3 times daily
3-4 years: 40-60 mL (1⅓-2 fl oz) 3 times daily
5-6 years: 70-90 mL (2⅓-3 fl oz) 3 times daily
7 years and older: 100-150 mL (3-5 fl oz) 3 times daily

Yarrow

Infusion: use 1 teaspoon of dried herb to 1 cup of boiling water. Let steep for 5 minutes, strain. Can be sweetened with honey or rice malt. Dilute with water if necessary.

DOSE

1-2 years: 15-30 mL (½-1 fl oz) 3 times daily
3-4 years: 40-60 mL (1⅓-2 fl oz) 3 times daily
5-6 years: 70-90 mL (2⅓-3 fl oz) 3 times daily
7 years and older: 100-150 mL (3-5 fl oz) 3 times daily

Dandelion Root

Decoction: use 1-2 teaspoons of chopped root to 1 cup of water, simmer covered for 5-10 minutes.

Can be sweetened with honey or rice malt. Dilute with water if necessary. Suitable for a digestive cause.

DOSE

1-2 years: 15-30 mL (½-1 fl oz) 3 times daily
3-4 years: 40-60 mL (1⅓-2 fl oz) 3 times daily
5-6 years: 70-90 mL (2⅓-3 fl oz) 3 times daily
7 years and older: 100-150 mL (3-5 fl oz) 3 times daily

Vervain

Infusion: use 1-1½ teaspoons of dried herb to 1 cup of boiling water. Let steep for 5 minutes, strain. Can be sweetened with honey or rice malt. Dilute with water if necessary.

DOSE

1-2 years: 15-30 mL (½-1 fl oz) 3 times daily
3-4 years: 40-60 mL (1⅓-2 fl oz) 3 times daily
5-6 years: 70-90 mL (2⅓-3 fl oz) 3 times daily
7 years and older: 100-150 mL (3-5 fl oz) 3 times daily

When stomach-ache is caused by indigestion with diarrhoea:

Chamomile

Infusion: use 1 teaspoon dried flowerheads to 1 cup of boiling water. Let steep for 5 minutes, strain. Can be sweetened with honey or rice malt. Dilute with water for smaller children.

DOSE

1-2 years: 20-40 mL (⅔-1⅓ fl oz) 3 to 4 times daily
3-4 years: 50-80 mL (1⅔-2⅔ fl oz) 3 to 4 times daily
5-6 years: 100-125 mL (3-4 fl oz) 3 to 4 times daily
7 years and older: 150-200 mL (5-6⅔ fl oz) 3 to 4 times daily

Marshmallow

Decoction: use 1-1½ teaspoons of chopped root to 1 cup of water, simmer covered for 5-10 minutes.
Infusion: use 2 teaspoons of dried leaf to 1 cup of boiling water, let steep for 10 minutes. Can be diluted with water.

DOSE

½-1 year: 15-30 mL (½-1 fl oz) 3 times daily
2-3 years: 40-50 mL (1⅓-1⅔ fl oz) 3 times daily
4-5 years: 60-80 mL (2-2⅔ fl oz) 3 times daily
6 years and older: 80-120 mL (2⅔-4 fl oz) 3 times daily

Slippery Elm bark

Use 2-3 teaspoons of powdered bark to ½ cup of hot water; this will form a paste that can be sweetened with honey or rice malt or mixed with fruit, porridge, etc.

DOSE

½-1 year: 2-4 teaspoons of the paste 3 times daily
2-3 years: 2-3 tablespoons of the paste 3 times daily
4-6 years: 4-6 tablespoons of the paste 3 times daily
7 years and older: 6-8 tablespoons of the paste 3 times daily

NOTE: Do not give the dried powder internally!

Calendula (Marigold)

Infusion: use 2 teaspoons of the dried flowerheads to 1 cup of boiling water. Let steep for 5 minutes, strain. Can be sweetened with honey or rice malt. Dilute with water if necessary.

DOSE

1-2 years: 15-30 mL (½-1 fl oz) 3 times daily
3-4 years: 40-60 mL (1⅓-2 fl oz) 3 times daily
5-6 years: 70-90 mL (2⅓-3 fl oz) 3 times daily
7 years and older: 100-150 mL (3-5 fl oz) 3 times daily

Cinnamon

Infusion: use ½ teaspoon of the crushed, dried bark quills to 1 cup of boiling water. Let steep for 5 minutes, strain. Can be sweetened with honey or rice malt. Dilute with water if necessary.

DOSE

1-2 years: 15-30 mL (½-1 fl oz) 3 times daily
3-4 years: 40-60 mL (1⅓-2 fl oz) 3 times daily
5-6 years: 70-90 mL (2⅓-3 fl oz) 3 times daily
7 years and older: 100-150 mL (3-5 fl oz) 3 times daily

Agrimony

Infusion: use 2 teaspoons of dried herb to 1 cup of boiling water. Let steep for 5-10 minutes, strain. Can be sweetened with honey or rice malt. Dilute with water if necessary.

DOSE

1-2 years: 15-30 mL (½-1 fl oz) 3 to 4 times daily
3-4 years: 40-60 mL (1⅓-2 fl oz) 3 to 4 times daily
5-6 years: 70-90 mL (2⅓-3 fl oz) 3 to 4 times daily
7 years and older: 100-150 mL (3-5 fl oz) 3 to 4 times daily

Meadowsweet

Infusion: use 1½-2 teaspoons of dried herb to 1 cup of boiling water. Let steep for 5 minutes, strain. Can be sweetened with honey or rice malt. Dilute with water if necessary.

DOSE

1-2 years: 15-30 mL (½-1 fl oz) 3 times daily
3-4 years: 40-60 mL (1⅓-2 fl oz) 3 times daily
5-6 years: 70-90 mL (2⅓-3 fl oz) 3 times daily
7 years and older: 100-150 mL (3-5 fl oz) 3 times daily

Homoeopathic Remedies

For stomach-ache, see Colic and Nausea.

Chinese Remedies

1 'Cold'

Sudden onset of pain. Aggravated by pressure or touch and eating. May also have nausea and vomiting. Limbs are cold. Likes warmth. May have fever. Complexion is darker than normal. Fingernails are red. Red vein at 'San Guan'. Loose stools. Urine is pale and copious. May have a runny nose with clear watery mucus.

LIANG FU WAN
XIANG SU SAN (if child also has a cold)
QIAN SHI BAI ZHU TANG (if also diarrhoea)
LING GUI ZHU GAN TANG (body is cold, pain relieved by warmth, no fever, tongue is pale, clear watery vomit, pale or white complexion)

2 'Deficiency'

Pain is dull and continuous. Relieved by pressure or touch and warmth. Eating causes discomfort. No appetite. Abdomen is cold and distended. Loose stools. Tiredness especially after eating. Tongue is pale and swollen with scalloped edges (i.e. tooth marks). Pale or yellowish complexion. Pale lips. Hair may be brittle with split ends. Eyes are dull. Speaks little. May sleep with eyes slightly open. May have a blue vein or bluish tint between the eyebrows. There may be a yellowish hue in the area between the eyelids and eyebrows and also the whites of the eyes.

XIANG SHA LIU JUN ZI TANG
HUANG QI JIAN ZHONG TANG (with cold hands and feet)

3 'Heat'

Strong colicky pain. Abdomen may appear or feel swollen. Pain aggravated by warmth, pressure or touch. Prefers cold food and drinks. Prefers light clothing or coverings. Red complexion. Red lips and tip of nose. Purple finger nails. Purple vein at 'San Guan'. May grind teeth when sleeping. Thirst. Constipation. Dark and scanty urine. Bad breath. May have sores in mouth and gums or bleeding gums. Tongue is redder than normal and there may be a crack down the middle. Tongue coating is thick and yellow. Pulse is more rapid than normal.

HUANG LIAN JIE DU TANG

4 'Phlegm' — 'Damp' Accumulation

Abdomen feels and appears swollen. Pain aggravated by pressure or touch and eating. Loss of appetite. Head and body feel heavy. Coughing or vomiting frothy mucus. Tiredness and depression. Complexion is yellowish. Sclera may also have a yellow hue. Loose stools. Tongue coat is thick and appears greasy.

BAN XIA XIE XIN TANG

5 'Food Retention'

Pain is persistent and colicky, and aggravated by pressure or touch and eating. Abdomen feels and may also look full and swollen. May also have belching (foul tasting and smelling) and vomiting. May be constipated at first, then foul smelling flatulence and diarrhoea which brings relief. Tongue has a thick coating and appears greasy. The area between the upper lip and nose may have a yellow or dark hue.

BAO HE WAN
REN SHEN JIAN PI WAN (weak constitution, chronic problem, chronic loose stools or diarrhoea, pale complexion, pale lips, dull eyes, pale tongue body, speaks little, poor appetite)

6 'Qi Stagnation'

Pain is spasmodic and changes location. Aggravated by pressure or touch and emotional upsets. Abdomen feels and may also appear to be full and swollen. Pain is temporarily relieved by belching and flatulence. Alternating constipation and diarrhoea. Tongue has a thin coating.

SI NI SAN (cold fingers and toes, rest of body warm, tongue red — not pale)
XIAO YAO SAN (pale complexion, pale lips, weakness, tiredness, tongue pale)
JIN LING ZI SAN (pain aggravated by hot food and drinks, tongue red)

Massage

There can be many reasons for a stomach-ache, from nervousness about school to worry about something in the future. If your child is old enough, while you give the massage have a chat with her about things that may be bothering her, which she may be having trouble verbalising. Place warm hot water bottle on child's tummy (comfortable to your wrist). Child may be more comfortable lying on one side or the other. Let her choose if she is able to.

1 Make thumb prints across the middle of each foot (centre line) and up to the base of the ball of the foot, work across the whole foot. Do this on both feet, making several passes.

2 Just below the ball of the foot in the soft instep on the left foot, press in with thumb or index finger. Toes should be relaxed or pulled towards the bottom of foot. Feel for any tight or tender spots and if you find one, hold and have the child take a breath then release it slowly.

SUNBURN

It is very important to protect young skins from the sun year-round. Hats all the time — for everybody — is the rule, plus sunscreens in summer. Make sure your child's hat provides protection for shoulders and back as well as heads and that the sunscreen is factor 15 sunblock. Babies younger than 12 months should not be exposed to direct sunlight for any length of time, especially in summer. Shield them with sunshades or umbrellas.

Most sunburn is first degree and quick action can help ease pain and avoid possible skin damage.

1 Immediate relief can be obtained by immersing the affected area in cold water for five minutes or so, or simply having a cool bath. Scattering a handful of oatmeal in the water is also soothing. Instead of immersion, you can just use a cool cloth, reapplying when it warms.
2 Apply Calamine lotion, Witch Hazel or Aloe Vera gel directly to the skin. Do not use oil substances such as baby oil, as these will seal in the heat.
3 Make sure the child drinks plenty of clear liquids.
4 Keep them totally out of the sun for a minimum of one week.

Home Remedies

- Add water to cornflour, arrowroot or bicarbonate of soda and make into a paste. Apply to burnt area. In about 10-15 minutes it will dry, crumble and fall off. Keep reapplying until heat disappears.
- Apply plain Acidophilus yoghurt directly to the burn.
- Use cucumber or potato slices to absorb the heat and to soothe.
- Apply Tea-Tree antiseptic cream for immediate relief; this helps prevent blistering. In severe cases apply pure Tea-Tree oil.
- Apply cool tea to burnt area.
- Apply a cooked potato poultice (see Appendix 7: Compresses, Poultices and Baths).

Herbal Remedies

Aloe Vera

Apply the fresh gel from the centre of a leaf to sunburn and other minor burns. If you don't grow an Aloe Vera plant you can buy products which are almost pure Aloe Vera gel in health food stores.

Marshmallow

Decoction: use 1-2 teaspoons of the dried, chopped root or 3 teaspoons of the dried leaf to 1 cup of water. Simmer 10 minutes covered, strain. Let cool down. Apply to affected area with a clean piece of cotton.

Potato flour

This has a cooling and soothing action and is excellent for sunburn.

Homoeopathic Treatment

Calendula cream is an excellent medicine for the quick and effective healing of sunburn. Causticum is useful as an internal medicine for the effect of severe sunburn.

CAUTION

Seek medical advice if the sunburn starts to blister and swell it is most probably a second degree burn and your doctor or hospital should be immediately consulted. Do not apply any lotions or peel the damaged skin.

SUNSTROKE/HEATSTROKE

Do not treat the body harshly by exposing it to undue ultra-violet rays for long periods of time as it is the fastest way to get sunstroke and skin cancer. Be aware of the danger that could occur if you don't take precautions with your children. Whenever you and your child go out in hot sun, use hats, sunblock and take plenty of liquids.

Sunstroke is not an uncommon condition, and young children are especially prone to it because their sweat glands are not fully developed. It is caused by the excessive loss of body fluids due to heat, which results in the rapid rise of body temperature. Due to the seriousness of this condition, take your child to the nearest medical practitioner or hospital immediately if sunstroke occurs.

Symptoms

- Thirst is likely to be the first symptom
- Loss of appetite
- General weakness
- Headache and ringing in the ears
- Dizziness

In severe cases other symptoms may include vomiting, diarrhoea, cramps, seizures, disorientation, and even unconsciousness.

Treatment

1 Call an ambulance or doctor.
2 Move the child into a cool spot.
3 Remove any restrictive or hot clothing.
4 Cool your child as quickly as possible. Splash with water, use a garden hose or immerse your child in a bath or pool. A helpful and effective method often used in the tropics is to cover your child with a wet sheet and direct a fan on to her. If your child is a small baby, place her in her crib and drape the cool sheets around her; then direct the fan onto her.
5 Give fluids.

Prevention

Like sunburn, prevention is the best cure for sunstroke. However, there are some ways to prevent this condition if you are in a situation where your child may be exposed to extreme heat.

1 Use a newspaper, magazine or something else to create a breeze.
2 Douse the child in cool water.
3 Have her drink many glasses of fluid.
4 Listen or watch the weather forecast before attempting an outing with small children. If the weather is going to be very hot, don't go.
5 Dress the children in light colours and avoid synthetic clothing.
6 Keep the body covered and wear a hat and apply sunblock.
7 Provide lots of cooling foods such as melons and salads as well as fruit-ices and juices.

SWOLLEN GLANDS

Symptoms

The main symptom is usually swelling itself, which can be anywhere from mild to extreme. Usually swollen glands or swollen lymph nodes, typically on the side of the throat or in the arm pits, indicate that the lymphatic system is dealing with intruding organisms, like an infection of some kind. Our bodies contain a wide variety of different glands which secrete anything from sweat to complex hormones that affect our basic emotions and daily functions. The swollen area may become red, sensitive to touch, painful upon swallowing, with accompanying fever. If the swelling persists for a few days there is very little cause for concern, but if the swelling persists for more than a few days, consult a qualified practitioner.

Causes

Most of the time the swelling that occurs is due to the fact that the body is trying to fight off an infection or illness in a nearby organ. Because the lymph glands produce white blood cells which are the body's first line of defence against invasion by foreign bodies, they often swell as a response to the job that they have to do to fight off these intruders.

Long-term swollen glands can also indicate a food allergy (see Allergies).

Home Remedies

- Apply a cold compress made with vinegar to ease the symptoms. (Add 250 mL/8 fl oz of vinegar to 2 cups of water.) Hold the compress in place with a scarf wrapped around the child's head.
- Prepare a sage leaf tea by steeping ½-1 teaspoon in a cup of boiling water. Cover and set aside for 5 minutes. Lemon rind may be added as well. Take ½ cup every 2-3 hours. Alternate with Echinacea tincture. (It may be sweetened with rice honey or barley malt.)

Herbal Remedies

Usually, swollen lymph nodes, typically on the sides of the throat or in the arm pits, indicate that the lymphatic system is dealing with intruding organisms, i.e. an infection. Swollen lymph nodes for only a few days is not cause for concern; however, if the swelling persists see a qualified practitioner.

Herbs like Calendula, Clivers and Fenugreek stimulate the lymphatic system.

Calendula (Marigold)

Infusion: use 2 teaspoons of the dried flowerheads to 1 cup of boiling water. Let steep for 5 minutes, strain. Can be sweetened with honey or rice malt. Dilute with water if necessary.

DOSE
1-2 years: 15-30 mL (½-1 fl oz) 3 times daily
3-4 years: 40-60 mL (1⅓-2 fl oz) 3 times daily
5-6 years: 70-90 mL (2⅓-3 fl oz) 3 times daily
7 years and older: 100-150 mL (3-5 fl oz) 3 times daily

Clivers (Cleavers)

Infusion: use 2 teaspoons of dried herb to 1 cup of boiling water. Let steep for 5 minutes, strain. Can be sweetened with honey or rice malt. Dilute with water if necessary.

DOSE
1-2 years: 15-30 mL (½-1 fl oz) 3 times daily
3-4 years: 40-60 mL (1⅓-2 fl oz) 3 times daily
5-6 years: 70-90 mL (2⅓-3 fl oz) 3 times daily
7 years and older: 100-150 mL (3-5 fl oz) 3 times daily

Fenugreek

Decoction: use 1 teaspoon of the crushed seeds to 1 cup of water. Simmer for 5 minutes, strain. Can be sweetened with honey or rice malt. Dilute with water if necessary.

DOSE
1-2 years: 15-30 mL (½-1 fl oz) 3 times daily
3-4 years: 40-60 mL (1⅓-2 fl oz) 3 times daily
5-6 years: 70-90 mL (2⅓-3 fl oz) 3 times daily

7 years and older: 100-150 mL (3-5 fl oz) 3 times daily

Homoeopathic Remedies

Where swollen glands are a chronic condition it should be referred to your homoeopathic practitioner.

Chinese Remedies

See Tonsillitis and Mumps

Massage

Swollen glands, see Sore Throat. Add:

1 Massage under each arm into the armpit and gently roll the swollen glands between your finger tips to soften and release. (Do not pinch.)
2 For swollen glands in the groin, push knee into chest and let leg fall open. These glands are located just inside and at the top of each leg. Do the same as above, massage in soft circles into the groin line and into the top of the leg.
3 Roll leg between both your hands as if you were rolling dough and gently shake the leg to loosen any tension being held there, too.

TEETHING

It is easy to assume that any and everything that occurs, whether it be a runny nose, slight irritability or sleeplessness can be due to teething. This may not be so. Teething is not a disease. Babies suffer from so many little ills that by the time you figure out what to do about one thing it has already been superseded by another!

When your baby's first teeth do finally decide to come in, it is a very individual process. On the average, the first teeth that begin to make an appearance at five or six months are the lower biting ones in front. If your baby is at least four or five months and doesn't have any teeth at all yet, and you are a concerned parent, give her some hard foods when she first starts to explore the world through her mouth, by putting anything and everything into it. Chewing food is great for the baby's jaw and the practice of feeding themselves with their own hands makes life easier later on.

Your baby's first tooth should look like a small bump and be visible under the gum for several days up to one or two weeks before it emerges. The back teeth (molars) will come through at about one to three years of age.

Symptoms

Included are: ear rubbing, loud bursts of crying for no apparent reason, clinging, slight fever, nasal discharge, dribbling from the mouth, green bowel movements, loose bowel movements, diarrhoea, insomnia, waking in the middle of the night, restlessness, irritability, red cheek or spot (looks like a pimple), will not settle easily to sleep, wakes frequently, not interested in food, wants more breast milk rather than food.

In oriental medicine the teeth, the stomach and digestive system are related so that when teething is happening digestion is hampered.

The best way to deal with teething problems is through the digestive system. Avoid too much fatty, rich food, spices and difficult to digest foods like heavy meats, raw vegetables, heavy breads and granola.

THINGS TO CHEW ON (WHEN SITTING UP ONLY)

Raw carrot or celery sticks, cucumber rings, raw apple rings, dried fruit, leather, teething rings, dolls' arms and legs, large chicken bones (cooked), hard crusts, rusks, smooth, large chop bones, peeled shallots, lemon wedges.

Home Remedies

Chamomile Tea

Combine 1 cup of boiling water with 1 teaspoon of dry Chamomile flowers or 1 tea bag in a cup. Strain and cool and sweeten it with rice honey or honey.

1 For babies
- Give 1-2 teaspoons every two hours.
- Soak a clean piece of muslin or cheesecloth in the tea. Cool in the fridge and give it to the baby to suck on.

2 For older children
- Give a cup to drink every two to three hours.

If you think that your child will tolerate a bandage try the following:

Place a teaspoon of Ground Cloves on the point described in the Massage section. Moisten it with a few drops of vinegar and cover with a bandage overnight. (This point is commonly used in acupuncture for gums and teething as an anaesthetic.)

Herbal Remedies

Both Chamomile and Catmint make excellent teething remedies.

Chamomile

Infusion: use 1 teaspoon dried flowerheads to 1 cup of boiling water. Let steep for 5 minutes, strain. Can be sweetened with honey or rice malt. Dilute with water for smaller children.

DOSE

1-2 years: 20-40 mL ($^2/_3$-$1^1/_3$ fl oz) 3 to 4 times daily

3-4 years: 50-80 mL (1²/₃-2²/₃ fl oz) 3 to 4 times daily
5-6 years: 100-125 mL (3-4 fl oz) 3 to 4 times daily
7 years and older: 150-200 mL (5-7 fl oz) 3 to 4 times daily

Catmint

Infusion: use 1 teaspoon of dried herb to 1 cup of boiling water. Let steep for 5 minutes, strain. Can be sweetened with honey or rice malt. Dilute with water if necessary.

DOSE

1-2 years: 15-30 mL (½-1 fl oz) 3 times daily
3-4 years: 40-60 mL (1¹/₃-2 fl oz) 3 times daily
5-6 years: 70-90 mL (2¹/₃-3 fl oz) 3 times daily
7 years and older: 100-150 mL (3-5 fl oz) 3 times daily

Homoeopathic Remedies

Chamomilla 30C is an excellent remedy for teething children, especially where they are in constant pain which expresses itself in great irritability, rage and restlessness. The child will often want to be carried.

One dose should be administered twice daily for up to three days.

Calcarea phos 6C (available as a tissue salt) is a useful medicine for slow teething and may be given in the tissue salt form three times daily for up to seven days.

Rheum 12C is very useful where the child is restless, irritable and has a sour odour during teething. A sour smelling diarrhoea in teething also indicates Rheum. The dose is twice daily for up to 3 days.

Massage

Locate a point on your child's hand by opening up the fingers and placing the thumb so that it lies parallel to the hand. The point is located on the back of the hand just next to the lower end of the crease where the thumb joins the hand.

Feel on your own hand for the spot that feels most sensitive, then try to find it on your child. Gently massage it with the tip of your finger vibrating it one to three minutes on each hand. (Do one hand at a time.)

While carrying or holding your baby:

1 Press at the base of all toes with tiny thumb prints, on the top and bottom of both feet. Also press softly below the toenails on each foot.
2 Rotate each toe on each foot.
3 Press thumb into the centre of the upper lip just below the nose. Hold with firm but gentle pressure. Do this in a playful way (with what could be a very fussy baby) using a cool wash cloth.
4 Place your fingertips on either side of nose and press down following along the cheekbones to the jaw joint (just beside and at base of ear). Make small circles with fingertips to soften tender spots.
5 Again make a game of massaging with small circles along jaw.
6 You can also massage inside your child's mouth on the gums, with your fingers, letting the baby bite down (assuming she doesn't have teeth yet) on your fingers. You can also use a cool wash cloth inside the mouth, pressing along the gums. Baby can bite down on this.
7 Hold hands on either side of face over jaws, directing calm energy between your hands into the child's gums.

THRUSH

Thrush is one of those nasty baby illnesses that are quite common. Though it has no dangerous side effects, it can still cause your child a certain amount of discomfort and is likely to occur again, once your baby has had it.

It is a mild fungus infection caused by a yeast-like organism. There are two types, monilia and candida.

Symptoms

Oral thrush is characterised by thick white 'clouds' or little spots in the mouth, on the insides of the cheeks and coating the tongue. Your child may have a milk coating on the tongue, but oral thrush is thicker and is difficult to scrape off. If you do rub it off, the underlying skin will bleed slightly and look inflamed.

It can make the mouth sore and will cause discomfort for the baby when feeding as well as general irritability.

Oral thrush can go through the gastrointestinal tract, coming out at the anus and infecting the nappy area. This can be distinguished from normal nappy rash as it has sharply demarcated borders with red pimple-like spots and inflamed skin. An easy way of recognising it is that it looks as if the baby has been burnt.

Causes

1 Can be caught from the mother during vaginal delivery. It then lies dormant in the baby for some time, finally appearing in the mouth.
2 Can be caused by antibiotics due to the removal of natural bacteria in the system.
3 May be caused by an excess amount of phlegm in the body, which encourages fungal growth.

Prevention

1 Check sterilisation if bottle feeding.
2 Mother should ensure that she does not have any vaginal thrush. This is characterised by excessive whitish vaginal discharge accompanied by irritation and soreness.
3 Give a small amount of cooled boiled water to the child after a feed. This washes out the milk and gives thrush fungus less to live on.

Home Remedies

1 Coat the inside of the baby's mouth with plain yoghurt (preferably goat's milk) after each feed. Dip your finger in the yoghurt and offer it to be sucked. Wash your finger afterward. Or paint the mouth with a cotton bud dipped in yoghurt. Or freeze small cubes of yoghurt and give them to the baby to suck. You will need to coat your nipples in yoghurt, too, if you are breast feeding. You must take care not to contaminate your yoghurt pot.
2 Dissolve 1 level teaspoon of baking soda in a cup of water. Take a cotton bud, and wipe the baby's cheeks, gums and tongue every time you nurse. You may prepare the solution fresh every day, and stir it up before using. It helps to bathe your nipples, after nursing, in a solution made from 4 teaspoons vinegar in a cup of water.
3 Normalise the bowel flora with Lactobacillus, Acidophilus or Bifidus, available in health food shops or from your naturopath.
DOSE
0-2 years: ¼ teaspoon twice daily
2-5 years: ½ teaspoon twice daily
5-7 years: ½ teaspoon twice daily
Over 7 years: ½-¾ teaspoon twice daily

Herbal Remedies

Mouth washes with one or more of the following herbs:

Calendula (Marigold)

Infusion: use 3-4 teaspoons of dried flowers to 1 cup of water. Let steep for 10 minutes, strain. Do not sweeten or dilute.

Echinacea

Decoction: use 1 teaspoon of dried root and rhizome to 1 cup of water, simmer covered for 5-10 minutes. Do not sweeten or dilute.

Golden Seal

Gargle and/or mouthwash: prepare as a decoction, using ½-1 teaspoon of dried roots and rhizome to 1 cup of water. Simmer covered for 10 minutes, strain. Do not sweeten or dilute.

Thyme

Infusion: use 1-2 teaspoons of dried herb to 1 cup of boiling water. Let steep for 5 minutes, strain. Do not sweeten or dilute.

Tincture of Myrrh or Propolis (if available)

Put 10 drops of the tincture in a little water and use as a mouthwash.

Homoeopathic Remedy

Oral thrush may be treated by prescribing **Sulphuric acid** 6C three times daily for up to three days.

Where this is a chronic condition it should be referred to your homoeopathic practitioner.

Chinese Remedies

1 'Excess'

Red complexion. Restlessness. Dry stool. Urine is dark and reduced in quantity. Purple vein at 'San Guan'. Fingernails are purple.

SAN HUANG XIE XIN TANG

2 'Deficiency'

Pale complexion with flushing in the malar region. Dry lips. No thirst. Emaciation. Diarrhoea. Urine is pale.

QIAN SHI BAI ZHU TANG

TONSILLITIS

Even though some doctors may try to convince you that removing your child's tonsils is the best way to go if they become infected too often, you would be wise to seek a second opinion. The tonsils are actually the way that your child's body fights and filters infections. It would be a rare case if tonsillitis was the signal to remove the tonsils. The tonsils intercept bacteria that enter the throat.

For years swollen or inflamed tonsils or even healthy ones have been the victims of unnecessary surgery. Now the evidence is pointing in the opposite direction. Hold on to them for as long as possible! They are part of the lymphatic system, which plays a large role in the body's defence against invading organisms. The adenoids and the tonsils are lymphoid tissues, which are the primary site of the body's immunologic activity against disease and are involved in fighting illness in the development of antibodies. So don't remove your child's first line of defence!

Symptoms

The tonsils become red, inflamed, swollen and painful rather suddenly. Your child may be having trouble swallowing and there may be a fever, cough or running nose with it too.

When the condition is chronic your child will get tonsillitis every week or two. She may feel that they are swollen all of the time, but they will rarely be painful in between bouts. She won't have much of an appetite and will complain of tiredness most of the time. If her swallowing is impaired, seek advice from a qualified practitioner.

Causes

When the immune system is weak, bacterial or viral infection sets in. Acute tonsillitis can be the result. Especially in the springtime these kinds of infections are more common. Perhaps the change in the weather is to blame, but

whatever the circumstances, the ears, eyes, nose and throat are usually infected as well.

Because tonsillitis affects the area of the throat which children use for speech and for the expression of their feelings and inner-most thoughts (hopefully), in chronic cases there may be some underlying cause such as the inability to express themselves vocally or verbally. If anger is not expressed and bottled up, very often problems in the throat area are likely to arise.

There are different reasons why your child gets tonsillitis:

1 Your child may find it difficult to fight off infections because her state of health is not strong enough.

2 Your child may be having recurrent bouts because of some inability to express herself emotionally. In this case you should try working with her to express herself as much as possible.

Herbal Remedies

Gargle with one or more of the following herbs (4 years and over):

Calendula (Marigold)

Infusion: use 3-4 teaspoons of dried flowers to 1 cup of water. Let steep for 10 minutes, strain. Do not sweeten or dilute.

Echinacea

Decoction: use 1 teaspoon of dried root and rhizome to 1 cup of water, simmer covered for 5-10 minutes. Do not sweeten or dilute.

Golden Seal

Gargle and/or mouthwash: prepare as a decoction, using ½-1 teaspoon of dried roots and rhizome to 1 cup of water. Simmer covered for 10 minutes, strain. Do not sweeten or dilute.

Sage

Gargle and/or mouthwash: prepare as an infusion using 1-2 teaspoons of dried herb or

5-6 teaspoons of chopped, fresh leaf to 1 cup of boiling water. Let steep for 10 minutes, strain. Do not sweeten or dilute.

Thyme

Infusion: use 1-2 teaspoons of dried herb to 1 cup of boiling water. Let steep for 5 minutes, strain. Do not sweeten or dilute.

Tincture of Myrrh or Propolis (if available)

Put 10 drops of the tincture in a little water and use as a gargle.

ALSO GIVE ONE OR MORE OF THE FOLLOWING HERBS INTERNALLY:

Echinacea

Echinacea stimulates the immune system. The use of the herb increases the chances that the infection will be dealt with quickly and effectively and reduces the risk of a chronic infection taking hold.

Decoction: use 1 teaspoon of dried root and rhizome to 1 cup of water, simmer covered for 5 minutes. Dilute with water if necessary. Can be sweetened with honey or rice malt.

DOSE
1-2 years: 10-15 mL (1/3-1/2 fl oz) 3 times daily
3-4 years: 20-30 mL (2/3-1 fl oz) 3 times daily
5-6 years: 40-50 mL (1 1/3-1 2/3 fl oz) 3 times daily
7 years and older: 60-100 mL (2-3 fl oz) 3 times daily

Calendula (Marigold)

Calendula is one of the best lymphatic agents. It is strongly indicated in tonsillitis.

Infusion: use 2 teaspoons of the dried flower-heads to 1 cup of boiling water. Let steep for 5 minutes, strain. Can be sweetened with honey or rice malt. Dilute with water if necessary.

DOSE
1-2 years: 15-30 mL (1/2-1 fl oz) 3 times daily
3-4 years: 40-60 mL (1 1/3-2 fl oz) 3 times daily
5-6 years: 70-90 mL (2 1/3-3 fl oz) 3 times daily
7 years and older: 100-150 mL (3-5 fl oz) 3 times daily

Clivers (Cleavers)

Clivers is another herb with specific action on the lymphatic system.

Infusion: use 2 teaspoons of dried herb to 1 cup of boiling water. Let steep for 5 minutes, strain.

Can be sweetened with honey or rice malt. Dilute with water if necessary.

DOSE
1-2 years: 15-30 mL (1/2-1 fl oz) 3 times daily
3-4 years: 40-60 mL (1 1/3-2 fl oz) 3 times daily
5-6 years: 70-90 mL (2 1/3-3 fl oz) 3 times daily
7 years and older: 100-150 mL (3-5 fl oz) 3 times daily

Homoeopathic Remedies

Apis mellifica 12C is useful where there is burning and stinging pain, redness and swelling of the tonsils. There may be a desire for cool things.

Baryta carb 12C is often indicated for chronically enlarged tonsils and the tendency for them to become inflamed when exposed to cold.

Use **Belladonna** 30C where the tonsils are red, swallowing is painful and the pain spreads to the ear. The child is usually thirsty for cold water in this situation. It may be associated with fever and flushing of the skin.

Hepar sulph 12C is most use for suppurating tonsils with sticking or splinter pains (as if a needle is passing through them). The pain often extends to the ear and cold air aggravates.

Mercurius 12C is required when the tonsils are suppurating (forming or discharging pus). The tongue is often swollen with scalloped edges from the imprint of the teeth. Salivation and sweat along with the thirst may be increased.

Dose: A dose three times daily for up to three days.

Chinese Remedies

1 Acute Tonsillitis

See Colds and Flu and Coughs for symptom pictures and treatments.

2 Chronic Tonsillitis

Frequently recurring tonsillitis is due to insufficient 'defensive energy' (i.e. lowered resistance), which is often due to a weakened digestive system.

XIAO CHAI HU TANG (to be taken for three to six months as a tonic)

Massage

See also Sore Throat and Swollen Glands. Use a small amount of oil (about the size of a five cent piece) warmed by rubbing your hands together briskly.

1 Massage in long firm downward strokes from base of ear along side of throat to base of neck.
2 Rotate big toe of each foot and press into the base of the big toe at the bottom of foot using your thumb or index finger
3 Press into the ball of the foot under the big toe and hold any tight or tender spots until they release or soften. Do this on both feet.
4 Press along the bottom of each foot at the base of each toe, again feeling for areas of sensitivity or tenderness. Hold for ten to thirty seconds. Circle and pull each toe lightly outward.

See also Appendix 7 and Colds and Flu.

VOMITING

All babies will from time to time bring up some food from their stomachs, hopefully not on you! This is usually referred to as 'vomiting'. If they do it once or twice there is really very little to be concerned about, as it occurs when food in the stomach cannot get to the intestines along the digestive tract. What happens is that your baby's stomach contracts, and the food comes up instead of going down.

The frequency of vomiting in children is often related directly to age. Infants vomit or spit up for all sorts of reasons, very often because they are overfed or because they are suffering from wind. Toddlers very often vomit, when something is 'bothering' them, as a symptom of an illness or when they have upset tummies. Older children vomit when they have tummy upsets or gastrointestinal infections, or overeat. These types of problems can usually be treated at home. But when vomiting is persistent, when it seems to be getting worse, when it is accompanied by severe and progressive abdominal pain, seek medical attention immediately.

Vomiting is often accompanied by nausea and as these are only symptoms and are often related to what is happening in the rest of the digestive system, it is best to consider the whole of your child's digestive pattern and treat accordingly.

Some Common Causes

1 Bringing up milk after a feed. This is called posseting and there is no cause for concern as almost all babies do it. It can be an indication of a weak stomach.

2 Food allergy or milk intolerance may lead to vomiting.

3 When infection is the cause of vomiting it's more than likely to be the result of a cold or flu and rarely continues for longer than twenty-four hours in babies and young children. May be replaced by diarrhoea.

4 Gastroenteritis, which is a gut infection.

5 Undigested food which may be too rich. Child usually experiences nausea before, may be emotionally unstable and complain of pain in the abdominal area.

6 Emotional excitement, over-stimulation or nervousness.

7 Constipation.

8 Weak digestion. Your child's digestion may be weak due to a long sickness or from a birth trauma. In this case the symptoms are undigested food, loose stools containing a lot of undigested food, lack of appetite and weight gain, occasional constipation and tiredness. Give small amounts of easily digested foods, encourage plenty of fresh air and exercise and regular meals.

9 Mucus can often accumulate in the stomach and interfere with digestion. The following symptoms may present themselves: not feeling 'right' days or hours before vomiting, may come about after a bout with whooping cough or as a reaction to the immunisation for it, colour of complexion is grey or pale, vomit has mucus-like quality to it or is watery. Avoid all mucus-forming foods and seek advice from a practitioner of your choice.

10 Heat. Usually occurs in a hot climate with such symptoms as thirst, insomnia, violent vomiting directly after a meal, no other symptoms, large appetite, red complexion and hot. Seek a practitioner's assistance for this complaint.

11 Poisons or medications.

Causes in the newborn

Two causes of vomiting in the newborn are infection and mechanical obstruction. These require professional assessment. If the baby also seems to have some sucking and swallowing difficulties, or if the vomiting is projectile in nature, professional advice should be sought.

SOME OTHER DANGER SIGNS

Persistent vomiting, green vomit, drowsiness, failure to suck well, failure to gain weight or failure to demand feed, fever, abdominal distension, failure to pass meconium in the first twenty-four hours, visible peristalsis, bulging fontanelle.

Causes of vomiting in the older child

- The most common are infection. Conditions that affect the gastrointestinal tract like appendicitis or gastroenteritis may present with vomiting rather than diarrhoea. Any other infection, such as ear infection, may also have the child vomiting. Treatment in this case must include treatment of the underlying cause.
- Childhood migraine (as early as six months of age) is another cause of nausea and vomiting in the child who has recurrent bouts of vomiting without fever. Headache may or may not accompany this. Food allergy or intolerance often accompanies this condition and may be the cause. Naturopaths commonly treat the liver in this condition.
- Stress and anger.
- Children do have sensitive and reactive digestive systems, so they will react quickly to food that is too rich for them, also to food that is contaminated in some way. Vomiting in this case is a helpful defence of the body. Some children who have poor secretion of digestive juices or poor gastric motility may be helped by a simple wholesome diet with herbs to stimulate digestion.
- Food allergy also can cause vomiting as the body tries to rid itself of the substance to which it is allergic.

What to look for to assess the situation

1 Is undigested food being vomited?
2 Is there mucus and what colour is it?
3 When does the vomiting occur?
4 Is the child constipated?
5 Are the stools yellow, brown, green, hard, soft?
6 Are there any other accompanying symptoms (pain, nausea, fever, chills)?
7 What is the child's facial colour like?
8 Does the child seem emotionally unstable and volatile at the drop of a hat?
9 If you are breastfeeding, assess yourself as well.

Travel sickness

- One of the best treatments for travel sickness is Ginger root. Ginger may be taken grated with lemon, honey and warm water to help the digestion and treat the nausea.
- Some children respond to vitamin B6 supplementation for the prevention of travel sickness.
- Children with problems of mucus congestion of the sinus and middle ear may be particularly susceptible to travel sickness. These problems should be treated for a better control of the situation.

See also Motion Sickness.

Home Remedies

Very often nausea is part and parcel of the process and so getting rid of the nausea is often helpful. If the child is old enough, get her to suck on a hard pit from dried fruit or a sweet lolly for thirty minutes or so. Best not to chew it. This can be followed up with sucking chipped ice and then progressively moving to clear liquids such as apple juice, weak tea, broth, or jellies (1 teaspoon every 10 minutes). If she keeps it down, try to increase the doses to a tablespoon every twenty minutes to 2 tablespoons every thirty minutes. This should stop the vomiting; if it does not, consult a medical practitioner. Increasing to readily digested foods such as cereals, soups, custards, puddings, soft-boiled eggs and pureed foods is the best way to reintroduce foods.

CAUTION

Seek medical attention if any of the following signs appear:

- **Vomiting is continuous for twenty-four hours or longer.**
- **Child becomes dehydrated.**
- **Pain in the lower right-hand side of the abdomen occurs.**
- **Temperature climbs above 40°C (104°F).**
- **Weight loss due to long term vomiting.**

Herbal Remedies

Dandelion root

Dandelion root stimulates the digestive functions and, in particular, the liver. If vomiting is caused by digestive deficiency, especially lack of bile, this herb is indicated.

Decoction: use 1-2 teaspoons of chopped root to 1 cup of water, simmer covered for 5-10 minutes. Can be sweetened with honey or rice malt. Dilute with water if necessary.

DOSE

1-2 years: 15-30 mL (½-1 fl oz) 3 times daily
3-4 years: 40-60 mL (1⅓-2 fl oz) 3 times daily
5-6 years: 70-90 mL (2⅓-3 fl oz) 3 times daily
7 years and older: 100-150 mL (3-5 fl oz) 3 times daily

Peppermint

Peppermint has a calming effect on the stomach but also prompts the gall bladder to secrete more bile. It is indicated when fatty foods cause vomiting.
Infusion: use ½-1 teaspoon of dried herb to 1 cup of boiling water. Let steep for 5 minutes, strain. Can be sweetened with honey or rice malt. Dilute with water if necessary.

DOSE

1-2 years: 15-30 mL (½-1 fl oz) 3 times daily
3-4 years: 40-60 mL (1⅓-2 fl oz) 3 times daily
5-6 years: 70-90 mL (2⅓-3 fl oz) 3 times daily
7 years and older: 100-150 mL (3-5 fl oz) 3 times daily

A few drops of pure Peppermint oil also may be dropped onto a spoonful of honey and taken directly.

Chamomile

This herb has a relaxing and soothing effect on the stomach. It is suitable if vomiting is caused by nervous tension, stress or acute stomach upset (gastritis).
Infusion: use 1 teaspoon dried flowerheads to 1 cup of boiling water. Let steep for 5 minutes, strain. Can be sweetened with honey or rice malt. Dilute with water for smaller children.

DOSE

1-2 years: 20-40 mL (⅔-1⅓ fl oz) 3 to 4 times daily
3-4 years: 50-80 mL (1⅔-2⅔ fl oz) 3 to 4 times daily
5-6 years: 100-125 mL (3-4 fl oz) 3 to 4 times daily
7 years and older: 150-200 mL (5-7 fl oz) 3 to 4 times daily

Fennel

Fennel has a calming and settling effect on the digestive tract.
Infusion: use ½-1 teaspoon of the dried seeds (best lightly crushed in a mortar) to 1 cup of boiling water. Let steep for 5 minutes, strain. Can be sweetened with honey or rice malt. Dilute with water if necessary.

DOSE

1-2 years: 15-30 mL (½-1 fl oz) 3 times daily
3-4 years: 40-60 mL (1⅓-2 fl oz) 3 times daily
5-6 years: 70-90 mL (2⅓-3 fl oz) 3 times daily
7 years and older: 100-150 mL (3-5 fl oz) 3 times daily

Homoeopathic Remedies

Where there is vomiting of milk in curds after breastfeeding **Antimonium crudum** 12C is indicated. It is also useful for vomiting after over-eating; exposure to heat and cold bathing.

Arsenicum album 12C may be used where vomiting is followed by great exhaustion. This may be accompanied by restlessness. It is often beneficial after food poisoning.

Where there is constant nausea with vomiting, pale face and a clean tongue **Ipecac** 12C is your medicine. It is the remedy of choice where the vomiting is brought on by over-indulgence in food.

Nux vomica 30C is indicated for the constant desire to vomit but efforts to do so only resulting in retching. Nausea mostly comes on in the morning. It is indicated where there has been over-indulgence in rich food or stimulants.

Veratrum album 30C is effective when there is violent vomiting and nausea aggravated by drinking and the least motion.

Other remedies including Aconite, Phosphorus and Pulsatilla (see section on description of medicines) may be used where the character of the symptoms and the temperament of the child are indicated.
Dose: Every half-hour when the vomiting is severe. Otherwise to be taken every two hours for up to one day and stop on marked improvement.

Chinese Remedies

1 Milk Retention in the Stomach

Vomiting of milk. Body is hot. Complexion is yellow. The skin is puffy. The pulse is rapid.
FU LING ZE XIE TANG

2 'Cold'

Due to over-eating cold or raw foods or too many foods with 'atmospheric energy'. Cold hands and feet. Pale lips and tongue. The vomited material is usually odourless and may contain undigested food from the previous meal. The pulse tends to be slow. The vein at 'San Guan' is red.

LING GUI ZHU GAN TANG

3 'Heat'

Due to over-eating foods with a hot 'atmospheric energy', such as oily, fatty or deep-fried food. The lips are red. The urine is dark and may have a red tint. The vomitus smells sour and appears watery. The body is hot. The mouth is dry and hot. Vomiting immediately after eating. The pulse is rapid. Purple vein at 'San Guan'.

SAN HUANG XIE XIN TANG

4 'Deficiency'

Due to weakness of the digestive functions. Continuous vomiting. Normal urination and defecation. Absence of thirst. Low energy. Dull eyes. Easily tired. Pale complexion. Pale lips and tongue. The eyes are slightly open during sleep. The pulse is slow.

LIU JUN ZI TANG
QIAN SHI BAI ZHU TANG (with diarrhoea or loose stools)
XIANG SHA LIU JUN ZI TANG (diarrhoea or loose stools, abdominal bloating and discomfort).

Massage

Just before a child vomits or in between sieges.

1 Just below the knee about one finger width toward the outside of leg (between tibia and fibula bone), press in and hold until point is no longer tender.
2 On back of leg in the centre of the calf press in and hold until tenderness subsides. Do these points on both legs.

WARTS

Witches and warts — the two seem to go together and children's fairytales are full of them. Warts are one of those mysterious afflictions that come and go and seem to be just as prevalent on children as on witches! Often associated with old folk remedies, everyone seems to know some way of getting rid of them. Providing they are not harmful, it's fun to try some of them, and who knows, they might even work.

Causes

Usually defined as a common benign viral skin infection, they could very well disappear when the body's immunologic mechanism is stimulated. The child herself produces the antibodies. These agents interfere with viral propagation or actually destroy the viruses outright.

Symptoms

Warts vary in their appearance depending on their location on the skin. They usually produce a thickening of the normal skin that is painless except over the sole of the foot. Over the foot, they appear as small 'seed-like' interruptions of normal skin lines.

Additional Facts

Some authorities believe that a wart develops when there is a lack of vitamin A in the skin. Dr Marvin Sandler, a podiatrist in Pennsylvania, used an injection of vitamin A on patients with plantar warts with excellent results.

Warts are on the increase, and W. M. Beeson, Ph. D., of the Department of Animal Sciences at Purdue University claims that our vitamin A food sources are being depleted because of synthetic nitrogen fertilisers. These are able to act on plants and limit the amount of vitamin A they contain. Another complication is that vitamin A is found most abundantly in fats, which most people are trying to avoid.

Prevention

Include lots of carrots, pumpkin, spinach, kale, leaf broccoli, apricots, sweet potatoes, parsley, asparagus, olives, peas, peaches, liver and green and red capsicums in the diet.

Home Remedies

1 Apply a bandaid continuously for about three weeks. This excludes air from the infected skin.
2 Place the inside of a banana peel on the wart and wrap it on. Repeat treatment regularly until wart has gone.
3 Vitamin A: use the oil capsules, ensuring that the oil is derived from fish or fish-liver. Break open the capsules and squeeze the liquid onto the wart. Rub it in and repeat daily. Children's warts should be gone in approximately one month. Do not take orally.
4 Castor oil/baking soda: mix castor oil into a thick paste together with the baking soda. Apply directly to the wart several times a day. Cover with a bandage, glove or sock.
5 Give your child a placebo, or simply encourage her to 'wish' them away. Try to believe yourself that it will work and tell your child. It has been documented that the power of suggestion for removing warts is very strong. The body's natural defence mechanisms are stimulated, quickening the normal process of removal.
6 Cover the wart with an unpeeled, grated potato. Cover with bandages and leave on 2-4 hours. Several hours later, repeat again and two times thereafter. It should soften and disappear within 5-7 days. *Do not leave on overnight.*

Orthodox Treatment

There are various forms of removal, including ointments containing 5 per cent salicylic acid. These are available from your chemist; however, their use is not recommended, as they can affect the surrounding skin. Lasers will also remove warts, but as well as the treatment being painful, the warts may often reappear or scars may be left.

Warts in children often spontaneously remit.

Herbal Remedies

Tincture of Thuja occidentalis applied *topically* to the wart daily for one to two weeks. The tincture is available from some health foods shops. *Do not give the tincture internally.*

Homoeopathic Remedies

Homoeopaths understand warts as a sign of a constitutional disorder and so should be treated by a professional practitioner with internal medicines.

Chinese Remedies

Seek professional advice — a Chinese herbalist can make up a powder for topical application.

WHOOPING COUGH

Whooping cough in Chinese paediatrics is known as the 'hundred days cough' because it often takes that long to heal. It is due to an infection by bacteria, and has an incubation period of seven to ten days. It mainly occurs in epidemics every six or seven years or so, and is extremely dangerous for babies under one year of age.

It mostly occurs in the late winter or early springtime, but certainly it can make its way into the environment anytime. Mostly transmitted through the air by coughing, sneezing or breathing, it affects the respiratory tract and causes the air passages to become plugged with mucus. More than half of all the children who contract this disease are under the age of two.

Why some children get whooping cough and others do not appears to be simply a matter of exposure. Another determining factor is if a child's lung energy is weak and she gets a cough, it will be more severe. She could have inherited the weakness through infectious diseases that occurred in the family, such as tuberculosis or asthma, or she may have had numerous bouts of coughs which automatically lower her resistance.

Symptoms

In the beginning its symptoms are hard to distinguish from the common cold: runny nose, sneezing, loss of appetite, listlessness, runny eyes, a slight cough and a low or no grade fever. This goes on for about two weeks, during which your child may develop a severe cough at night and the disease progresses to the second stage. Now the cough becomes paroxysmal and your child may not be able to catch her breath. Her colour may change to a purple or bluish hue. The cough may be provoked by a tickle in the throat or lying down, and she has pains in her ribs when coughing. At the end of each bout of coughing there is a whooping sound, which accounts for the name of the disease.

Vomiting may also accompany the coughing spell. Thick, slimy mucus may be brought up with vomiting in between. Sometimes there is a small amount of bleeding in between from the mouth or nose and bloodshot eyes. She may also cry before the cough in anticipation of it and the pain associated with it and may gasp with each whoop.

Another symptom may appear such as cramping in the toes and fingers as they are clenched during the coughing bouts. Usually this occurs in the middle of the night. Drinking boiled, warm water often helps. This stage may last anywhere from two to three months.

In the third stage the cough gradually subsides, the whoop becomes less severe, and it becomes looser and more productive. Some children may experience a rattling cough, but may be too weak to bring up the phlegm. Others may have a dry cough, that is persistent and harsh and finally others may not be able to bring up the mucus despite feeling it in the chest. This stage may also last one to two months depending upon the child. However, all children will be weak due to the stress and strain put on the body from the coughing and vomiting.

Infected children can transmit the disease to others for about one month after the appearance of the first symptoms.

General Care

There is no specific treatment that your doctor can offer you, other than antibiotics, to which whooping cough responds well. There are also many natural remedies that have been quite successful over the years. Along with the ones recommended in the treatment section, acupuncture coupled with Chinese herbs works well. (See resource list for organisations providing lists of acupuncturists.)

Keep calm, and by all means keep your child in the same room as you. She will not feel as frightened and you will be more secure as well.

If this is not possible, be sure to leave the doors open to both rooms, and leave a light on at all times. Be prepared with a bucket, towels, and a face cloth and boiled warm drinking water by the bed. Make sure that she sleeps in a semi-upright position, chest down and with her head to one side if possible to avoid the danger of choking on vomit in the middle of the night. Make sure that you and your child get adequate rest during the day to make up for the loss of sleep during the night.

Dietary guidelines

- Serve warm soups and stews with lots of vegetables in them.
- Avoid all raw and cool and cold foods.
- Avoid all mucus-forming foods.
- Serve more foods during the day and less in the evening.
- Do not serve orange juice, as this may cause vomiting.
- Try apple, pear or honey drinks.

Home Remedies

All stages: Leave a glass with some purified water and a few drops of Bach Rescue Remedy in it beside the bed to support your child in remaining somewhat calm.

Stage Two: Try a bath with dried Thyme. Place a handful of dried Thyme in an old sock. Put this in the bath water and bathe in the usual manner. Rub ointment into the chest and back. Apply a Garlic poultice to the feet (see page 130) to expel the phlegm. Only leave on for short periods at a time as blisters can form if left on for too long.

Herbal Remedies

Whooping cough should be treated by a qualified practitioner.

Thyme is regarded as the best Western herb for the condition, but other expectorants such as Licorice, Elecampane and Mullein may be included in the treatment.

Thyme

Infusion: use 1 teaspoon of dried herb to 1 cup of boiling water. Let steep for 5 minutes, strain. Can be sweetened with honey or rice malt. Dilute with water if necessary.

DOSE
1-2 years: 15-30 mL (½-1 fl oz) 3 times daily
3-4 years: 40-60 mL (1⅓-2 fl oz) 3 times daily
5-6 years: 70-90 mL (2⅓-3 fl oz) 3 times daily
7 years and older: 100-150 mL (3-5 fl oz) 3 times daily

Licorice

Decoction: use ½ teaspoon chopped Licorice root to 1 cup of water. Simmer covered for 10 minutes.

DOSE
1-2 years: 20 mL (⅔ fl oz) 3 times daily
3-4 years: 30-50 mL (1-1⅔ fl oz) 3 times daily
5-6 years: 60-80 mL (2-2⅔ fl oz) 3 times daily
7 years and older: 100-120 mL (3-4 fl oz) 3 times daily

Elecampane

Decoction: use 1-1½ teaspoons of chopped root to 1 cup of water, simmer covered for 5-10 minutes.

DOSE
1-2 years: 15-30 mL (½-1 fl oz) 3 times daily
3-4 years: 40-60 mL (1⅓-2 fl oz) 3 times daily
5-6 years: 70-90 mL (2⅓-3 fl oz) 3 times daily
7 years and older: 100-150 mL (3-5 fl oz) 3 times daily

Mullein

Infusion: use 2 teaspoons of the dried leaves or ½ teaspoon of the dried flowers to 1 cup of boiling water. Let steep for 5-10 minutes, strain. Can be sweetened with honey or rice malt.

DOSE
1-2 years: 15-30 mL (½-1 fl oz) 3 times daily
3-4 years: 40-60 mL (1⅓-2 fl oz) 3 times daily
5-6 years: 70-90 mL (2⅓-3 fl oz) 3 times daily
7 years and older: 100-150 mL (3-5 fl oz) 3 times daily

Homoeopathic Remedies

Drosera is a great remedy for whooping cough and should be administered in the 30C potency three times daily. You may also refer to other medicines in the general Cough section. Where your selected medicine is not quickly effective in controlling the cough professional assistance should be sought.

Chinese Remedies

1 'Cold'

Low fever. Coughing up thin white mucus in moderate to copious amounts. Loss of appetite. Fingertips are pale. Tongue is pale with a white coating. The pulse is slow. Red vein at 'San Guan'.

XIAO QING LONG TANG

2 'Heat'

Red complexion. The mouth is dry and hot. The fingertips are purple or blue-green. The vein at 'San Guan' is purple. Nose bleeds. Coughing up blood or mucus streaked with blood. Tongue is red with a dry yellow coating. The pulse is rapid.

QING FEI YI HUO TANG

3 'Deficiency'

Weak cough with small amount of mucus. Pale lips. Pale fingertips. Bouts of coughing are frequent and of short duration. The tongue is pale. Quiet, low voice.

BU FEI TANG

4 Chronic or prolonged disease

Fatigue. Loss of appetite. Diarrhoea or loose stools. Poor digestion. Bloating after meals.

XIAO CHAI HU TANG taken together with BAN XIA XIE XIN TANG

5 Aftermath of prolonged disease

Weakness. Fatigue. Pale complexion with flushing of the malar area. Shortness of breath on mild exertion. Dry mouth. Tongue is dry and red with little coating. Pulse is rapid.

MAI MEN DONG TANG
Liquid extract of AMERICAN GINSENG

Massage

See Bronchitis and add:

1 Press with thumb all across the ball of both feet. Press deeply up from the ball of the foot to the base of the big toe. This works the bronchial area as well.

2 Press around the base of the big toe and make thumb prints from the base of big toe to the top of the toe. Rotate each toe on both feet.

3 Press into the centre of the ball of each foot and hold for ten to thirty seconds. Release pressure. Repeat six times.

Appendices

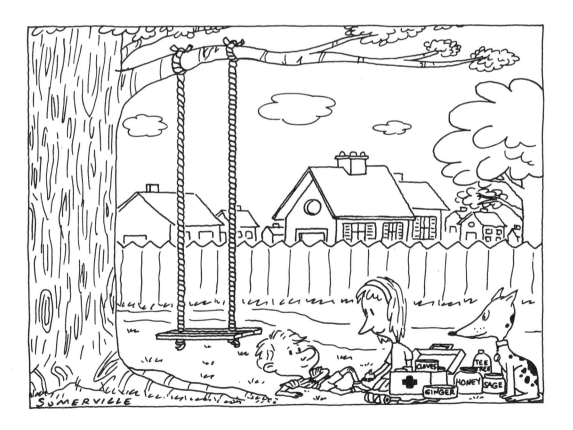

APPENDIX 1 —
SCALE OF INTERVENTION

Children become ill very quickly and recover very quickly. So you must learn to decide which illnesses you have to worry about and which ones you don't. First decide whether or not any of the following vital functions is impaired:
- State of consciousness — has it changed? Is your child conscious? Is she making sense? Check pupils for dilation and equal size.
- Is she having trouble breathing? Has her colour changed to bluish or pale?
- Is she drinking liquids? Is she vomiting constantly? Is she urinating? Or is she having chronic diarrhoea?

If your child experiences severe disturbances of any of these vital functions, call a medical practitioner immediately. If these functions are not impaired, it is possible you can afford to wait and see.

The medical intervention scale is set up from 10-100. Ten is the least likely to need intervention and 100 needs immediate intervention.

Abdominal pain

constipation — can be a symptom of a more serious bowel disorder	20
diarrhoea — may require medical intervention if it doesn't respond to simple measures within twenty-four to forty-eight hours, especially in hot weather	60

Allergy

sneezing — eliminate obvious cause (food, dust, etc)	20
cough — can be a symptom of asthma, or an inhaled foreign body — it does require medical intervention if it is persistent	70
rash — remove obvious cause — if it persists longer than twenty-four hours seek medical attention	60
headache — if it persists for longer than twelve hours or is combined with sensitivity to light and/or vomiting	80

Asthma — see Allergy

Bed-wetting — not treated until seven years of age	10
Bites	
snake	100
spider	100
Bleeding	
if it persists for more than an hour	100
if it is bleeding profusely	100
if it stops	10
Boils	10
Bronchitis — seek medical intervention	80
Bumps and bruises — first aid	10
Burns — first-degree only	10
Burns — second and third-degree	100
Chickenpox	10
Choking — parent must perform life saving measures	100
Colds	
nasal congestion	10
sore throat accompanied by fever	50
sore throat — no fever	10
Colic — if persistent for more than three hours seek medical intervention as it may be something other than colic	50
Conjunctivitis	10
Constipation — see abdominal pain	
Convulsions — first aid intervention then seek medical attention	100
Cough — see Allergy	
Cradle cap	10
Crying — very persistent or lasting more than three hours	100
Cuts and grazes	10
Dehydration	100
Diarrhoea — see Abdominal pain	
Earache — with fever	80
Earache — no fever	20
Eczema — chronic rather than acute	20
Electric shocks	100
Emergencies — artificial resuscitation	100
Eye injuries	80
Fever — over 39°C (102°F) and not coming down with home remedies	100
Fever — under 39°C (102°F) can wait six	

to twelve hours before intervention	80
Flatulence	20
Foreign bodies	
eye (if not easily removed)	100
ear (if not easily removed)	100
nose (if not easily removed)	100
swallowed — contact a doctor for advice depending on object swallowed	30
Fractures and dislocations	100
German measles	10
Head injuries	
loss of consciousness	100
no loss of consciousness	20
Hyperactivity	80
Infections, skin — if there is no response to first aid measures within several days	20
Measles	20
Motion sickness	10
Mouth ulcers	10
Mumps	20
Nappy rash	10
Nausea	20
Nose bleeds — for more than thirty minutes if bleeding profusely	100
Phlegm	30
Pneumonia	
viral	30
bacterial	100

Poisoning — treat immediately at home then take child to a medical practitioner	100
Rashes — if the cause is not obvious, for example, nappy rash take the child to a medical practitioner if the rash persists for longer than twenty-four hours	50
Sleeping habits — if patterns change considerably or insomnia develops for three or more days	50
Sore throat	40
Splinters — glass or metal	100
Stings	100
Stomach-ache — if it wakes the child at night persistently	80
Sunburn	10
sunstroke	100
Swollen glands — if persists for more than three days	80
Teething	10
Teeth knocked out	100
Thrush	10
Tonsillitis	70
Travel sickness — see Motion sickness	
Vomiting — if persistent for longer than twelve hours	50
Warts	10
Worms	
threadworm	10
tapeworm	50

APPENDIX 2 — FIRST FOODS

For infants from six to eight months

Brown Rice Milk

(Makes 4 cups or 1 qt.)
100 g (3½ oz) short grain, organically grown brown rice
1 L (4 cups) purified water

- Soak rice in the water for several hours.
- Bring rice and water to the boil in a heavy, covered sauce-pan.
- Simmer 2-3 hours, or pressure cook 1 hour.
- Strain through muslin.
- Add a few drops of rice honey to taste if necessary.
- Dilute to the desired consistency.

Oat Milk

100 g (3½ oz) whole oats, organically grown
(4 cups) purified water

- Combine oats and water in a heavy pot, bring to the boil, lower heat and simmer, covered, for 1-2 hours or until oats are soft. (You can soak overnight to hasten the cooking time. In this case you'll need more liquid.)
- Skim or strain off the top liquid. Use in any recipe requiring milk, such as sauces, soups, custards or desserts.

Grain Mix

2 tablespoons of a combination of cooked rice, oats, barley or millet
½ teaspoon unroasted tahini
1 tablespoon steamed pumpkin, carrot or cauliflower

- Sieve, purée or mash depending upon the age of the infant.

Kuzu Soup

½ cup oat milk (see above)
1 teaspoon of rice honey
2 teaspoons kuzu diluted in 1 tablespoon cold water

- Bring oat milk and rice honey to the boil.
- Stir in kuzu and continue to mix until thickened.
- Serve without seasoning.

Kuzu is a gluten-free plant starch with thickening properties and is particularly suited for weak digestion.

Vegetable Soup

In enough cold filtered water to cover, add a variety of vegetables such as pumpkin, carrot, potato and parsley. Bring to the boil, cover and simmer for 15-20 minutes or until the vegetables are tender. Serve as is, mash or purée.

APPENDIX 3 — ANTIBIOTICS CHART

DISEASE/ILLNESS	USE OF ANTIBIOTICS
Common cold	no
Whooping cough	yes, will not help the already infected child yes, will stop child spreading infection
Chest infections (croup, pneumonia)	80-90 per cent no 10-20 per cent yes, doctors may disagree as these illnesses are the hardest to judge
Urinary infections	yes, but should be diagnosed and laboratory tested
Gastroenteritis	no, could worsen condition if it is viral in origin yes, only a few exceptions to this rule if the gastroenteritis is bacterial in origin
Ear infections	yes, 90 per cent need treatment due to bacterial infection, may prevent complications
Measles, mumps	no, in majority of cases
Chicken pox	yes, only if complicated by bacterial infection
Tonsillitis	no, for more than 50 per cent of infections yes, for the rest, depending on cause
Scarlet fever	yes, great danger of complications
Very ill baby	probably, but doctors must be sure of diagnosis — usually only after tests

APPENDIX 4 — NATURAL MEDICINE KITS FOR HOME AND TRAVEL

Natural Medicine Kits for Home and Travel

The beauty of using natural medicine in your home and when you are travelling with your family is that you can take more responsibility for healing and also share what you have learned in the way of knowledge and experience with your friends and relatives.

Not long after you begin treating your family with natural medicines, you will find that you are on your way to building an abundant supply of natural medication. So when your child does become ill you may already have the necessary remedies to make the job just that much easier. You will also find yourself quickly developing a network of friends who also use natural medicines. You may find that you can call on them to help you out if you don't have just the remedy you need.

When you travel it's comforting to know that you can be prepared for most eventualities and will be able to take care of your family when the need arises.

If you are putting together a kit for the first time, consider the following points:

- Which type of healing are you particularly attracted to?
- What kinds of practitioners are available in your immediate vicinity?
- What natural medicines are most readily available to you?

- Consider your child's history of illness and what complaints run in your family.
- Go through the A-Z of complaints and see if you can find a pattern of symptoms that matches your child's previous illnesses, for example, respiratory tract complaints or gastric complaints.
- Compile a list of remedies that are recommended for these complaints. This is the beginning of your home medicine kit.
- After you have chosen the kinds of remedies that you feel most comfortable with, consult a practitioner of your choice and ask her what she would recommend as a starting kit for home use. I prefer to have a selection of different kinds of treatments on hand so that in case my children don't want to take one, there is an alternative.
- It is best to keep your home medicine kit and first aid kit together to be prepared for any eventuality — I have two sets, one in the house and one in the car. Make sure that you store your homoeopathic preparations away from light and strong-smelling substances such as eucalyptus oil.

If you have already had experience with using natural therapies you may already have the basic remedies at your fingertips. In this case you may want to add to your kit some of the following suggestions. They have been particularly useful to my family.

Home Medicine Kit

Homoeopathic Remedies

Aconite
Apis Mellifica
Arnica
Arsenicum
Belladona
Cantharis
Chamomilla
Ferrum Phos.
Gelsemium
Hepar Sulph
Hypericum
Ledum
Nat Mur
Nux Vomica
Pulsatilla

Herbal Remedies

Echinacea
Thyme
Yarrow

Sage
Elder Flowers
Licorice Root
Chamomile
Catmint

Chinese Remedies

Ban Xia Xie Xin Tang
Gan Mai Da Zao Tang
Lui Jun Zi Tang
Long Dan Xie Gan Tang
Shen Ling Bai Zhu San
Yin Qiao San

Home Remedies

Arnica Ointment
Calendula Ointment and Tincture
Aloe Vera Gel
Eucalyptus Oil
Tea-Tree Oil
Miso (see Appendix 10)
Kuzu (see Appendix 10)
Bancha Tea (see Appendix 10)

For further information about the remedies suggested for the home and travel medicine kit please consult the various Materia Medicas in each section.

Travel Kit

A complete first aid kit (see Appendix 5) together with the following homoeopathic remedies.

Aconite

For the first signs of cold, fever and flu. Ailments which come on suddenly, especially after exposure to cold dry winds. The effects of fright and shock.
Recommended potency: 30C

Apis Mellifica

For the effects of bites and stings and other afflictions where there is hot swelling.
Recommended potency: 12C

Arnica

Important for injuries to soft parts leading to bruising, concussion or haemorrhage. The effects of strain or over-exertion.
Recommended potency: 30C

Belladonna

A remedy for fevers and inflammations characterised by sudden onset and flushing of the face. Throbbing headaches.
Recommended potency: 30C

Cantharis

Important for burns and scalds and urinary tract infections associated with burning pains.
Recommended potency: 30C

Chamomilla

Used for painful ailments which are accompanied by irritability and restlessness. Teething and fevers with one red cheek.
Recommended potency: 30C

Hypericum

A primary remedy for injury to sensory nerves or for injury to parts rich in nerves, such as fingers, toes, spine, brain and tail bone.
Recommended potency: 30C

Nat. Mur

For the first signs of colds accompanied by running nose and sneezing.
Recommended potency: 30C, 2 tablets ½ hourly

APPENDIX 5 — FIRST AID KIT

Bandages

Adhesive bandages for small wounds.

Sterile gauze and adhesive strapping for larger wounds.

Crepe bandages to use as pressure bandages.

Large sterile piece of material sealed in a plastic bag that has not been opened, for covering serious wounds or burns in emergencies.

Cotton tips, cotton wool, swabs and cotton balls, for cleaning wounds.

Instruments

Tweezers
Needles and matches for sterilising
Scissors
Eye bath
Thermometer
Safety pins

Gels, Creams, Ointments and Tinctures

Aloe Vera Gel for burns and skin irritations.

Arnica ointment for bruises, sprains and muscle soreness.

Calendula ointment for open wounds and grazes.

Olbas oil made from essential oils of wintergreen, eucalyptus, juniper, peppermint, cajuput and clove — for insect bites, muscles soreness, burns and bruises.

Tea-Tree ointment and oil for burns, insect bites, infections, open wounds.

Bach Rescue Remedy for shock, stress and panic.

Hypericum — relieves pain from superficial bruising and wounds.

Ipecac syrup from the cephaelis ipecacuanha plant, to induce vomiting in case of poisoning.

Ginger capsules to relieve motion sickness and for general cases of nausea and vomiting.

Honey to stop bleeding.

Sage (powdered) to stop bleeding.

Emergency first aid book — the most current available edition from a society such as The Red Cross.

It is useful to have two kits. One for your house and one for your car.

APPENDIX 6 — FRIENDLY BACTERIA

Our gastrointestinal tract is home to millions of 'friendly bacteria'. They play a variety of roles, from controlling acne to acting as anti-cancer factors.

Types of Friendly Bacteria

Lactobacillus acidophilus — most prominent in the small intestine.

Bifidobacteria — major inhabitant of the gastrointestinal tract. The type of food given to an infant seems to determine the balance between these healthy bacteria and unhealthy bacteria. Breastfed babies have a much higher level of healthy bacteria than bottlefed babies.

Foods to enhance bifidobacteria: vegetables, whole grains, fruits, pulses and yoghurt containing *lactobacillus bulgaricus and streptococcus thermophilus.*

Things that disturb the amount of bifidobacteria in infants and children: immunisation, antibiotics, chronic constipation, diarrhoea, sudden changes in diet or weather and some common infections.

Lactobacillus bulgaricus — important yoghurt culture, not a 'natural' resident of the gastrointestinal tract but enhances both the above bacteria.

Streptococcus thermophilus — important yoghurt culture (see above).

Both of these are used to make yoghurt, but are usually only present in very small quantities in commercially produced yoghurt.

The Advantages of Friendly Bacteria

- Useful in the treatment of eczema, allergies, headache/migraine, many bowel problems, thrush, food poisoning, urinary tract infections.
- Help control harmful yeasts such as Candida
- Manufacture B vitamins and folic acid
- Help control cholesterol
- Help develop healthy digestive tracts in growing babies
- Allow the digestion of milk-based foods
- Enhance the immune system
- Protect against the negative effects of radiation and toxic pollution

Supplementation for Sick Infants and Children

- Pregnant or women breastfeeding should take ½ to 1 teaspoon Bifidobacterium infantis daily before meals in purified water. (Do not use tap water as the chlorine in it will kill all friendly bacteria.)
- In infants supplement with Bifidobacterium infantis. (When not available you can use Lactobacilius acidolphilus.) This particular strain is suitable for children up to seven years of age. Any other kind of supplement should only be given if it has the approval of a doctor or health care professional.
- Doses for children should be stirred into unchilled purified water and drunk immediately, forty-five minutes before a meal. (For quantities see specific complaints.)

Information obtained from:
Chaitow, L. and Trenev, N., *Probiotics: The revolutionary 'friendly bacteria' way to vital health and well-being.*

APPENDIX 7 – COMPRESSES, POULTICES AND BATHS

Compresses, Poultices and Baths

Compresses

Compresses are external applications to the body using water or other liquids as a base and adding or infusing other substances. A wrapper is used to secure and seal the healing properties in place. Wrappers for compresses should be made from materials that are porous and soft, such as cheesecloth or muslin.

Cold Compress

A cold compress has an anti-inflammatory, calming effect, reduces both local heat and circulation. Apply at the height of an inflammation.

Immerse a cotton towel, piece of linen, or some other porous, natural material, in cold water. You can float ice-cubes in the water or wrap them in the compress. Fold it several times until it is a suitable size and place directly on the affected area. Change the compress regularly when it starts to get warm.

For stimulating inflammation. This compress is essential at the beginning of an inflammation when the body's defences are reacting slowly. It is applied cold in the same way as above, but when it starts to become warm, leave the compress in place. When the warmth becomes intense, cover it with a hot water bottle to enhance the warming process. Once the body is improving, switch over to cold compresses.

Hot Compress

For primarily relieving pain. Use two porous cloths in succession, so that treatment can be constant. Immerse the first cloth in very hot water, and wring it out well. Lay it on the affected part of the body, changing the compress every few minutes or as it starts to cool. Cover the compress with a wool cloth to help retain the heat. Continue the application for approximately 30 minutes unless otherwise specified.

Ginger Compress

Stimulates blood and body fluid circulation, for chills, fatigue, body aches. Finely grate fresh ginger. Place it in a cotton sock, piece of cheesecloth or muslin. Secure the top to form a bag. Immerse the bag in hot, not boiling water, turn off the heat and press the bag with a wooden spoon so that the ginger juice flows into the water. Dip a towel in the water, squeeze out the excess until the towel is dry, fold and apply it to the affected area following the procedures for a Hot Compress.

Clay Compress

For inflammatory relief, infection and swelling in cases of insect stings (for stings, the compress should be replaced hourly), disorders of metabolism and congestion in the tissues and muscles.

Apply the clay compress and use only sterilised clay. (This can be purchased or you can sterilise it yourself by heating the clay in the oven for 1 hour, then pulverising it.) Mix the pulverised clay into a paste together with vinegar and water. It should be about the same consistency as an ointment. Spread it onto a cloth approximately the same size as the body part to be treated, and apply the compress. Clay mixture can also be applied directly to the affected part. The clay mixture should dry out and will simply crumble off. The remaining clay can be wiped or washed off. Apply warm olive oil after treatment to lubricate the skin.

For applications to large body parts or the whole of the body, apply the paste approximately 2 cm (¾ inch) thick and wrap with a dry sheet or blanket. Follow the rest of the procedures as above.

Cottage Cheese Compress

For fever to the head and pneumonia to the chest and lung areas. In a bowl place cottage cheese, milk and a few drops of vinegar. Stir until the mixture thickens. Spread onto a cotton or linen cloth and apply. If desired the mixture can be applied directly to the affected part. Wrap a sheet or blanket around the compress and leave on until the cottage cheese has dried and starts to crumble. Replace.

Green Vegetable Compress

For infection, bruises, swelling, fever, earache. Blend or chop and mash leaves into a paste. Mix with a little flour if too watery. Place mashed greens onto a piece of cheesecloth or cotton material to form a layer about 2 cm (¾ inch) thick. Apply to afflicted area and change every 2-3 hours or when it becomes warm.

Tofu/Green Vegetable Compress

For fever, inflammation, earache. Chop or blend several leaves of spinach or cabbage. Mash about 250 g (8 oz) fresh tofu and a 2 cm (¾ inch) piece of freshly grated ginger until it is a paste, combine with vegetables and apply as above.

Tofu Compress

For fever. Squeeze the water from 250 g (8 oz) of fresh tofu. Mash it and add 30 g (1 oz) flour and a 2 cm (¾ inch) piece of fresh ginger, grated. Mix together and apply directly to the forehead or the back of the neck.

Sesame Oil and Ginger Compress

To improve circulation and nerve reactions, and relieve aches and pains. Mix equal amounts of fresh ginger and sesame oil. Dip a piece of cloth into this mixture and rub vigorously onto the affected area.

Poultices

Poultices are similar to compresses but they are warmer and continue to retain their warmth longer. They are applied to relieve a variety of ailments from congestion and inflammations, to the draining of pus.

Potato Poultice (uncooked)

For boils, and drawing pus. Mix grated, raw potato with a 2 cm (¾ inch) piece of fresh ginger, grated. Spread it 2 cm (¾ inch) thick on gauze and apply directly to the skin. Change every four hours.

Onion Poultice

For earache. Dry fry a finely chopped onion for a few seconds until hot. Wrap in a cloth and apply behind the ear. Bind to head with bandage.

Potato Poultice (cooked)

For eczema, sunburn, reducing puffiness. Boil unpeeled potatoes. When cooked, mash them. Place between two layers of linen or cotton gauze and apply to the affected area. Make sure that the application is not too hot by testing it on your cheek. Wrap in a sheet or towel and remove when cold.

Mustard Poultice

For coughs and chest congestion. Add hot water to dry mustard in a bowl and stir the mixture well. Place this mixture onto a paper towel, fold it over itself, and put it between two towels. Apply this to the affected area. Do not let the mustard touch the skin as it can burn. Leave for 10-15 minutes to create heat.

Hot Salt Poultice

For diarrhoea and the chills of fever. Roast salt in a dry frying pan until it becomes hot. Wrap it in thick cotton or put it into a pillowcase and wrap a towel around it. Allow the poultice to cool a little before applying it to the abdomen. Change when the pack becomes cool.

Flaxseed Poultice

For abscesses and inflammation. Boil 2-4 handfuls of flaxseed (linseed meal can be used instead) in water, stirring constantly until it has formed a thick paste. Spread between two pieces of linen or cotton and fold. Make sure the poultice is not too hot before applying. Cover poultice with a sheet or blanket, and remove when cool.

Fenugreek Poultice

For small external complaints and boils. Place 2-3 handfuls of fenugreek powder in cold water and bring to the boil, stirring constantly. Apply as above.

Bath Therapy

Sometimes it is more appropriate to give your child a bath as a way of administering a natural remedy rather than by mouth or massage. Because water has a soothing as well as therapeutic effect, it is an easy way to get certain substances absorbed into the body, either directly through the skin or by way of inhalation.

Adding herbs to the bath water helps the body to absorb the vital elements that may be missing at the time into the blood for easy distribution. Baths are especially good for itchy skin, eczema, colds, acute and chronic coughing, and chronic bronchitis.

Preparation

It is best to brew your bath mixtures before adding them to the bath water.

- Combine the herbs or other plant materials with cold water in an enameled, glass or clay saucepan, (no metal).
- Bring to the boil and simmer for 4-5 minutes for flowers, or soft materials; 10-15 minutes for roots, barks, or twigs.
- Set aside and steep 3-4 minutes, covered.
- Strain and pour into the bath water.

SUGGESTED MATERIALS

Chamomile flowers. Use 125 g (4 oz) for a child under the age of three, 250 g (8 oz) from three to seven years, and 500 g (1 lb) for over the age of seven. For inflammation, cleaning wounds, itchy skin, eczema and catarrhal conditions.

Thyme. Use the same amounts as for chamomile flowers. For acute and chronic coughing.

Rice, wheat or oat bran. For inflammation of the skin. Especially effective for hives, eczema and hypersensitive skin. Use 500 g (1 lb) for children under three, 750 g (1½ lb) from 3-7, and 1 kg (2 lb) from 7-12 years. Place the bran in a cotton sock, cheesecloth or muslin. Tie it into a bag and bring it to the boil in a large pot of water. Press the bag until a milky liquid comes out. Add all the boiled water and bran to the bath water. Gently wash your child's skin.

Oatmeal bath. Wrap 3-4 cups (15-20 oz) of oatmeal in a piece of cheesecloth, muslin or sock. Add this to the bath water. Use as above.

All of the above may be used as footbaths as well. Decrease the amount by half for each age group.

Rescue remedy bath. Add 2-3 drops of Bach Rescue Remedy to the bath water.

APPENDIX 8 — CHINESE MEDICINE

Tongue Diagnosis

In the Chinese herbal Materia Medica, the tongue is described as 'red', 'pale', 'dark', etc. This is meant to indicate a shade of colouring more intense or pronounced than normal. It is therefore advisable to familiarise yourself with the normal colouring of your child's tongue, fingernails, ears, etc., so that you are better able to observe the changes that occur when the child becomes ill (or preferably before an illness becomes apparent). It is also helpful to observe the tongues, complexions, pulses, etc., of other children, in order to gain an appreciation of the normal variation of these factors both in health and disease.

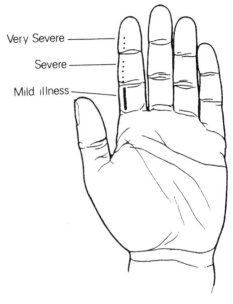

Very Severe

Severe

Mild illness

Normal Pulse Rates

AGE	RATE	
Years	Beats per breath	Beats per minute
0-1	9-10	120-140
1-3	8	116-120
4	5-7	110
5-10	5-6	90

Inspecting the Vein at 'San Guan'

Hold the baby's left hand with your left hand and observe the left index finger's palmar surface. Rub the finger from its junction with the palm to the tip, using your right thumb. Do this seven or eight times. You may also apply a few drops of water while you are doing this to make it easier to see the vein. If hardly any vein appears this is considered normal.

When the child is sick, a vein will be visible, usually within the segment between the crease opposite the knuckle and the crease of the adjacent finger joint. If the vein extends beyond this crease into the middle or to the top segment the disease is a serious one and professional treatment should be sought.

In approximately 30 per cent of normal, healthy children, this vein is visible (according to a recent study in China), so you should practise observing this vein on your child while healthy, just as it is also a good practice to become familiar with your child's normal pulse rate. Then you will be better able to judge the changes that occur when your child becomes ill.

Chinese Herbs

The formulas recommended are granulated extracts which can be mixed into your child's food and are easier to take than decoctions (which usually have an unpleasant taste and smell).

Please note that the dosage of prepared Chinese herbal formulas is normally ¼ adult dose for children under 2 years old, ⅓ adult dose for children 2-5 years old, ½ adult dose for children 5-7 years old and ⅔ adult dose for children 7-15 years old.

FORMULA (Pin Yin)	COMMERCIAL NAME
BAI SHAO GAN CAO TANG ('SHAO YAO GAN CAO TANG')	Paeonia and licorice combination
BAN XIA XIE XIN TANG	Pinellia combination
BAO HE WAN	Protect the harmony
BU FEI TANG	Tonify the breath
CHUAN PEI MO	Relieve the cough
DA CHENG QI TANG	Major order of Qi
ER CHEN TANG	Citrus and pinellia combination Two cured decoction
FU LING ZE XIE TANG	Poria and water plantain formula
GAN MAI DA ZAO TANG	Licorice and jujube combination Licorice and jujube decoction
GE GEN TANG	Kudzu formula
GUI PI TANG	Ginseng and longan combination Ginseng and longan combination
GUI ZHI TANG	Cinnamon combination Cinnamon twig decoction
HUANG LIAN JIE DU TANG	Coptis and scute combination Coptis decoction to relieve toxicity
HUANG QI JIAN ZHONG TANG	Astragalus combination
HUO XIANG ZHENG QI TANG ('HUO XIANG ZHENG QI SAN')	Dispel turbidity powder
JIN FANG BAI DU SAN	Schizonepeta and leoebu uriella powder
JIN GUI SHEN QI WAN	Pill from golden cabinet
JIN LING ZI SAN	Melia toosendan powder
LI ZHONG WAN	Ginseng and ginger combination Regulate the middle
LIANG FU WAN	Galangal and cyperus pill
LING GUI WEI GAN TANG	Poria, cinnamon, schisandra and licorice
LING GUI ZHU GAN TANG	Attractylodes and hoelen combination Poria, cinnamon, attractylodes and licorice
LIU JUN ZI TANG	Six major herb combination Six gentlemen decoction
LIU MO TANG	Six milled formula
LIU WEI DI HUANG WAN	Rehmannia six formula Six ingredient pill (rehmannia six)
LONG DAN XIE GAN TANG	Gentiana longdanca decoction
MA ZI REN WAN	Apricot seed and linum formula Mazi seed pill
MAI MEN DONG TANG	Ophiopogon combination Ophiopogon formula
MU XIANG SHUN QI SAN	Saussurea sooth the Qi
QIAN JIN NEI TUO SAN	'Formula worth 1000 gold coins'

FORMULA (Pin Yin)	COMMERCIAL NAME
QIAN SHI BAI ZHU TANG	Attractylodes and arrowroot formula
QING XIN CHA	Cool the heart tea
QING FEI YI HUO TANG	Cool and suppress the fire
QING WEI SAN	Clear the heat
REN SHEN BAI DU SAN	Ginseng powder to overcome influences
REN SHEN JIAN PI WAN	Ginseng spring tonic pill
SAN HUANG XIE XIN TANG	Coptis and rhubarb combination Purge heat
SAN ZI YANG QIN TANG	Three seed decoction to nourish one
SANG JU YIN	Morus and chrysanthemum combination Morus and chrysanthemum decoction
SHA SHEN MAI MEN DONG TANG	Glehnia and ophiopogon formula
SHAO YAO TANG	Paeonia decoction
SHEN LING BAI ZHU SAN	Ginseng and attractylodes formula Ginseng-attractylodes formula
SHENG MA GE GEN TANG	Cimicifuga and arrowroot formula
SI JUN ZI TANG	Four major herb combination Four gentlemen
SI NI SAN	Bupleurum and chih-shih (zhi shi) formula Four anti-adverse powder
TENG HUA BAI DU SAN	Formula to cleanse and detoxify
TIAN WANG BU XIN DAN	Emperor's heart tonic pill
TUO LI XIAO DU YIN	Gleditsia formula to dispel the poison
WU LING SAN	Hoelen five formula Hoelen five powder
WU WEI XIAO DU YIN	Five ingredients to relieve toxins
XIANG RU SAN	Elsholtzia powder
XIANG SHA LIU JUN ZI TANG	Cardamom — the six noble decoction
XIANG SHA YANG WEI TANG	Nourish the stomach formula
XIANG SU SAN	Cyperus and perilla formula Cyperus and perilla leaf formula
XIAO CHAI HU TANG	Minor bupleurum combination Minor buplerum
XIAO JIAN ZHONG TANG	Minor cinnamon and paeonia combination Restoring the middle
XIAO QING LONG TANG	Minor blue green formula
XIAO YAO SAN	Bupleurum and tang kuei (dang gui) formula The ease powder
XIE BAI SAN	Morus and lycium formula
('XIE FEI SAN')	Purge the lung heat
XING SU SAN	Apricot kernel and perilla leaf formula
XUAN DU FA BIAO TANG	Formula to eliminate and disperse toxin

FORMULA (Pin Yin)	COMMERCIAL NAME
YIN QIAO SAN	Lonicera and forsythia formula Honeysuckle and forsythia
YUE JU WAN	Free restraint
ZHI GAN CAO TANG	Baked licorice combination Baked licorice decoction
ZHI TUO CHUANG YI FANG	Formula to heal sores on the head
ZHU YE SHI GAO TANG	Bamboo leaf and shigao

Acupressure Treatments

The application of pressure, rubbing or kneading of certain 'Acupuncture' points is often an extremely effective way to relieve discomfort and assist your child in the healing process.

In China, acupressure combined with various specialised massage techniques is referred to as 'Infant Tuina' and is widely used as a substitute for acupuncture in treating children below the age of six. Following are a few of the most powerful acupoints which can be safely applied to your child. The ones selected are useful in treating: headaches; fever; coughs and colds; digestive problems (such as vomiting, diarrhoea or loss of appetite); enuresis (bedwetting); over-excitement (ie. for calming and sedating); general weakness and low energy.

Hegu (Colon 4)

Location: In the fleshy area between the thumb and first finger, about half-way between the knuckle of the first finger and the junction of the metacarpal bones of the thumb and first finger.
Uses: Common cold; headache; diseases of the eyes, ears, nose and face in general; coughing; acute asthma attack; fever; pain in general.
Method: Press with finger or thumb on dorsal surface, supporting with thumb or finger of same hand on palmar surface. Hold with firm yet gentle pressure for about one second, then release for one second. Repeat 50 to 100 times. Treat both sides.

Yangchi (Triple Burner 4)

Location: With the hand laying flat, palmar surface down, it is at the midpoint of the wrist crease in a small depression.
Uses: Headache; fever; constipation; common cold; tonsillitis.
Method: Finger or thumb pressure as for HEGU (Colon 4). Treat both sides.

Neiguan (Pericardium 6)

Location: On the inside (ie. palm side) of the upper arm, in line with the middle of the wrist-crease, three finger-widths (use your child's first three fingers for measurement) away from the wrist-crease. Have the arm laying flat with the palm facing up. It is in-between the two tendons that are visible when the child makes a fist and then raises the hand by flexing the wrist.
Uses: Restlessness; anxiety; irritability; insomnia; nausea; vomiting; poor appetite.
Method: Either have the child's arm lying palm up on a firm surface or hold the arm with your thumb on the point and supporting with your fingers on the outside of the forearm. Apply pressure and release with finger or thumb, as for HEGU (Colon 4), 50 to 100 times. Do both sides.

Taiyuan (Lung 9)

Location: With the palm facing up, the point is found at the base of the thumb in a slight depression at the thumb end of the wrist-crease.
Uses: Cough with mucus for example flu, bronchitis, asthma, whooping cough.
Method: Apply pressure with thumb or first finger. Use either press and release (as for HEGU — Colon 4), or use rotation. Do both sides, 50 to 100 repetitions on each.

Yintang

Location: On the face midway between the two eyebrows.
Uses: Restlessness; anxiety; irritability; insomnia; headache; nasal congestion.
Method: (a) Using thumb or finger moistened with oil or water gently rub from the point upwards to the hairline. Repeat 30 to 50 times.
(b) Using both thumbs or two fingers moistened with oil or water gently rub from the point moving outwards across the eyebrows, follow-

ing the line of the eyebrows. Repeat 30 to 50 times. (This is also helpful for eye diseases.)

Taiyang

Location: At the temple about 2.5 cm (1 inch) behind a point midway between the outer 'corner' of the eye and the tip of the eyebrow; in the fleshy area behind the bony orbit (eye socket).

Uses: Restlessness; anxiety; irritability; insomnia; headache; fever.

Method: Using middle and index fingers together apply gentle pressure and rotate in an anti-clockwise direction for right hand side, clockwise for left. Fingers may be moistened with oil or water. Repeat 30 to 50 times on each side.

Yingxiang (Colon 20)

Location: At the side of the nostril.

Uses: Nasal congestion.

Method: Place both index fingers beside each nostril, middle of the tip of each finger level with the base of the nose. Press at a slight angle towards sinuses (i.e. slightly upwards). Press as for HEGU (Colon 4). Repeat 30 to 50 times.

Zhongwan (Conception 12)

Location: On the upper abdomen, half-way between the navel and the xiphoid process (the little piece of cartilage that forms the base of the sternum and protrudes downwards from the junction of the ribs in the middle).

Uses: Digestive disorders, for example, vomiting, diarrhoea, poor appetite.

Method: Apply moderate pressure to the point with thumb or palm of hand. Massage in a circular motion for five minutes. May be followed by massaging the upper border of the abdomen, just below the ribs, using both thumbs or index fingers. Begin at the xiphoid and move from the centre outwards, following the line of the ribs. Repeat 100 to 200 times. Fingers may be moistened with oil or water.

Fengmen (Bladder 12) and Feishu (Bladder 13)

Location: On the upper back, midway between the spine and the inside edge of the sapula (shoulder blade). The first point is level with the lower end of the second thoracic vertebra; the second point is level with the lower end of the third thoracic vertebra. To find the first thoracic vertebra, have your child sit up and drop the head forward. The vertebra that sticks out at the base of the neck is the last cervical (neck) vertebra. The one below it is the first thoracic ('T1'); below this is the second thoracic vertebra ('T2'), and so on.

Uses: Cough; colds; flu; asthma.

Method: Applying pressure to both points using two fingers or thumb, you may (a) press and release as for HEGU (Colon 4), 50 to 100 times, or (b) gently rotate, 50 to 100 times, or (c) massage in a downwards and outwards direction towards the shoulder blade, 50 to 100 times. Do both sides.

Pishu (Bladder 20)

Location: In the central area of the back, the same distance from the spine as the last two points, level with the lower end of the 11th thoracic vertebra. To help locate this point, the bottom tip of the shoulder blade is level with the seventh thoracic vertebra.

Uses: Digestive problems, for example, vomiting, diarrhoea, poor appetite; low energy; overall weakness.

Method: Placing two fingers or the thumb on the back so that they can apply pressure to this point and one directly below it (in line with the lower end of the 12th thoracic vertebra). Treat as for HEGU (Colon 4) 50 to 100 times. Do both sides.

Shenshu (Bladder 23)

Location: In the lower part of the back, the same distance from the spine as the previous point, in line with the midpoint between the top of the hip bone and the bottom of the last rib.

Uses: Bed-wetting; weakness; low energy.

Method: Apply pressure and release as for HEGU (Colon 4), using finger or thumb, 50 to 100 times on both sides.

Zusanli (Stomach 36)

Location: On the outer side of the upper part of the calf. Run your hand down the upper part of the tibia immediately below the kneecap at the front of the calf. There is a round 'knob' of bone at the top of the tibia before you get to the straight edged shaft of the bone. The point is level with the junction between these two sections, where the outer edge of the bone becomes straight, and is one 'finger-width' (of your child's finger) away from the bone.

Uses: Digestive disorders, for example, vomiting, diarrhoea, poor appetite; general weakness; low energy; anaemia; excessive mucus production.

Method: Apply pressure using finger or thumb. Use either the press-release technique (as for HEGU — Colon 4) or continual rotation. Repeat 50 to 100 times. Do both sides.

San Yinjiao (Spleen 6)

Location: On the inside of the lower part of the calf, one hand-width (your child's hand) above the tip of the inner ankle bone, one finger width (your child's hand) away from the edge of the bone in the fleshy section between the bone and the upper part of the achilles tendon.
Uses: Bed-wetting; digestive disorders: general weakness; low energy.
Method: Moisten thumb or finger with oil or water and massage in an upwards direction using moderate pressure. Begin the movement a little below the point and finish just above it so that you cover 2 to 3 cm (1–1½ inches). Repeat 50 to 100 times, being careful not to damage the skin. Do both sides.

Zhaohai (Kidney 6)

Location: Directly beneath the inner ankle bone.
Uses: Bed-wetting; pharyngitis; tonsillitis; insomnia.
Method: Apply pressure and release using finger or thumb as for HEGU (Colon 4). Repeat 50 to 100 times. Do both sides.

Notes on Applying Acupressure

Select three to five different points for each treatment session. This usually means that you will be treating six to ten points, as most of them occur at corresponding positions on both sides of the body.

Make sure that both you and your child are in a comfortable position that also allows easy access to the point or points that you are treating. You may find that you need to change positions in order to get to different points, for example, if you have selected some points on the front of the body and some on the back. The time spent applying acupressure is usually from fifteen to twenty minutes. It is generally done once daily but may be done more frequently in acute conditions.

The precise location of a point is not as critical when applying acupressure as it is when practising acupuncture. The extremely small width of the acupuncture needle makes it very important to be minutely accurate in finding and stimulating the exact spot. When using thumbs and fingers, on the other hand, you are applying the stimulation over a much larger area, and such a high degree or accuracy is not necessary. Generally the points are to be found in small hollows or depressions and there is usually a distinctive 'feel' of the tissues at an acupoint.

Practise regularly both on yourself and your child. You will then become aware that many of the points are quite tender and often become more so when the body is weak or ill. You will also find that your accuracy and ability to locate the points improves and you have at your disposal a simple and very effective method to relieve discomfort and to promote well-being.

APPENDIX 9 — THE ENERGETIC PROPERTY OF FOOD

FOOD	Hot	Warm	Neutral	Cool	Cold
Almond		<			
Apple					<
Arrowroot				<	
Asparagus					<
Barley					<
Banana			<		
Bay Leaf		<			
Beef		<			
Beets		<			
Black Date		<			
Bread			<		
Broad Bean		<			
Brown Rice		<			
Brown Sugar		<			
Buck Wheat					<
Butter		<			
Button Mushroom		<			
Cabbage		<			
Carrots					<
Cashew Nut		<			
Celery				<	
Chestnut		<			
Cherry		<			
Chicken		<			
Chinese Cabbage					<
Chinese Greens					<
Coconut		<			
Coconut Milk		<			
Coriander		<			
Coriander Seed		<			
Corn				<	
Crab					<
Duck					<
Dill Seed		<			
English Spinach				<	
Fennel		<			
Fruit Juice			<		
Garlic		<			
Ginger		<			
Grapefruit					<
Green Beans					<
Green Onion		<			

FOOD	Hot	Warm	Neutral	Cool	Cold
Green Pepper	<				
Ham		<			
Hazelnut		<			
Honey				<	
Kidney		<			
Leek		<			
Lemon Rind		<			
Lentils					<
Lettuce					<
Liver		<			
Malt		<			
Malt Sugar		<			
Mangos					<
Millet					<
Mung Bean		<			
Mushrooms		<			
Mussels		<			
Nutmeg		<			
Oats					<
Parsnips					<
Peach					<
Peanut		<			
Pear					<
Peas					<
Pearl sago		<			
Pickles		<			
Pineapple				<	
Pine Nuts		<			
Pork					<
Prawn				<	
Pumpkin		<			
Rabbit		<			
Red Date		<			
Red Pepper		<			
Rice				<	
Rosemary		<			
Rye					<
Salt					<
Seaweed					<
Sesame Seed					<
Sheeps Milk		<			
Shrimp		<			

FOOD	Hot	Warm	Neutral	Cool	Cold
Silver Beet					<
Soybean					<
Spearmint		<			
Spinach		<			
Sprouts					<
Strawberry		<			
Squash		<			
Sunflower Seeds					<
Sweet Basil		<			
Sweet Potato		<			
Sweet Rice		<			
Tamari				<	
Tangerine Peel				<	

FOOD	Hot	Warm	Neutral	Cool	Cold
Taro Potato		<			
Tea					<
Tofu					<
Veal		<			
Vinegar		<			
Walnuts		<			
Water (drinking)					<
Watermelon					<
Wheat					<
White Beans					<
Whole Wheat			<		
Yams					<
Zucchini					<

APPENDIX 10 — FOOD GLOSSARY

Bancha tea: made from small twigs from the tea plant, this excellent tea may be taken frequently as it is very low in tannin and caffeine and works as a buffer-solution in the stomach, neutralising over-acidic or alkaline conditions.

Kuzu: a white starch made from the root of the kuzu (kudzu-) vine. It can be used as a thickening agent. Medicinally it is used to help the stomach and the intestines work well and has a cooling effect.

Miso: a fermented soybean paste, miso is high in protein and beneficial to the digestive and circulatory systems.

Tofu: called 'meat without a bone' in Asia, tofu is soybean curd. It is high in protein and low in fat and cholesterol. It has a cooling effect on the body.

APPENDIX 11 — COMMON ORTHODOX MEDICINES AND THEIR SIDE-EFFECTS

This appendix is designed to help you understand the possible side-effects of some commonly prescribed or over-the-counter orthodox medications. The list is by no means exhaustive, covering only some childhood illnesses. Generic drugs are listed using their most widely recognized brand names. In many cases there are other brands available. The side-effects refer specifically to the generic drug.

Dietary recommendations for the illnesses are provided when appropriate. These are only guidelines. Listen to what your child has to say about food and try to support his cravings by choosing good quality food. For example, if your child asks for something sweet, make up a drink or dessert from naturally sweet ingredients, without adding extra sugar and refined food. Children usually know what they need in taste, not quality!

Abdominal Pain

Orthodox Medicine

Common brand names: Panadol, Tylenol
Generic name: Paracetamol

Side-effects

See Colds and Flu

Dietary Recommendations

Before: Natural foods that may be the cause of abdominal pain include tomatoes, cucumber, oranges, apricots, prunes, peaches, plums, raspberries, grapes and allergenic foods.
During: Depends on diagnosis

Allergy — Stings, Bites and Medically Prescribed Drugs

Orthodox Medicine

Common brand name: Cortone Acetate
Generic name: Cortisone Acetate

Side-effects

Mild hirsutism (excessive growth of hair on the body where hair is not found), moon face and temporary muscular weakness may occur. Sodium and potassium imbalance may follow high doses, leading to sodium retention, potassium depletion and increased blood sugar levels.

Allergy — All Others

Orthodox Medicine

Common brand names: Phenergan, Prothazine
Generic name: Promethazine

Side-effects

The most common adverse reactions are pronounced sedative effects and confusion and disorientation. Other adverse reactions include lassitude, fatigue, incoordination, tinnitus, problems with eyeball movement, double vision, insomnia, excitation, nervousness, euphoria, hysteria, tremors, seizures, catonic-like states, decreased number of white blood cells, low blood platelet count, gastrointestinal side-effects may include loss of appetite, nausea, vomiting, constipation or diarrhoea.
Serious or life-threatening reaction: coma, death.
Contraindications: Hypersensitivity to the drug; patients who have received large doses of central nervous system depressants and/or comatose; solar dermatitis has been reported in patients with eczema or rheumatic tendencies; the product should not be used in jaundiced patients.
Precautions: Caution is advised in patients with cardiovascular disease, impaired liver function, acute or chronic respiratory impairment or bladder neck obstruction. Promethazine may cause drowsiness and may potentate the effects of alcohol. It should not be used by pregnant women or those likely to become pregnant. Neither is it known whether it has a harmful effect on a breastfed newborn.

Dietary Recommendations

Before: Avoid excessive amounts of sugar, salt, refined carbohydrates and fat. Avoid foods containing preservatives, artificial flavourings and colourings.

During: Follow dietary suggestions as prescribed by practitioner and follow the suggestions for 'Before'.

Asthma

Orthodox Medicine 1

Common brand names: Ventolin, Proventil, Albuterol
Generic name: Salbutamol

Side-effects

A fine tremor of skeletal muscle has been reported in some patients when salbutamol is administered orally or inhaled, and in about 20 per cent of patients receiving it by injection, the hands being the more obviously affected. A few feel tense. These effects are dose related and caused by a direct action on skeletal muscle.

Increases in heart rate may occur in patients after administration of respirator solution, nebules or injection. In patients with pre-existing rapid heartbeat, especially those in status asthmatics, the heart rate tends to fall after injection, respirator solution or nebules as the condition of the patient improves.

With higher doses than recommended, or in patients unusually sensitive to this group of drugs, dilation of blood vessels may occur. Other reactions which may occur are headaches, nausea, palpitations and sensations of warmth. Slight pain or stinging may occur after injection.

Contraindications: Hypersensitivity to any of the ingredients. The most common adverse reactions are gastric irritation, nausea, vomiting, palpitations and tremor. More serious side-effects such as a grossly abnormal heartbeat and convulsions may also appear rarely.

Dietary Recommendations

Before, During and After: Avoid mucus-forming foods. Under 12 months avoid heavy foods such as unyeasted wholemeal breads and undercooked wholegrains and refined sugar, food colourings and chemical additives, especially sulphites. See also Allergy.

Orthodox Medicine 2

Common brand names: Slo-Phyllin, Theolair
Generic name: Theophylline

Side-effects

The incidence and severity of particular side effects depends on the doses and rate of administration. At recommended therapeutic doses, the frequency of side effects is minimal.

Contraindications: Nuelin should not be used where hypersensitivity is known.

Precautions: Monitoring plasma levels of individual patients is recommended for dosage determination. Theophylline should be administered with caution to patients with cardiac disease or hyperthyroidism. Theophylline clearance decreases in patients with pneumonia and acute feverish episodes. Side-effects are dependent upon the dosage. It should not be administered concurrently with other drugs in the same group. Theophylline crosses the placenta, and the effect on the foetus is unknown. It is excreted in breast milk, and dosage to the mother should be minimised to avoid toxicity to the infant.

Orthodox Medicine 3

Common brand names: Bricanyl, Brethine
Generic name: Terbutaline

Side-effects

More common: Tremor, nervousness, increased heart rate, palpitations.

Less common: Cardiovascular — abnormal beats; gastrointestinal — nausea, vomiting, bad taste, diarrhoea; general — sweating; musculo-skeletal — muscle twitching, cramps; central nervous system — drowsiness, headache, dizziness; dermatological — rash.

Serious or life-threatening reactions: Overdose may produce significant fluctuations in the heart beat and hypotension.

Contraindications: Known hypersensitivity to this group of drugs.

Precautions: Caution is advised when terbutaline is administered to patients with irregular heartbeat rhythms. In some patients, doses have been reported to cause some changes in an electrocardiograph (ECG) test result but the exact significance is not known. Due to the blood glucose increasing effects, extra blood glucose controls are initially recommended with diabetic patients. Though no adverse effects in pregnant women have been reported, care is recommended in the first three months of pregnancy.

Orthodox Medicine 4

Common brand name: Delta-Cortex
Generic name: Prednisolone

Side-effects

The side-effects associated with the use of corticosteroids such as prednisolone in the large doses necessary to produce a therapeutic response result from the excessive action on body sodium/potassium balance. Excessive action on other aspects of metabolism, including the action on tissue repair and healing, and an inhibitory effect on the secretion of corticotrophin by the anterior pituitary gland also occur. Disturbance of sodium and potassium and water balance is manifest in sodium retention with abnormal infiltration of the tissues with fluid, and the increased excretion of potassium with the development of potassium deficiency.

Other metabolic effects include mobilisation of calcium and phosphorous with osteoporosis and spontaneous fractures, nitrogen depletion and hyperglycaemia with accentuation or precipitation of the diabetic state. The insulin requirements of diabetic patients are increased and appetite is often increased.

The effect on tissue repair manifests as peptic ulceration with haemorrhage and perforation, delayed wound healing and increased liability to infection, including sepsis, fungal and viral infections. Large doses may produce symptoms typical of hyperactivity of the adrenal cortex, with moonface, buffalo hump, flushing, striane and acne, sometimes leading to a fully developed Cushing's Syndrome. These symptoms are usually reversed if the administration of the hormone is discontinued immediately, but this may be dangerous.

Growth retardation in children has been reported, and in this respect cortisone is only one-tenth as potent as prednisone and prednisolone. Other toxic effects included mental and neurological disturbances and intercranial hypertension. Infections may be masked since corticosteroids have marked anti-inflammatory and antipyretic properties, and may also cause a reduction in the number of circulating white blood cells. Muscular weakness is an occasional side effect of most corticosteroids, particularly when taken in large doses.

Contraindications: There are no known contraindications in children.
Precautions: Corticosteroids should be used with caution in the prescience of infectious diseases and renal failure.

Withdrawal of corticosteroids should always be gradual, because sudden withdrawal can precipitate a hypertensive crisis due to lack of cortisone.

Dietary Recommendations

Before: Asthma attacks are often triggered by an allergy to artificial colourings and flavouring, and foods like bitter apples, oranges and tomatoes. Mucus-producing foods should also be eliminated from the child's diet. Babies and toddlers should be given easily digested foods. Refined sugar should be avoided. Also eliminate dairy products, bananas, avocadoes and tofu. Avoid meat, fish, eggs, chocolate, salt, tap water, soybeans and peas. Restrict grains and potatoes.
During: Black beans, onions, black pepper, cardamom, ginger and garlic are usually beneficial for respiratory complaints.

Bites and Stings

Orthodox Medicine

Common brand names: Phenergan, Prothazine
Generic name: Promethazine Hydrochloride
Common brand names: Amoxil, Amoxicillin
Generic name: derivative of Penicillin

Side-effects

Contraindications: Should be avoided if a history of allergic reactions to penicillins is known.
Precautions: Serious and occasionally fatal hypersensitivity reactions have been reported. The use of medications such as Amoxil and Moxacin can lead to the development of severe colitis, which can be fatal. If significant diarrhoea occurs, discontinue the medication.

Safety for use in pregnancy has not been established, therefore the drug should not be used in pregnant women or those likely to become pregnant. There is also a possibility of superinfections occurring and this drug should not be taken by patients with sore throat or pharyngitis.

Boils

Orthodox Medicine

Common brand name: Bactroban
Generic name: Mupirocin

Side-effects

Hypersensitivity to any of the components.

Dietary Recommendations

Before: Boils may occur when there is a build up of rich fatty foods such as peanuts, eggs, chicken and milk in the body.
During: Fresh vegetables and fruit, and vitamin and mineral supplements, may help to eliminate boils.
After: Less fatty, greasy foods.

Bronchitis

Orthodox Medicine

Common brand names: Amoxil, Amoxicillin
Generic name: derivative of Penicillin

Side-effects

See Bites and Stings

Dietary Recommendations

Before: Avoid too much rich, fatty mucus-forming foods.
During: Honey and pear can both be eaten to moisten the lung. White radish is helpful in resolving phlegm in children over three years of age, as can walnut kernel.
After: More fruits, grains, vegetables and preservative-free foods.

Bumps and Bruises

Orthodox Medicine

Common brand name: Wintergreen Oil
Generic name: Methyl Salicylate

Side-effects

Hypersensitivity to any of the components.

Burns and Scalds

Orthodox Medicine

Common brand name: Silvadene
Generic names: Silver Sulfadazine, Chlorohexane Digluconate

Side-effects

Hypersensitivity to any of the components.

Colds and Flu

Orthodox Medicine — Fever

Common brand names: Panadol, Tylenol
Generic name: Paracetamol

Orthodox Medicine — Nasal Congestion

Common brand names: Sudafed, Sinutab, Cenafed
Generic names: Pseudophedrine, Hydrochloride

Side-Effects of Paracetamol

Dyspepsia, nausea or allergic reactions have been rarely reported.
Precautions: Paracetamol should be administered with caution to patients with hepatic or renal dysfunction. Soluble tablets should be used with caution if restricted salt intake is indicated.
   Paracetamol is also excreted in breast milk, but does not appear to present a risk to the nursing infant.

Side-effects of Pseudophedrine

Side-effects are uncommon. In some patients pseudophedrine may occasionally cause insomnia. Other ephidrine-like symptoms may occur, such as nervousness, tremor, vertigo, headache, tachycardia, palpitations, sweating or flushing.
Contraindications: Individuals who have previously exhibited intolerance to pseudophedrine.
Precautions: As pseudophedrine stimulates the sympathetic nervous system, it should be used with caution in patients taking other similar drugs such as decongestants. Safety in pregnancy has not been established.

Dietary Recommendations

Before: Avoid over-eating, refined sugar, artificial additives, preservatives and food colourings and fat.
During: During a cold or fever, light vegetable soup, thin porridge, noodles or diluted fruit juice are useful. Black bean and green mung bean soup both fight infection. Fresh ginger and chrysanthemum flower tea are both helpful in providing relief from a cold.
After: Strengthening soups and stews with chicken and/or fish stock and lots of vegetables, garlic, ginger and a small amount of well-cooked barley or rice.

Colic

Orthodox Medicine

Common brand names: Bentyl, Byclomine
Generic names: Dicyclomine Hydrochloride, Simethicone

Side-effects

None have been reported for this product. However, administration of dicyclomine hydrochloride in other preparations has been associated in rare reports, mostly with children under 2 months, with breathlessness, breathing difficulties, convulsions, variable pulse rate, muscle hypotonia and loss of consciousness. The onset of these symptoms have been variable, sometimes within minutes of administration and lasting up to 20 to 30 minutes. Dry mouth, thirst and dizziness may occur; also rarely reported have been fatigue, sedation, blurred vision, rash, constipation, anorexia, nausea, vomiting, headache and painful urination.
Contraindications: Sensitivity to dicyclomine; obstructive diseases of the gastrointestinal tract; voluntary muscle fatigue (particularly in the eye).
Precautions: Should be used with caution and only on medical advice on children under 3 months. Infacol should only be administered when the infant is quiet, alert and upright.

Dietary Recommendations

Before: Eliminate from your child's diet, and from your own if you are breastfeeding, cold foods such as bananas, lettuce and yoghurt, and 'windy' foods such as cucumbers, cabbage, brussel sprouts, lettuce, garlic, legumes, turnips, green peppers, onions and beans. These foods are difficult to digest and may be a leading cause of colic. Goat's milk or soya milk may be easier for the child to digest, and cow's milk can be made more digestible by simmering it for 15 minutes with half an onion.
During: Wild cherry and quince are also helpful to eliminate colic as are dill and fennel tea.
After: Same as 'Before'.

Conjunctivitis

Orthodox Medicine

Common brand names: Chloromycetin, Chloroptic S.O.P.
Generic name: Chloramphenicol

Side-effects

Should irritation occur, use should be discontinued as this may indicate an allergic reaction.
Contraindications: Patients allergic to any of its constituents.
Precautions: As with other antibiotic preparations, prolonged treatment may result in the overgrowth of nonsusceptible organisms.

Dietary Recommendations

During: Avoid rich, fatty and allergic foods.

Constipation

Orthodox Medicine

Common name: Suppositories — Ducolax, Coloxyl
Generic name: Bisacodyl

Side-effects

Soreness in the anal region can be caused by a leakage of the suppository base. Often this is due to failure to insert the suppository sufficiently high into the rectum.
Contraindications: Apart from acute surgical abdomen, where any laxative is contraindicated, there are no known contraindications to bisacodyl.

Dietary Recommendations

Before: For children under 3 years of age, provide similar-sized meals at the same time each day, avoiding snacks. They should eat food which is easy to digest. Avoid excesses of greasy, fatty foods, brown bread, bran muesli and too many raw vegetables.
    Over the age of 3, a diet high in fibre, fruits, vegetables and beans is good, and small amounts of animal food, mainly fish.
During: Foods that help relieve constipation in babies and toddlers — maple syrup, fig syrup, stewed prune juice, fresh pears; for older children — figs, prunes, slippery elm, bananas, pears, licorice root, tomatoes, rhubarb, buttermilk, honey, wheat, oatbran taken with fluid, apples, whey powder, yoghurt, apricots.
After: Same as 'Before'.

Convulsions

Orthodox Medicine

Common brand name: Dilantin (the only brand available in Australia)
Generic name: Phenytoin Sodium

Side-effects

The central nervous system is the most common place where manifestations of Dilantin therapy are encountered. These include involuntary jerky movement of the eyeball, defective muscle control, slurred speech and mental confusion. Cases of dizziness, insomnia, transient nervousness, motor twitching and headache have also been reported. These side effects may disappear by continuing therapy at a reduced dosage.

Dilantin may cause nausea, vomiting and constipation. To prevent gastric irritation due to alkalinity, Dilantin should be taken with at least half a glass of water. Also administer during or following meals to prevent gastric irritation.

Dermatological manifestations sometimes associated with fever have included rashes resembling those found in scarlet fever or measles. The latter case is the most common with other types of dermatitis being more rare. Generally, rashes are more common in children. More serious forms which may be fatal have been reported and they include bullous exfoliative dermatitis, bruises, sores or rash.

Some fatal haemopoietic (concerned with the production of blood) complications have occasionally been reported in association with the administration of phenytoin. Included in these are spontaneous bruising and prolonged bleeding after injury, a decreased number of white blood cells, and suppression of bone marrow function. Although anaemia has occurred, these are more a consequence of folic acid deficiency.

Inflammation of the gum occurs frequently and its incidence may be reduced by good oral hygiene, including gum massage, frequent brushing and dental care. Occasionally, inflammation of the arteries and excessive hair growth in abnormal regions as well as potentially fatal cases of toxic hepatitis and liver damage may occur.

Contraindications: Patients with a history of hypersensitivity to this group of drugs.

Precautions: The main site of biotransformation of Dilantin is the liver, so patients with impaired liver function, or those gravely ill, may show early signs of toxicity on standard doses. In some individuals, the rate of Dilantin metabolism has been slower than normal. This may be due to enzymatic unavailability or defective induction methods. Phenytoin has been associated with reversible lymph node hyperplasia, and if lymph node enlargement occurs in patients on Dilantin, substitituion of another anticonvulsant drug is necessary.

Dilantin should be discontinued if a skin rash appears. If the rash is exfoliative or purple, use of the drug should not be resumed. If the rash is mild, therapy can be resumed after the rash has completely disappeared. There have been some reports suggesting a possible association between the use of anticonvulsant drugs and birth defects.

Dietary Recommendations

Before: Avoid mucus-producing foods and hot foods, avoiding all red meat.
After: Diet should be based on grains, beans and fruit, with small amounts of white meat. Same as 'Before'.

Cough and Bronchitis

Orthodox Medicine

Common brand name: Benadryl Expectorant
Generic names: Diphenhydramine Hydrochloride, Dextromethorphan Hydrobromide, Phenylephrine Hydrochloride, Ammonium Chloride, Sodium Citrate Glycerol, Sucrose, Glucose, Alcohol

Side-effects

Precautions: This preparation may cause drowsiness, nausea, vomiting and rapid heartbeat.

Dietary Recommendations

Before: Avoid mucus-producing foods such as cow's milk, cheese, roasted peanuts, sugar and bananas, and soy products.
During: Vegetable stews, chicken soup and cooked fruit. Avoid nuts, fatty foods and mucus-producing foods.
After: More vegetables and fruits, less fatty foods and sugar. Chicken and fish soups.

Earaches

Orthodox Medicine

Common brand names: Amoxil, Amoxicillin
Generic name: derivative of Penicillin

Side-effects

Contraindications: Should be avoided if a history of allergic reactions to penicillins is known.

Precautions: Serious and occasionally fatal hypersensitivity reactions have been reported. The use of Amoxil or Moxacin can lead to the development of severe colitis, which can be fatal. If significant diarrhoea occurs, discontinue the medication.

Safety for use in pregnancy has not been established, therefore the drug should not be used in pregnant women or those likely to become pregnant. There is also a possibility of superinfections, such as candida, occurring.

Dietary Recommendations

Before: A diet full of rich and spicy foods may cause heat to accumulate in the body, which may lead to earache. Also avoid mucus-producing foods. Animal fats, for example those in dairy foods, meat, poultry and eggs, as well as the intake of cool, cold or frozen foods (like icecream) can also cause earache.
During and after: Same as 'Before'. Light on fatty foods and cold foods.

Eczema

Orthodox Medicine

Common brand names: Lanacort-5, Corticaine
Generic name: Hydrocortisone

Side-effects

Contraindications: Patients with tuberculosis or viral infections of the skin, fungal or bacterial infections; also, patients with hypersensitivity to any of the ingredients.
Precautions: Prolonged treatment (more than 4 weeks) of extensive areas in infants and young children should be avoided. Prolonged use in pregnancy and during breastfeeding should also be avoided.

Dietary Recommendations

Before: Food allergies which may cause eczema include eggs, chicken, honey, saturated fats and mucus-producing foods. Avoid the over-consumption of fats and oils, animal foods and vegetable oils. An excessive intake of refined sugars, corn syrup, honey and fruit, or baked flour products can also contribute to eczema. Avoid soy, peanut, chocolate and potato.
During: The breastfed baby's intake of food should be limited. The baby should be burped properly after feeds. Ensure she does not go to sleep immediately after eating. The breastfeed-

ing mother should avoid cheese, cow's milk, roasted peanuts, red meat, and greasy, rich and spicy meals. Most bottlefed babies with eczema find it difficult to digest cow's milk. In weaned babies and toddlers, consider a change from cow's milk to goat's milk or soya milk. Avoid cheese, peanuts, orange juice, prawns and shellfish. Serve regular, small meals, avoid snacks. Half a teaspoon of linseed oil mixed into the food each day may help heal the condition.
After: Follow suggestions for 'Before' and 'During'.

Eye Injuries

Orthodox Medicine

Common brand names: Chloromycetin, Chloroptic S.O.P.
Generic name: Chloramphenicol

Side-effects

See Conjunctivitis

Fever

Orthodox Medicine

Common brand names: Panadol, Tylenol
Generic name: Paracetamol

Side-effects

See Colds and Flu

Dietary Recommendations

During: So that the child's energy is not used to digest food, food should be sparsely consumed until 12 hours after the fever has subsided. Rich, fatty and heat-producing foods should especially be avoided. A drink of lemon and honey in warm water may be given at all times. 1 cup of fluid should be consumed each hour.
After: Babies should be given very weak sweet water and then diluted milk or fruit juice after a fever has subsided. Older children can start with a small amount of light vegetable broth, soup, porridge or a piece of toast. If your child is very weak, beef tea or the juice from a stew can be used to replenish their energy.

Headaches

Orthodox Medicine

Common brand names: Panadol, Tylenol
Generic name: Paracetamol

Side-effects

See Colds and Flu

Dietary Recommendations

During: Check to see if a food allergy is the cause. Avoid fatty and spicy foods, preservatives, food colourings, chocolate and sugar.
After: Same as 'During'.

Hyperactivity

Orthodox Medicine

Common brand name: Phenobarbital
Generic name: Phenobarbitone

Side-effects

Drowsiness.
Contraindications: Pathological changes and photosensitivity in nervous and muscular tissue, hyperkinetic children, severe hepatic or renal impairment.
Precautions: Respiratory insufficiency. Prolonged use may lead to physical dependence and tolerance.

Dietary Recommendations

During: Such behavioural problems can be attributed to allergies to gluten, an excess of sugar or artificial colourings and flavourings. Give regular meals, and do not overfeed. Avoid foods which are hard to digest, cut down on milk and eliminate artificial additives from the diet.

Motion Sickness

See Nausea

Nausea

Orthodox Medicine

Common brand names: Maxolon, Reglan
Generic name: Metoclopramide Hydrochloride

Side-effects

The most frequent adverse reactions to Maxolon are restlessness, drowsiness, fatigue and lassitude which occur in approximately 10 per cent of cases. Less frequently, insomnia, headache, dizziness, nausea or bowel disturbances may occur. A single instance of supraventricular tachycardia following intramuscular administration has been reported.

Although uncommon in normal dosages, muscular reactions have been reported. These include spasm of the facial and jaw muscles, rhythmic protrusion of the tongue, spasm of the eye muscles including problems with eyeball movement, unnatural positioning of the head and shoulders and extreme extension of the body in muscle spasm. There may be a generalised increase in muscle tone. The majority of reactions usually disappear within 48 hours of withdrawal of the drug, however, close observation is required.
Contraindications: Maxolon should not be used whenever stimulation of gastrointestinal motility might be dangerous, for example, in the presence of gastrointestinal haemorrhage, mechanical obstruction or perforation. Maxolon is contraindicated in patients with a known sensitivity to the drug. The drug should only be used in pregnancy if clearly needed. It is excreted in milk and although it is not known whether Maxolon has a harmful effect on newborns, it is only recommended if the benefits to the mother outweigh any possible risk to the baby.
Precautions: The symptomatic relief provided by Maxolon may delay recognition of a serious disease. It should not be prescribed until diagnosis has been established.

This drug should not be given to children unless a clear indication has been established for its use, because of the higher incidence of aversion in this age group.

Dietary Recommendations

Before: Give small amounts of easily digested foods; regular meals (every 2 hours for children under 4 years of age) and very little sugar.
During: See Nausea.
After: Same as 'Before'. Avoid rich foods.

Parasites

Orthodox Medicine

Common brand names: Antiminth, Reese's Pinworm
Generic name: Pyrantel Embonate

Side-effects

Anorexia nervosa, nausea, vomiting, abdominal discomfort or cramps, diarrhoea, headache, dizziness, drowsiness, insomnia, fatigue and rash have been frequently reported. Minor abnormalities of liver function have occasionally been associated with treatment.

Contraindications: It is recommended that Combantrin should not be administered to children with acute liver disease. Use of Combantrin should be avoided in pregnancy where possible.

Dietary Recommendations

During: Raw fruits, refined foods, nuts and flour products should be avoided until the condition improves. Pumpkin, squash or sunflower seeds, roasted without salt, can be used as snacks.

After: Reduce sugar, flour and refined food intake.

Phlegm/Mucus

Orthodox Medicine

Common brand names: Sudafed, Sinutab, Cenafed
Generic names: Pseudophedrine, Hydrochloride

Side-effects

See Colds and Flu

Dietary Recommendations

Before: Avoid too much cow's milk, cream, butter, cheese, roasted peanuts, more than one orange per week for children, bananas or excessive sugar.

During: Garlic, onions, watercress, horseradish and umeboshi plums (Japanese pickled plums) tend to reduce mucus production.

After: Combine 'Before' and 'During'.

Pneumonia

Orthodox Medicine

Common brand names: Amoxil, Amoxicillin
Generic name: derivative of Penicillin

Side-effects

See Bites and Stings

Dietary Recommendations

During: Patients should be given warm vegetable or chicken broth, thin porridge and light dhal soup. Both garlic juice and garlic syrup can be used to treat pneumonia. 20 mL (1 tablespoon) of juice containing 5 per cent garlic can

be taken 4 times a day. Garlic syrup containing 10 per cent garlic should be taken every 4 hours, 15 to 20 mL each time. One-quarter of this dose should be administered for children 2 to 5 years old, one-third for those 5 to 7 and one-half for 7 to 12 year olds.

After: Strengthening soups and stews made from chicken or fish with miso, noodles, grains and vegetables with garlic and ginger.

Rashes/Skin Irritations

Orthodox Medicine

Common brand name: Aureomycin Cream (the only brand available in Australia)
Generic name: Chlortetracycline

Dietary Recommendations

Before: Rashes can occur as a result of too much meat, sugar or fruit juice, or a food allergy. The child should eat lots of fresh foods and avoid red meat, spicy and fatty foods, sugar, fruit juice and preservatives and food colourings.

During and after: Same as 'Before'.

Stomach-ache

Orthodox Medicine

Common brand names: Panadol, Tylenol
Generic name: Paracetamol

Side-effects

See Colds and Flu

Dietary Recommendations

Before: Stomach-aches often occur as a result of the consumption of restrictive foods such as eggs, poultry, fish, salt, meat and baked foods. The over intake of cool/cold foods or drinks, raw fruit, oily foods, sweeteners, spices or vegetables such as tomatoes and potatoes may result in stomach-ache, as can overeating or lack of chewing. The two main dietary causes of stomach-ache in children are caused by food intolerances, cow's milk being one of the most common. Children who have not previously had salt included in their diets should not be introduced to it at this stage.

During: If the child is asking for food, helpful foods include light soups such as pearl barley and vegetable soup and miso soup. Green, leafy vegetables are also beneficial in treating stomach-ache. Fresh ginger, tangerine peel and

radish can be effective in treating stomach-ache.
After: Same as 'Before'.

Sunburn

See Burns and Scalds

Teething

Orthodox Medicine

Common brand names: Panadol, Tylenol
Generic name: Paracetamol

Side-effects

See Colds and Flu

Dietary Recommendations

During: Chamomile tea, breast milk (most babies don't want to eat).

Thrush

Orthodox Medicine

Common brand names: Mycelex, Lotrim
Generic name: Clotrimazole

Side-effects

Precautions: It is usually well tolerated. Avoid contact with eyes. Capable of interacting with DNA of living cells, indicating possible carcinogenicity. Reported cases of patients who have developed necrotic (localised tissue death) skin reactions after application. And approximately 1 per cent who develop oral ulceration after treatment for oral candidiasis.

Dietary Recommendations

During: For mother if breastfeeding — avoid sugar, too many fermented foods, dairy products and alcohol. Take Lactobacillus as recommended by practitioner.

Tonsillitis and Sore Throat

Orthodox Medicine 1

Common brand names: Amoxil, Amoxicillin
Generic name: derivative of Penicillin

Side-effects

See Bites and Stings

Orthodox Medicine 2

Common brand name: Betadine (gargle)
Generic name: Povidone-iodine

Side-effects

Contraindications: History of sensitivity to iodine containing products.
Precautions: In the very rare event of local irritation or sensitivity, discontinue use.

Dietary Recommendations:

Before: Avoid 'heating' foods.
During: Provide Chamomile tea, boiled water, stewed fruit and fruit juice, green and yellow vegetables, grains, beans and white meat.
After: Avoid mucus-producing and 'heating' foods.

Travel Sickness

See Nausea

Vomiting

Sea Nausea

Whooping Cough

Orthodox Medicine

Common brand names: E-Mycin, Ery-Tab
Generic name: Erythromycin

Side-effects

The most frequent side effects of erythromycin preparations are gastrointestinal, such as abdominal cramping and discomfort, and are dose related. Nausea, vomiting and diarrhoea occur infrequently with oral doses. During prolonged or repeated therapy, there is a possibility of over-growth of nonsusceptible bacteria or fungi. If this occurs the drug should be discontinued and appropriate therapy instituted. Allergic reactions, including hypersensitivity to a foreign protein which may lead to bronchial problems and death have been reported. There have been reports of reversible hearing loss occurring chiefly in patients receiving high doses of erythromycin.
Contraindications: Patients with known hypersensitivity to loss antibiotic. Severely impaired hepatic function.

Precautions: This appears to be principally degraded and excreted by the liver. There have been reports of transient hepatic dysfunction, with or without jaundice, occurring in patients receiving oral erythromycin products.

Dietary Recommendations

During: Mucus-producing foods should be avoided, as should raw and cold foods. The daily intake of warm vegetable soup will aid the body's natural protection. Main meals should be at breakfast and lunch, as this lessens the chance of vomiting at night, when the coughing is most prevalent. Avoid citrus juice. Diluted apple juice or honey should be given instead. *After:* Strengthen the system with soups and stews made with miso and rice, vegetables, beans, noodles, mushrooms, chicken, fish or lamb.

INDEX